Cervical Cancer: From Etiology to Prevention

Cancer Prevention – Cancer Causes

Volume 2

Cercival Cancer:
From Etiology to Prevention

Edited by

Thomas E. Rohan, M.B.B.S., Ph.D.

Professor Chairman,
Department of Epidemiology and Population Health,
Albert Einstein College of Medicine,
Bronx, New York, U.S.A.

and

Keerti V. Shah, M.D., Dr.P.H.

Professor,
Departments of Molecular Microbiology and Immunology,
Johns Hopkins Bloomberg School of Public Health,
Baltimore, Maryland, U.S.A.

Foreword by Harald zur Hausen, M.D., D.Sc.

KLUWER ACADEMIC PUBLISHERS
DORDRECHT / BOSTON / LONDON

A C.I.P. Catalogue record for this book is available from the Library of Congress.

ISBN 1-4020-1410-4

Published by Kluwer Academic Publishers,
P.O. Box 17, 3300 AA Dordrecht, The Netherlands.

Sold and distributed in North, Central and South America
by Kluwer Academic Publishers,
101 Philip Drive, Norwell, MA 02061, U.S.A.

In all other countries, sold and distributed
by Kluwer Academic Publishers,
P.O. Box 322, 3300 AH Dordrecht, The Netherlands.

Printed on acid-free paper

To Our Wives,
Rosa and Farida

Contents

Contributors

E. Neely Atkinson, Ph.D.
Department of Biomathematics, The University of Texas M. D. Anderson Cancer Center, Houston, TX

F. Xavier Bosch, M.D., M.P.H.
Servei d'Epidemiologia i Registre del Càncer Institut Català d'Oncologia, Barcelona, Spain

Jack Cuzick, Ph.D.
Cancer Research UK , Dept. of Epidemiology, Mathematics and Statistics, Wolfson Institute of Preventive Medicine, London, UK

Patti E. Gravitt, M.S., Ph.D.
Department of Epidemiology, Johns Hopkins Bloomberg School of Public Health, Baltimore, MD

Michele Follen, M.D., Ph.D.
Center for Biomedical Engineering, The University of Texas M. D. Anderson Cancer Center, Houston, TX

Robert A. Hiatt, M.D., Ph.D.
Division of Cancer Control and Population Sciences, National Cancer Institute, NIH, Bethesda, MD

Harald zur Hausen, M.D., D.Sc.
Deutsches Krebsforschungszentrum, Heidelberg, Germany

Jon F. Kerner, Ph.D.
Division of Cancer Control and Population Sciences, National Cancer Institute, NIH, Bethesda, MD

Laura A. Koutsky, Ph.D.
Department of Epidemiology, University of Washington, Seattle, WA

Laimonis A. Laimins, Ph.D.
Department of Microbiology – Immunology, Feinberg School of Medicine, Northwestern University, Chicago, IL

Morris Ling, B.A.
Department of Pathology, The Johns Hopkins Medical Institutions, Baltimore, MD

Douglas R. Lowy, Ph.D.
Laboratory of Cellular Oncology, National Cancer Institute, NIH, Bethesda, MD

Frank L. Meyskens, Jr., M.D.
Chao Family Comprehensive Cancer Center, University of California–Irvine, Irvine, CA

Anthony B. Miller, M.B., F.R.C.P.
Division of Clinical Epidemiology, Deutsches Krebsforschungszentrum, Heidelberg, Germany

Stephen T. Oh, Ph.D.
Department of Microbiology – Immunology, Feinberg School of Medicine, Northwestern University, Chicago, IL

Electra D. Paskett, Ph.D.
School of Public Health/Comprehensive Cancer Center, Ohio State University, Columbus, OH

Thomas E. Rohan, M.B.B.S., Ph.D.
Department of Epidemiology and Population Health, Albert Einstein College of Medicine, Bronx, NY

Mack T. Ruffin IV, M.D., M.P.H.
Department of Family Medicine, University of Michigan, Ann Arbor, MI

John T. Schiller, Ph.D.
Laboratory of Cellular Oncology, National Cancer Institute, NIH, Bethesda, MD

David Schottenfeld, M.D.
Department of Epidemiology, School of Public Health, The University of Michigan, Ann Arbor, MI

Keerti V. Shah, M.D., Dr.P.H.
Department of Molecular Microbiology and Immunology, Johns Hopkins Bloomberg School of Public Health, Baltimore, MD

Mark H. Stoler, M.D.
Robert E. Fechner Laboratory of Surgical Pathology, Department of Pathology, University of Virginia Health System, Charlottesville, VA

Raphael P. Viscidi, M.D.
Department of Pediatrics, Johns Hopkins School of Medicine, Baltimore, MD

Mary Ellen Wewers, Ph.D., R.N., M.P.H.
College of Nursing and School of Public Health/Comprehensive Cancer Center, Ohio State University, Columbus, OH

Rachel L. Winer, M.P.H.
Department of Epidemiology, University of Washington, Seattle, WA

T.-C. Wu, M.D., Ph.D.
Departments of Pathology, Oncology, Obstetrics and Gynecology, and Molecular Microbiology and Immunology, The Johns Hopkins Medical Institutions, Baltimore, MD

Preface

In the last few years there has been enormous progress in terms of our understanding of the etiology and pathogenesis of cervical cancer, particularly with respect to the role of human papillomaviruses. These advances have opened up new avenues for the prevention of this disease, one of the most common cancers in women, both through the refinement of existing technologies for cervical cancer control and through the development and evaluation of new technologies. This book was motivated by the perceived need to make knowledge of these advances accessible to a wide audience. To this end, we have been assisted by scientists working in a wide range of disciplines that are pertinent to the epidemiology and prevention of cervical cancer, and who have contributed reviews of its descriptive and analytical epidemiology, and of approaches to cervical cancer prevention and control through public health policy, education, screening, chemoprevention, and vaccine development.

The book is divided into 5 sections. Section 1 lays the foundation for the remainder of the book with chapters that address the histological classification of cervical neoplasia (i.e., cervical cancer and its precursors) and the natural history of the disease. Section 2 focuses on infection with human papillomaviruses. It commences with chapters on the biology and molecular basis of the effects of human papillomavirus infections, and concludes with chapters on methods for the detection of human papillomaviruses and on the epidemiology of infection with these viruses. Section 3 describes the etiology of the two main histological types of cervical neoplasia, namely squamous cell carcinoma and adenocarcinoma. Section 4 considers approaches to cervical cancer prevention, including risk reduction through educational means; screening using Pap smears, HPV detection, and other methods; chemoprevention; and preventive and therapeutic vaccination. The final section of the book, Section 5, contains a chapter addressing policy issues relevant to the implementation of preventive measures, and it also considers barriers to the implementation of such measures and strategies to surmount those barriers.

Given its scope, the book should appeal not only to oncologists, primary care practitioners, and public health professionals working on the policy implications of scientific developments, but also to basic scientists, pathologists, epidemiologists, and graduate students in cancer-related fields who want to gain an understanding of the topic.

We are grateful to Professor Harald zur Hausen, a major contributor to the understanding at a fundamental level of the role of human papillomaviruses in causing cervical cancer, for writing the foreword for the book, and we thank our colleagues whose excellent contributions made the book possible. We were helped enormously with the myriad tasks associated with production of the book by our assistants, Olga Mendoza and Joy Mays. We appreciate the contribution of Jaime Stone and Angela Coraccio at Harvard, who prepared the camera-ready versions of the chapters, and we also appreciate the help and advice that we received from the editorial staff at Kluwer, namely Cristina Miranda Alves dos Santos, Melania Ruiz, and Marianne Janssen.

Thomas E. Rohan, M.B.B.S., Ph.D.
Bronx, New York

Keerti V. Shah, M.D., Dr.P.H.
Baltimore, Maryland

September, 2003

Foreword

A Brief History of Human Papillomavirus Research

Harald zur Hausen, M.D., D.Sc.
Deutsches Krebsforschungszentrum, Heidelberg, Germany

We are presently looking back to more than 100 years of papilloma and papillomavirus research. It is still relatively poorly recognized that McFadyean and Hobday in England started tumorvirus research in 1896 by demonstrating the cell-free transmission of canine warts. In 1907 this was followed by the more frequently quoted cell-free transmission of human warts by Ciuffo in Italy. Warts of course were not considered as authentic tumors at that time. It is therefore not too surprising that the subsequent cell-free transmission of chicken leukemia by Ellermann and Bang in Copenhagen (1908) and of chicken sarcoma by Rous in New York (1911) received much more attention by the scientific community.

In spite of a limited number of studies on papillomas and their viral etiology in subsequent decades, it took almost 80 more years before this field found broad interest, particularly in medicine. This resulted from the demonstrated relationship between specific papillomavirus infections and cancer of the cervix. It is, however, fair to say that the recent surge in activities in papillomavirus research has four (initially relatively independent) historical roots: *(i)* studies on papilloma development in cattle, *(ii)* in rabbits, *(iii)* in a rare human hereditary condition (epidermodysplasia verruciformis), characterized by an extensive verrucosis and the subsequent development of cancer in warts located at sun-exposed sites, and *(iv)* from the search for a viral etiology of cancer of the cervix. Although started from different initial observations, all four types of studies fertilized the subsequent progress and stimulated specific experimental approaches. In a brief outline of pioneering work performed in these four areas, I will briefly try to characterize some of the early major advances made in these fields:

The infectious origin of bovine warts was initially demonstrated in Brazil (Magelhaes, 1920). Interest in these types of frequently giant papillomas developed from early studies of Olson and Crook who showed that transmission of these viruses to another species, horses, resulted in the induction of sarcoids. These invasively growing, but non-metastasizing tumors were also noted in domestic horses under natural conditions. Thus, their experimental induction suggested an origin from transspecies transmission of bovine papillomavirus, much later proven by molecular analyses (Lancaster et al., 1978). The Olson group made another striking observation, namely the induction of bladder tumors in cattle by bovine papillomavirus (BPV) infection (Olson et al., 1959). Only four years later two additional publications by Black et al. (1963) and Thomas and colleagues (1963) demonstrated the transforming activity of BPV preparations for bovine fetal and murine cells. This permitted for the first time the application of tissue culture studies to papillomavirus research and profoundly influenced progress in subsequent years.

The development of molecular biology and of DNA cloning techniques in the 1970s and application of this technology to the BPV system resulted in the characterization of parts of the BPV genome as responsible elements for tissue culture transformation (Lowy et al., 1980). Shortly thereafter BPV 1 represented the first fully sequenced papillomavirus type (Chen et al., 1982).

The interest in bovine papillomavirus studies continues until today. This is mainly based on the ease of using some of the most prevalent BPV types (BPV 1 and 2) in tissue culture studies to understand the mechanisms of viral genome persistence, as well as the expression pattern of specific viral genes. In addition, the use of viral BPV DNA in shuttle vectors and the episomal persistence of this DNA greatly increased the number of studies of these virus types.

Retrospectively, the impact of BPV research on the papillomavirus field originated mainly from analysis of BPV-caused cell transformation, from the dissection of the viral genome and from the structural and functional characterization of individual viral genes and gene products. The obtained data facilitated in particular early studies on human papillomavirus infections.

A second root of papillomavirus research, substantially influencing cancer research in general terms, goes back to the identification of papillomas and their infectious origin in wild cottontail rabbits in the early 1930s by Shope (1933). After successful transmission of this infection to domestic rabbits, Rous and Beard (1934) soon noted that in the latter animals the initial papillomas frequently converted into squamous cell carcinomas. Occasionally malignant conversion occurred also in the natural host, the cottontail rabbit. In a number of ingenious studies by the Rous group, synergistic effects between viral and chemical carcinogens were observed. Rous developed the concept of tumor initiation by analyzing this system (e.g., Rous and Kidd, 1938; Rous and Friedewald, 1944). He conceptually preceded his contemporaries by several decades, but the importance of his work was only acknowledged in 1966, when he received the Nobel award. In 1961, Ito and Evans showed that purified DNA of the cottontail rabbit papillomavirus (CRPV) was able to induce squamous cell carcinomas in rabbits, thus directly revealing the carcinogenicity of a viral genome.

The research by Peyton Rous was not specifically driven by his interest in the infectious agent of rabbit papillomas. He wanted to understand the mechanisms of cancer induction. The frequent progression of rabbit papillomas into squamous cell carcinomas provided him with a most useful model to analyze steps in cancer development and to understand the synergistic effects of different classes of carcinogens. Interestingly, the rabbit papillomavirus system found comparatively little attention in the subsequent period. The PubMed bibliography today lists only 189 titles for the cottontail rabbit papillomavirus, in contrast to 1085 titles for bovine papillomaviruses, 389 for epidermodysplasia verruciformis, and 5895 for genital papillomavirus infections.

The analysis of human papillomatous lesions and their relationship to virus infections and carcinogenesis had a much slower start. Since the cell-free transmission of human warts, their infectious etiology was clearly established. Yet, warts were mainly regarded as a cosmetic nuisance and not considered to be of significant medical interest.

A gradual change of this view originated from the description of a syndrome published in 1922 by Lewandowsky and Lutz in Basel. They described a hereditary condition, characterized by an extensive verrucosis, which they named epidermodysplasia verruciformis. At sun-exposed sites of those patients, at the forehead, the face, the back of the hands and arms some of these papillomatous lesions converted into squamous cell carcinomas. In 1946 Lutz and subsequently Jablonska and Millewsky (1957) proved the viral etiology of these warts in autoinoculation experiments. Schellender and Fritsch (1970) and Ruiter and van Mullem (1970) were particularly intrigued by the restriction of squamous cell carcinoma development to sun-exposed sites. It was mainly the merit of Stefania Jablonska in Warsaw, Poland, to point to a possible role of the papillomavirus particles seen in these warts as causal factors for the subsequent development of squamous cell cancers of the skin (Jablonska et al., 1972). In collaboration with the Paris group of Gérard Orth, both groups successfully demonstrated the presence of novel types of papillomaviruses, most frequently HPV 5, within epidermodysplasia verruciformis lesions and within squamous cell carcinoma biopsies of those patients (Orth et al., 1978; 1979).

Although HPV 5 represents the first human papillomavirus infection regularly detected in cutaneous squamous cell cancers of these patients, the rarity of the syndrome, the difficulties in obtaining sufficient clinical materials for extensive studies, and the absence of tissue culture lines from these carcinomas were probably the reasons for a limited interest in this condition. Even more than 25 years after the initial discovery of HPV 5 and related viruses most questions relating to their etiological role and to the mechanism of their interaction in infected host cells in the course of carcinogenesis still remain open. Only in more recent years the study of cutaneous papillomavirus infections and their relationship to non-melanoma skin cancer in immunosuppressed and immunocompetent patients is finding increasing attention.

A fourth track of papillomavirus research resulted in the identification of specific HPV types as causative agents for cancer of the cervix, other anogenital cancers, and a subset of oropharyneal carcinomas. Our group started these investigations in search for a viral etiology of cancer of the cervix. After finding Epstein-Barr virus DNA in a 'virus-free' Burkitt lymphoma cell line (zur Hausen and Schulte-Holthausen, 1970) and in biopsies from Burkitt's lymphoma and nasopharyngeal cancer (zur Hausen et al., 1970), we used the same techniques in attempts to detect herpes simplex type 2 (HSV 2) DNA in biopsies from cervical cancer. By the end of the 1960s and during the 1970s serological studies suggested a role of HSV 2 in this cancer (Rawls et al., 1968; Naib et al., 1969). Our failure to find traces of HSV 2 DNA in these cancer biopsies prompted considerations to look for potential other infectious candidates causing this cancer, since its epidemiology provided good reasons to suspect an infectious etiology.

A number of anecdotal reports on malignant conversion of genital warts (condylomata acuminata), scattered in the medical literature of the preceding 100 years, caught our attention. This resulted in the speculation on a possible causal role of papillomavirus infections for cervical cancer and led to initial attempts to characterize the viral DNA in genital warts (zur Hausen et al., 1974; 1975; zur Hausen 1976; 1977). These and other studies had the early consequence of discovering the heterogeneity of the papillomavirus family (Gissmann and zur Hausen 1976; Orth et al., 1977; Gissmann et al., 1977), presently counting close to 100 fully sequenced genotypes (de Villiers, 1994; and personal communication). Although the eventual isolation of HPV DNA from genital warts, labeled as HPV 6 (Gissmann and zur Hausen, 1980), and from laryngeal papillomas (HPV 11) two years later (Gissmann et al., 1982) did not yield positive data for these viruses in cervical cancer, the use of their DNA in hybridization experiments, performed under conditions of reduced stringency, permitted the subsequent cloning of HPV 16 (Dürst et al., 1983) and of HPV 18 (Boshart et al., 1984), the two papillomavirus types most frequently found in cervical cancer. The following years resulted in a burst of activities. These included, among numerous other observations,

- the demonstration of a specific expression pattern of the viral E6 and E7 genes in the respective carcinoma tissue (Schwarz et al., 1985; Yee et al. 1985);

- the immortalization of human keratinocytes by high risk HPV, expressing the E6 and E7 genes (Dürst et al., 1987; Pirisi et al., 1987);

- the interaction of E6 and E7 proteins with various cellular proteins, initially particularly with pRb and p53 (Dyson et al., 1989; Werness et al., 1990);

- the direct demonstration that E6 and E7 proteins are responsible for the malignant phenotype of cervical carcinoma cells (von Knebel Doeberitz et al., 1992; 1994);

- and large scale epidemiological studies identifying high-risk HPV types as the major risk factor for cervical cancer (Muñoz et al., 1992; Bosch et al., 1995).

Today the practical consequences of these studies become more and more apparent: gaining an order of magnitude as diagnostic approaches to validate early precursor lesions of cervical cancer and the development of preventive vaccines with the potential to prevent one of the major cancers of women are no longer unrealistic fantasies (reviewed in zur Hausen, 2002). The recent demonstration of an effect of a virus-like particle vaccine preventing persistent infection by HPV 16 and early precursor lesions of cervical cancer (Koutsky et al., 2002) impressively underlines this potential. Thus, besides hepatitis B vaccine, another cancer-preventive vaccine will soon become available.

It is likely that papillomavirus research is still going to expand in the future: the role of these virus infections in at least some subsets of other anogenital and oropharyngeal cancers has substantially gained in substance during the past few years (IARC Report). In addition, an interesting mode of an *indirect* contribution to carcinogenesis (zur Hausen, 1999) by certain cutaneous papillomavirus types preventing apoptosis in UV-damaged cells becomes increasingly apparent (Jackson et al., 2000; 2002).

In this book, Drs. Rohan and Shah have produced a comprehensive treatment of the evidence relating to cervical cancer etiology and prevention. They have done so by assembling a team of leading cervical cancer researchers who have addressed the biology and natural history of human papillomavirus infection and cervical cancer, as well as the etiology of cervical cancer, approaches to its prevention, and the policy issues relating to implementation of preventive strategies. The book is very timely in that it synthesizes the substantial advances in knowledge of these topics that have taken place in recent years, advances that put us on the threshold of a new era in cervical cancer prevention and control.

REFERENCES

Black PH, Hartley JW, Rowe WP, et al. Transformation of bovine tissue culture cells by bovine papilloma virus. Nature 1963;199:1016-8.

Bosch FX, Manos MM, Muñoz N, et al. Prevalence of human papillomavirus in cervical cancer: a worldwide perspective. J Natl Cancer Inst 1995;87:796-802.

Boshart M, Gissmann L, Ikenberg H, et al. A new type of papillomavirus DNA, its presence in genital cancer and in cell lines derived from genital cancer. EMBO J 1984;3:1151-7.

Chen EY, Howley PM, Levinson AD, et al. The primary structure and genetic organization of the bovine papillomavirus (BPV) type 1 genome. Nature 1982; 299: 529-34.

Ciuffo G. Innesto positivo con filtrate di verruca volgare. G Ital Mal Venereol 1907;48:12-17.

de Villiers EM. Human pathogenic papillomaviruses: An update. Curr Topics Microbiol Immunol 1994; Springer Verlag, Berlin-Heidelberg, 86: 1-12.

Dürst M, Gissmann L, Ikenberg H, et al. A papillomavirus DNA from a cervical carcinoma and its prevalence in cancer biopsy samples from different geographic regions. Proc Nat Acad Sci USA 1983;80:3812-5.

Dürst M, Dzarlieva-Petrusevska RT, Boukamp P, et al. Molecular and cytogenetic analysis of immortalized human primary keratinocytes obtained after transfection with human papillomavirus type 16 DNA. Oncogene 1987;1:251-6.

Dyson N, Howley PM, Münger K, et al. The human papillomavirus-16 E7 oncoprotein is able to bind to the retinoblastoma gene product. Science 1989;243:934-7.

Ellermann V, Bang O. Experimentelle Leukämie bei Hühnern. Centralbl F Bakt Abt 1 (Orig) 1908;46:595-609.

Gissmann L, Diehl V, Schultz-Coulon H, et al. Molecular cloning and characterization of human papillomavirus DNA from a laryngeal papilloma. J Virol 1982;44:393-400.

Gissmann L, Pfister H, zur Hausen H. Human papilloma viruses (HPV): Characterization of four different isolates. Virology 1977;76:569-80.

Gissmann L, zur Hausen H. Human papilloma viruses: physical mapping and genetic heterogeneity. Proc Nat Acad Sci USA1976; 73:1310-3.

Gissmann L, zur Hausen H. Partial characterization of viral DNA from human genital warts (condylomata acuminata). Int J Cancer 1980;25:605-9.

IARC Monographs on the Evaluation of Carcinogenic Risks to Humans. Human Papillomaviruses. Vol. 64, 1995.

Ito Y, Evans CA. Induction of tumors in domestic rabbits with nucleic acid preparations from partially purified Shope papilloma virus and from extracts of the papillomas of domestic and cotton tail rabbits. J Exp Med 1961;114: 485-91.

Jablonska S, Dabrowski J, Jakubowicz K. Epidermodysplasia verruciformis as a model in studies on the role of papovaviruses in oncogenesis. Cancer Res 1972;32:583-9.

Jablonska S, Millewski B. Zur Kenntnis der Epidermodysplasia verruciformis Lewandowsky-Lutz. Dermatologica 1957;115:1-22.

Jackson S, Ghali L, Harwood C, Storey A. Reduced apoptotic levels in squamous but not basal cell carcinomas correlates with the detection of cutaneous human papillomavirus. Brit J Cancer 2002; 87: 319-3213

Jackson S, Harwood C, Thomas M, Banks L, Storey A. Role of Bak in UV-induced apoptosis in skin cancer and abrogation by E6 proteins. Genes Dev 2000; 14: 3065-73.

Koutsky LA, Ault KA, Wheeler CM, et al. A controlled trial of a human papillomavirus type 16 vaccine. N Engl J Med 2002;347:1645-51.

Lancaster WD, Olsen C. Demonstration of two distinct classes of bovine papilloma virus. Virology 1978;89:371-9.

Lewandowsky F, Lutz W. Ein Fall einer bisher nicht beschriebenen Hauterkrankung (Epidermodysplasia verruciformis). Arch Dermatol Syph (Berlin) 1922;141:193-203.

Lowy DR, Dvoretzky I, Shober R, et al. In vitro tumorigenic transformation by a defined subgenomic fragment of bovine papilloma virus DNA. Nature 1980;287:72-4.

Lutz W. A propos de l'epidermodysplasie verruciforme. Dermatologica 1946 ;92,30-43.

Magelhaes. Verruga dos bovideos, Brasil-Medico 1920;34:430-1.

McFadyean J, Hobday F. Note on the experimental "transmission of warts in the dog". J Comp Pathol Ther 1898;11: 341-4.

Muñoz N, Bosch FX, de Sanjose S, et al. The causal link between human papillomavirus and invasive cervical cancer: a population-based case-control study in Colombia and Spain. Int J Cancer 1992;52:743-9.

Naib ZM, Nahmias AJ, Josey WE, et al. Genital herpetic infection: association with cervical dysplasia and carcinoma. Cancer 1969;23:940-5.

Olson C, Cook RH. Cutaneous sarcoma-like lesions of the horse caused by the agent of bovine papilloma. Proc Soc Exp Biol Med 1951;77:281-4.

Olson C, Pamukcu AM, Brobst DF, et al. A urinary bladder tumor induced by a bovine cutaneous papilloma agent. Cancer Res 1959;19:779-82.

Orth G, Favre M, Croissant O. Characterization of a new type of human papillomavirus that causes skin warts. J Virol 1977;24: 108-20.

Orth G, Jablonska S, Jarzabek-Chorzelska M, et al. Characteristics of the lesions and risk of malignant conversion as related to the type of the human papillomavirus involved in epidermodysplasia verruciformis. Cancer Res 1979;39:1074-82.

Orth G, Jablonska S, Favre M, et al. Characterization of two new types of HPV from lesions of epidermodysplasia verruciformis. Proc Nat Acad Sci USA 1979;75:1537-41.

Pirisi L, Yasumoto S, Fellery M, et al. Transformation of human fibroblasts and keratinocytes with human papillomavirus type 16 DNA. J Virol 1987; 61:1061-6.

Rawls WE, Tompkins WA, Figueroa ME, et al. Herpesvirus type 2: association with cancer of the cervix. Science 1968;161:1255-6.

Rous P. A sarcoma of the fowl transmissible by agent separable from tumor cells. J Exp Med 1911;13: 397-411, 1911.

Rous P, Beard JW. Carcinomatous changes in virus-induced papillomas of the skin of the rabbit. Proc Soc Exp Biol Med 1934;32:578-80.

Rous P, Friedewald WF. The effect of chemical carcinogens on virus-induced rabbit papillomas. J Exp Med 1944;79:511-37.

Rous P, Kidd JG. The carcinogenic effect of a papillomavirus on the tarred skin of rabbits. I. Description of the phenomenon. J Exp Med 1938;67:399-422.

Ruiter M, van Mullem PJ. Behaviour of virus in malignant degeneration of skin lesions in epidermodysplasia verruciformis. J Invest Dermatol 1970;54:324-31.

Schellender F, Fritsch F. Epidermodysplasia verruciformis. Neue Aspekte zur Symptomatologie und Pathogenese. Dermatologica 1970;140:251-9.

Schwarz E, Freese UK, Gissmann L, et al. Structure and transcription of human papillomavirus type 18 and 16 sequences in cervical carcinoma cells. Nature 1985;314:111-4.

Shope RE. Infectious papillomatosis of rabbits. J Exp Med 1933;58:607-27.

Thomas M, Banks L. Inhibition of Bak-induced apoptosis by HPV-18 E6. Oncogene 1998; 17:2943-53.

Thomas M, Levy JP, Tanzer J, et al. Transformation in vitro de cellules de peau de veau embryonnaire sous l'action d'extraits acellulaires de papillomes bovins. Compt Rend Acad Sci (Paris) 1963;257:2155-8.

von Knebel Doeberitz M, Rittmüller C, zur Hausen H, et al. Inhibition of tumorigenicity of cervical cancer cells in nude mice by HPV E6-E7 antisense RNA. Int J Cancer 1992; 51: 831-4.

von Knebel Doeberitz M, Rittmüller C, Aengeneyndt F, et al. Reversible repression of papillomavirus oncogene expression in cervical carcinoma cells: consequences for the phenotype and E6-p53 and E7-pRB interactions. J Virol 1994;68:2811-21.

Werness BA, Levine AJ, Howley PM. Association of human papillomavirus types 16 and 18 E6 proteins with p53. Science 1990;248:76-9.

Yasumoto S, Burckhardt AL, Doninger J, et al. Human papillomavirus type 16 DNA induced malignant transformation of NIH3T3 cells. J Virol 1986;57:572-7.

Yee C, Krishnan-Hewlett Z, Baker CC, et al. Presence and expression of human papillomavirus sequences in human cervical carcinoma cell lines. Am J Pathol 1985; 119:361-6.

zur Hausen H. Condylomata acuminata and human genital cancer. Cancer Res 1976;36:530.

zur Hausen H. Human papilloma viruses and their possible role in squamous cell carcinomas. Current Topics in Microbiol. Immunol 1977;78:1-30.

zur Hausen H. Papillomaviruses and cancer: from basic studies to clinical application. Nature Rev Cancer 2002;2:342-50.

zur Hausen H. Viruses in human cancers. Millenium Rev. 2000, Europ J Cancer 1999;35: 1174-81.

zur Hausen H, Gissmann L, Steiner W, et al. Human papilloma viruses and cancer. In: Clemensen J, Yohn DS, eds. Bibliotheca Haematologica 1975; 43:569-71.

zur Hausen H, Meinhof W, Scheiber W, et al. Attempts to detect virus-specific DNA sequences in human tumors: I. Nucleic acid hybridizations with complementary RNA of human wart virus. Int J Cancer 1974;13:650-6.

zur Hausen H, Schulte-Holthausen H. Presence of EB virus nucleic acid homology in a "virus-free" line of Burkitt tumor cells. Nature (London) 1970;227:245-8.

zur Hausen H, Schulte-Holthausen H, Klein G, et al. EBV DNA in biopsies of Burkitt tumours and anaplastic carcinoma of the nasopharynx. Nature (London) 1970; 228: 1056-8.

Introduction

Thomas E. Rohan, M.B.B.S., Ph.D.
Department of Epidemiology and Population Health, Albert Einstein College of Medicine

Keerti V. Shah, M.D., Dr.P.H
Department of Molecular Microbiology and Immunology, Johns Hopkins Bloomberg School of Public Health

It is estimated that about 15.6% of all cancers worldwide, or about 1.45 million cases annually, are attributable to infections (Pisani et al 1997). A cancer of infectious origin may be preventable by immunization against the etiologic agent, as is already evident in the decreasing incidence of hepatocellular carcinoma following immunization against the hepatitis B virus (Chang et al., 1997). Recent advances in our understanding of the causes of cervical cancer have raised the possibility that a reduction in the incidence of this disease might be accomplished through similar means.

Cervical cancer is a major cause of morbidity and mortality worldwide. Each year, approximately 470,000 women are diagnosed with the disease and about 230,000 die from it, making it the second most common cancer amongst women (Parkin et al., 2001). Given its importance, cervical cancer has been subjected to intensive investigation in order to identify its causes, and to develop and improve methods for preventing and controlling it.

Epidemiologic studies conducted several decades ago provided clues to the role of sexual activity in the etiology of cervical cancer. In particular, cervical cancer rates were noted to be low in Catholic nuns (Fraumeni et al., 1969) and in other religious groups (Boyd and Doll, 1964; Cross et al., 1968). Furthermore, risk of cervical cancer was observed to be increased in women who married at young ages (Boyd and Doll, 1964) and who therefore initiated sexual activity relatively early in life (Terris et al., 1967), and it was also observed to be increased in association with the number of sexual partners that a woman had had (Terris et al., 1967). Attributes of the male partners of women who develop cervical cancer were found also to be related to risk, given the increased risk of cervical cancer observed in the wives of men with penile cancer (Martinez, 1969), the increased risk of cervical cancer in the wives of men previously married to cervical cancer patients (Kessler, 1977), and the higher number of sexual partners reported by the husbands of women with cervical cancer than by the husbands of women without the disease (Buckley et al., 1981). Observations such as these helped to generate the concept that a sexually transmitted agent might be involved in the etiology of cervical cancer.

Early efforts to identify a sexually transmissible agent focused on herpes simplex virus type 2 (Rawls et al., 1968). However, the case for a primary role for this virus was weakened considerably when cervical tumors failed to show consistent evidence of HSV 2 DNA and protein (Park et al., 1983), and when the results of a large cohort study of Czechoslovakian women did not show a significantly increased risk of cervical neoplasia in association with HSV 2 serology at enrolment (Vonka et al., 1984; Schiffman et al., 1996).

Interest in the possible role of human papillomaviruses (HPV) in the etiology of cervical cancer was spurred by the discovery of HPV DNA in cervical tumors (zur Hausen et al., 1974), and at about the same time, by the observation by pathologists that the earliest precursor lesion of cervical cancer, low grade cervical dysplasia, was associated with HPV infection (Meisels et al., 1982). Subsequently, the immortalizing ability of HPV DNA and of the encoded viral oncogenes was demonstrated (Pirisi et al., 1987; Münger et al., 1989; zur Hausen, 2002). Over the course of the last decade, epidemiologic studies have shown that the association between the presence of HPV DNA in cervical specimens and risk of cervical neoplasia (both squamous cell carcinoma and adenocarcinoma) is one of the strongest ever observed in the study of human cancer etiology (Bosch et al., 2002). In addition, experimental investigations have provided insight into the mechanisms underlying the association, thereby helping to confirm the causal role of HPV infection in the development of cervical cancer (zur Hausen, 2002). Indeed, HPV is considered to be a necessary cause of cervical cancer, the first etiological agent to be given this designation for a human cancer (Bosch et al., 2002). While necessary, HPV infection alone is not sufficient to cause cervical cancer, indicating that progression from persistent (rather than transient (Burk,1999)) HPV infection to cervical neoplasia is likely to require exposure to other factors (so-called cofactors). Candidate cofactors include cigarette smoking, use of oral contraceptives, high parity, and infection with other sexually transmitted diseases (Castellsague et al., 2002), but research in this area is still at a relatively early stage.

Identification of the causal role of HPV infection in cervical carcinogenesis has made prevention of the disease a real possibility. Prevention of HPV infection through modification of sexual behavior presents enormous challenges, although some sex and AIDS education programs have been shown to delay the initiation of intercourse and reduce its frequency, to reduce the number of sexual partners, and to increase the use of condoms (Kirby et al., 1994; Rock et al., 2000). However, current efforts directed towards the development of vaccines designed to prevent HPV infection (Koutsky et al., 2002) and to prevent progression of existing HPV infections and neoplastic lesions (Moniz et al., 2003) represent more realistic prospects. Chemopreventive agents which target HPV transcription (Rösl et al., 1997) or which operate by other means (Rock et al., 2000) might also find application eventually.

The natural history of cervical cancer is now reasonably well understood. Essentially, it begins with disruption of the normal maturation of the epithelium of the transformation zone of the cervix (Franco and Ferenczy, 2002) leading to progressively more advanced grades of pre-invasive cervical neoplasia, known as cervical intraepithelial neoplasia (Richart, 1980), or equivalently, squamous intraepithelial lesions (Solomon et al., 2002). If such lesions are not treated, some will progress to involve the full thickness of the cervical epithelium (carcinoma in situ), and subsequently will break through the basement membrane and become invasive. Progression from an initial HPV infection to carcinoma in situ has been estimated to take more than 17 years on average (Ylitalo et al., 2000), and progression from carcinoma in situ to invasive cancer has been estimated to take an average of about 13 years (Gustafsson and Adami, 1989).

The long time course required for the development of cervical cancer renders it amenable to secondary prevention by screening. Specifically, the Papanicolaou test, in which exfoliated cells collected from the cervical transformation zone are examined microscopically, allows detection of cervical lesions at a relatively early stage in the natural history of cervical cancer; if followed by appropriate treatment, the course of the disease can be arrested. However, the conventional Pap smear has relatively low sensitivity, so that a substantial proportion of women who develop cervical cancer have adequate recent screening histories (Sasieni et al., 1996). More recently, with identification of the central role of HPV infection in the development of cervical neoplasia, use of HPV testing as an adjunct to or replacement for Pap screening has been suggested as a means of improving detection (Kulasingam et al., 2002), and such approaches are currently undergoing active evaluation. Indeed, screening based on HPV testing alone may be particularly suitable in resource-poor settings (Kuhn et al., 2000).

The developments outlined above have led to considerable optimism that the public health burden of cervical cancer can be reduced substantially in the coming years. However, important health policy issues remain, and they differ between developed and developing countries (Goldie, 2002). In developed countries, the main issues relate to how to ensure that the clinical benefits of state-of-the-art technologies are maximized. In contrast, in developing countries, the main issue currently (in the absence of an established HPV vaccine) is how to establish effective cervical cancer screening programs where it has not been possible to implement cervical cytology-based screening, given that resources are limited and that there are many competing priorities.

Our aim in this book has been to expand upon the themes introduced here. It is our hope that in doing so we have assembled an up-to-date resource that will be of use to those interested in cervical cancer etiology and prevention.

REFERENCES

Bosch FA, Lorincz A, Muñoz N, et al. The causal relation between human papillomavirus and cervical cancer. J Clin Pathol 2002;55:244-65.

Boyd JT, Doll R. A study of the etiology of carcinoma of the cervix uteri. Br J Cancer 1964;18:419-34.

Buckley JD, Harris RWC, Doll R, et al. Case-control study of the husbands of women with dysplasia or carcinoma of the cervix uteri. Lancet 1981;2:1010-5.

Burk RD. Pernicious papillomavirus infection. N Engl J Med 1999;341:1687-8.

Castellsague X, Bosch FX, Muñoz N. Environmental co-factors in HPV carcinogenesis. Virus Res 2002;89:191-9.

Chang MH, Chen CJ, Lai MS et al. Universal hepatitis B vaccination in Taiwan and the incidence of hepatocellular carcinoma in children. N Engl J Med 1997; 336: 1855-1859.

Cross HE, Kennel EE, Lilienfeld AM. Cancer of the cervix in an Amish population. Cancer 1968;21:102-8.

Franco EL, Ferenczy A. Cervix. In: Franco EL, Rohan TE, eds. Cancer precursors: epidemiology, detection, and prevention. New York: Springer-Verlag, 2002, 249-86.

Fraumeni JF Jr., Lloyd JW, Smith EM, et al. Cancer mortality among nuns: Role of marital status in etiology of neoplastic disease in women. J Natl Cancer Inst 1969;42:455-68.

Goldie SJ. Health economics and cervical cancer prevention: a global perspective. Virus Res 2002;89:301-9.

Gustafsson L, Adami HO. Natural history of cervical neoplasia: consistent results obtained by an identification technique. Br J Cancer 1989;60:132-41.

Kessler II. Venereal factors in human cervical cancer: evidence from marital clusters. Cancer 1977;39:1912-9.

Kirby D, Short L, Collins J, et al. School-based programs to reduce sexual risk behavior: a review of effectiveness. Public Health Rep 1994;109:339-60.

Kuhn L, Denny L, Pollack A, et al. Human papillomavirus DNA testing for cervical cancer screening in low-resource settings. J Natl Cancer Inst 2000;92:818-25.

Kulasingam SL, Hughes JP, Kiviat NB, et al. Evaluation of human papillomavirus testing in primary screening for cervical abnormalities. JAMA 2002;288:1749-57.

Martinez I. Relationship of squamous cell carcinoma of the cervix uteri to squamous cell carcinoma of the penis among Puerto Rican women married to men with penile carcinoma. Cancer 1969;24:777-80.

Meisels A, Fortin R. Condylomatous lesions of the cervix and vagina. 1. Cytologic patterns. Acta Cytol 1976;20:505-9.

Moniz M, Ling M, Hung CF, et al. HPV DNA vaccines. Front Biosci 2003;8:D55-68.

Mηnger K, Phelps WC, Bubb PM, et al. The E6 and E7 genes of human papillomavirus type 16 are necessary and sufficient for transformation of primary human keratinocytes. J Virol 1989;63:4417-23.

Park M, Kitchener HC, Macnab JC. Detection of herpes simplex virus type-2 DNA restriction fragments in human cervical carcinoma tissue. EMBO J 1983;2:1029-34.

Parkin DM, Bray FI, Devesa SS. Cancer burden in the year 2000. The global picture. Eur J Cancer 2001;37:S4-S66.

Pirisi L, Yasumoto S, Fellery M, et al. Transformation of human fibroblasts and keratinocytes with human papillomavirus type 16 DNA. J Virol 1987;61:1061-6.

Pisani P, Parkin DM, Munoz N, Ferlay J. Cancer and infection: estimates of the attributable fraction in 1990. Cancer Epidemiol Biomark Prev 1997;6:387-400.

Rawls WE, Tompkins WA, Figueroa ME, et al. Herpesvirus type 2: association with carcinoma of the cervix. Science 1968;161:1255-6.

Richart RM. The patient with an abnormal Pap smear: screening techniques and management. N Engl J Med 1980;320:332-4.

Rock CL, Michael CW, Reynolds RK, et al. Prevention of cervix cancer. Crit Rev Oncol Hematol 2000;33:169-85.

Rösl F, Das BC, Lengert M, et al. Antioxidant-induced changes of the AP-1 transcription complex are paralleled by a selective suppression of human papillomavirus transcription. J Virol 1997;71:362-70.

Sasieni PD, Cuzick J, Lynch-Framery E. Estimating the efficacy of screening by auditing smear histories of women with and without cervical cancer. Br J Cancer 1996;73:1001-5.

Schiffman MH, Brinton LA, Devesa SS, et al. Cervical cancer. In: Schottenfeld D, Fraumeni JF Jr., eds. Cancer epidemiology and prevention, 2nd ed. New York: Oxford University Press, 1996, 1090-1116.

Solomon D, Davey D, Kurman R, et al. The 2001 Bethesda System. Terminology for reporting results of cervical cytology. JAMA 2002;287:2114-9.

Terris M Wilson F, Smith H, et al. The relationship of coitus to carcinoma of the cervix. Am J Public Health 1967;57:840-7.

Vonka V, Kanka J, Hirsch I, et al. Prospective study on the relationship between cervical neoplasia and herpes simplex type-2 virus. II. Herpes simplex type-2 antibody presence in sera taken at enrollment. Int J Cancer 1984;33:61-6.

Ylitalo N, Sorensen P, Josefsson AM, et al. Consistent high viral load of human papillomavirus 16 and risk of cervical carcinoma in situ: a nested case-control study. Lancet 2000;355:2194-8.

zur Hausen H, Meinhof W, Scheiber W, et al. Attempts to detect virus-specific DNA sequences in human tumors: I. Nucleic acid hybridizations with complementary RNA of human wart virus. Int J Cancer 1974;13:650-6.

zur Hausen H. Papillomaviruses and cancer: from basic studies to clinical application. Nature Rev Cancer 2002;2:342-50.

Section 1

BIOLOGICAL BASIS

Chapter 1

The Pathology of Cervical Neoplasia

Mark H. Stoler, M.D.
Robert E. Fechner Laboratory of Surgical Pathology, Department of Pathology, University of Virginia Health System

INTRODUCTION

Cervical cancer and its precursors are defined by their pathology. For the purposes of this discussion, the pathology of cervical neoplasia is essentially the pathology of HPV-associated disease. In this chapter, the goal is to present the histopathology of this spectrum of HPV-associated disease, together with the correlated manifestations of the major lesions identified on Pap smear. During the presentation, the terminology used in various cytologic and histologic classification schemes is commented on, emphasizing the current usage trends in the United States that are driven mainly by the cytology classification system, the 2001 Bethesda System (TBS) (Solomon et al., 2002). While the molecular pathogenesis of cervical neoplasia including the role of human papillomaviruses (HPV) is detailed elsewhere (see Chapter 4), some elements will also be touched upon here as this well understood model of human epithelial carcinogenesis directly influences current classification concepts (Stoler, 1997).

In order of decreasing clinical occurrence, the pathology of the uterine cervix can mainly be divided between infectious/inflammatory processes, epithelial neoplasms, and a variety of relatively uncommon mesenchymal proliferations, many of which are similar throughout the rest of the female genital tract. The mesenchymal tumors and most of the infectious and inflammatory or reactive lesions will not be covered here. For a more comprehensive treatment of cervical pathology the reader is referred to any of several major works on gynecologic pathology (Fu, 2002; Kurman et al., 2002).

Obviously, interest in cervical pathology is primarily justified by the morbidity and mortality caused by cervical epithelial cancers and their precursors (Stoler, 2000a). Worldwide, cervical cancer is the first or second most common cancer of women. In the U.S., there are approximately 13,000 cases of cervix cancer per year and about 4500 associated deaths. In unscreened populations, the annual cervical cancer incidence ranges from 30 to $40/10^5$ to as high as $100/10^5$, compared to the current U.S. rate of approximately $5/10^5$. Hence, screening has effected up to a 90% reduction in the incidence of cervical cancer, directly attributable to the efficacy of cytologic screening. Coincident with the decrease in invasive cancer, there has been a dramatic increase in the frequency and attendant costs of detection and treatment of the precursors of cervix cancer. In the United States about five hundred thousand high-grade precursors and 2-3 million cases of low-grade lesions are referred for colposcopic assessment each year. The attendant costs for management of these lesions, by some estimates, is 3-6 billion dollars.

1   SPECIMEN TYPES

For the non-pathologist reader, some commentary on the types of specimens processed in pathology laboratories and some of the pitfalls associated with each specimen is appropriate background, since the pathologic interpretation defines the clinical management.

1.1   Pap smear

The Papanicolaou smear (Pap smear or Pap) is a microscopic examination of cells collected from the uterine cervix. Originally, it did not involve direct sampling, but rather was a collection of naturally exfoliated cells from the vaginal vault. Today it refers to an examination of cells directly collected from the cervix using a variety of devices aimed at optimizing collection of cells from the transformation zone (see section 3.2). Classically, the cells are directly smeared on slides, fixed with 95% ethyl alcohol and stained in such a way that nuclear and cytologic detail is optimized for microscopic examination. The average Pap smear slide contains between 50,000 and 300,000 cells. Depending on the condition of the patient, a significant proportion of these cells may be inflammatory cells and/or red blood cells. In contrast, DNA analysis of the average Pap collection demonstrates that more than a million nucleated cells are routinely collected in a good sample (Peyton et al., 1998). Thus, as little as 5% of the sample may actually make it onto the slide, and with the traditional Pap sampling method, this is not a random subset of the total sample collected.

Hence, not all Pap smears are equal in their sensitivity, specificity or clinical performance (Stoler, 2000a, Stoler, 2000b). Pre-analytic variables include the skill of the collector, the type of sampling device(s), the cervical anatomy and the quality of the slide, including smear thickness and cellular preservation or fixation. Indeed, simple but major early advances included the conversion from a vaginal pool specimen to direct cervical sampling, an improved differential staining technique and the training of a highly skilled workforce of dedicated cytotechnologists. These have combined to bring about the current situation; a Pap test so good that the general population unrealistically expects it to be perfect. Yet worldwide, there is great variation in Pap smear quality mostly because of sampling device variation. Historically, the most frequent type of cervical sampling device has been the modified Ayre spatula, alone or in combination with some form of endocervical sampler, most often a cotton tipped applicator. With current interest in adequate sampling, cytobrush samples of the endocervix have been popularized. Combined with a spatula sample, these brushes often provide an abundant endocervical sample. Of course, overzealous or inappropriate use of the brush can be problematic, as the endocervical sample may overwhelm the smear and depending upon the degree of cervical eversion entirely miss the transformation zone (T-zone), rather sampling the high endocervix or lower uterine segment. With such specimens there is a tendency to over-diagnose endocervical cell abnormalities. Clinically, the brush may be associated with some degree of discomfort and bleeding. Several years ago, the Unimar Cervex-Brush™ was introduced in the U.S. Popular in Europe, this device which is affectionately known as the "broom", is designed to simultaneously sample the ecto- and endocervix, addressing the issues of sampling, single slide preparation, and decreasing the risk of air-drying artifact (Hutchinson et al., 1991; Pfenninger et al., 1992). As with all cervical sampling procedures, clinical attention to detail is the most important factor in adequate sampling. The broom must be rotated 4-8 times to collect an adequate sample. It also may not be appropriate for a minority of patients with either cervical stenosis or unusual anatomy.

In the last decade, laboratory control of many of the pre-analytic variables has been facilitated by the development of liquid based thin layer technology (Sherman et al., 1998). The attractions of thin layer technologies include improvements in sampling, fixation, staining and background. In essence, most of the variables in slide quality are removed from the realm of the sample collector and placed under more stringent control within the laboratory. The entire sample is placed directly into a vial of liquid fixative, optimizing fixation. Randomization of the sample through mixing and liquid suspension ensures a more representative sampling on the slide submitted for screening. Optimization of fixation and staining helps to minimize uncertainty and equivocal diagnosis. A tremendous advantage of liquid based methods is that they allow other tests e.g., HPV testing, to be performed on the residual sample, which statistically should be representative of the cells seen on the slide (Peyton et al., 1998).

1.2   Cervical biopsy

Cervical biopsies are generally small pieces of tissue removed from the cervix to confirm a cytologic or histologic diagnosis. Biopsies may be performed in a non-directed manner, as opposed to systematically sampling each quadrant; most frequently they are taken under colposcopic guidance. Historically, many clinicians considered colposcopic biopsy the gold standard of diagnosis. Yet today we know that there is significant observer variability in colposcopic skill and biopsy placement such that the biopsy may not represent the true severity of the pathology (Cinel et al., 1990; Stoler and Schiffman, 2001). This is especially important when the cytology suggests a high-grade lesion and the biopsy is less than high grade. In such a case, conization may be required to resolve the discrepancy and insure that the patient is adequately treated for a potential cancer precursor.

1.3   Cone biopsy

The term cone biopsy or conization refers to a cone shaped excision of the cervix encompassing the transformation zone. The pathology thus displayed is the gold standard for cervical diagnosis short of examination of tissues obtained after hysterectomy. Conization is often both a diagnostic as well as a therapeutic procedure. Conizations vary in size and extent depending upon cervical anatomy, patient age and desire for fertility and surgical technique. Loop electrosurgical excision procedures (LEEP) are increasingly replacing traditional conization as well as other forms of local ablative therapies. Regardless of surgical technique the goal of the procedure is complete excision of the transformation zone with adequate margins of normal ectocervix and endocervix to allow a thorough pathologic assessment of the entire area of the cervix at risk. As with smaller biopsies, the quality of the surgeon, the patient's anatomy, and the skill of the pathologist all can affect the accuracy of this assessment (Howe and Vincente, 1991; Irvin et al., 2002).

1.4   Hysterectomy

Hysterectomy is removal of the uterus usually with the cervix en bloc. The type of hysterectomy will vary depending upon the pathology. For treatment of cervical cancer, radical hysterectomy with pelvic lymph node dissection is performed for patients of suitable stage, usually clinical stage IB. However, many patients are treated by primary radiation therapy, either alone or in combination with chemotherapy, after the diagnosis is established by clinical examination and biopsy.

2   ANATOMY

The cervix is the most caudal portion of the uterus where it fuses with the vagina. The cervix measures 2.5-3.0 cm in length, 2-2.5 cm. in diameter, and the vaginal portion that usually appears convex, is delimited by the anterior and posterior vaginal fornices (Kurman et al., 1992). Depending upon parity, the centrally located external os is either slit-like or circular and the endocervical canal ends at the internal os where the isthmus or lower uterine segment begins.

The major sites of lymphatic drainage, which relate to pathways of metastatic spread, are the external iliac, internal iliac, common iliac and sacral nodes through anterolateral, lateral and posterolateral collecting trunks that follow the main vascular and ligamentous supports of the cervix.

Embryologically, the cervix, as is most of the upper female genital tract, is a mesodermal derivative of the Muellarian ducts. The source of the reserve cells that give rise to the mucosal epithelium is still debated, although most feel that they are stromally derived. The stroma induces differentiation into a variety of epithelia: squamous, mucinous and tuboendometrial (ciliated) cells well as argyrophilic (neuroendocrine) cell types.

3   HISTOLOGY

3.1   Epithelial types

There are four main types of epithelium present in the normal cervix (Figures 1-4). The ectocervix is lined by native squamous epithelium. Microscopically this epithelium can be divided into basal, intermediate, and superficial zones. Normally there is no stratum granulosum or stratum corneum. The squamous epithelium proliferates under, among other things, estrogen stimulation, which also causes glycogen accumulation. Cell proliferation is normally limited to the basal zone. Studies have shown that the basal or first parabasal cell divides and one cell maintains the basal population while the other migrates upward and differentiates in a highly controlled manner.

Prior to menarche there is usually a sharp demarcation between the native squamous epithelium and the endocervical glands. While not true glands, the ridges of the endocervix are lined primarily by a mucinous columnar epithelium admixed with ciliated (tubal) cells. The usual maximal depth of extension of the endocervical glands is 5 mm. Histochemical studies demonstrate a minor population of neuroendocrine (argyrophilic) cells in the endocervix.

3.2   Transformation zone

The transformation zone (T-zone) is the area in which squamous metaplasia of the endocervical glands occurs. Metaplasia is defined as the replacement of one cell type with another cell type. Colposcopically and histologically, the T-zone is defined as the zone between the original and current squamocolumnar junctions. The process of squamous metaplasia is most active during late fetal life, adolescence, and pregnancy. It is obviously related to hormonal, physical, and inflammatory stimuli. The origin of metaplastic epithelium is thought to be the subcolumnar reserve cell capable of multiphasic differentiation. The transformation zone is the most frequent site for detection of cervical cancer and its precursors. The reason for this is not well defined but may be as simple as the fact that the basal cells are both exposed and actively proliferating at this junctional site. Indeed analogous squamocolumnar junctions at other body sites like the rectum, larynx, and nasal cavity demonstrate similar susceptibility to HPV infection.

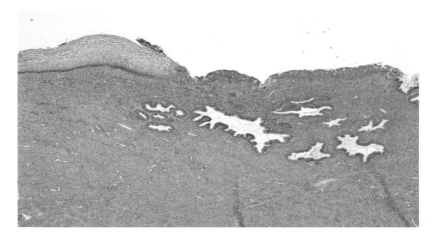

Figure 1. Low power image of the cervical transformation zone. The stratified native ectocervical mucosa is to the left. The original squamocolumnar junction is just at the point where the endocervical glands are evident. In the right half of the image the first several endocervical glands are covered by immature squamous metaplasia, and then near the right corner of the image, the squamous metaplasia ends, thus defining the upper end of the transformation zone.

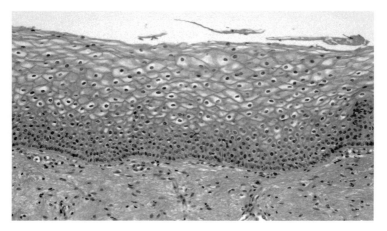

Figure 2. A low power image of normal ectocervical squamous mucosa demonstrating stratification of the epithelium and orderly squamous maturation.

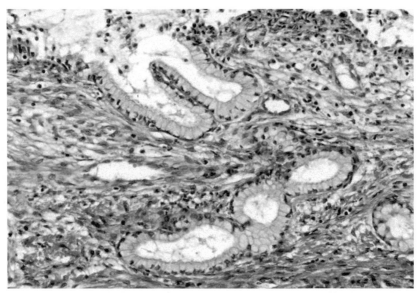

Figure 3. Normal endocervical glands are lined by a simple columnar mucus-secreting epithelium.

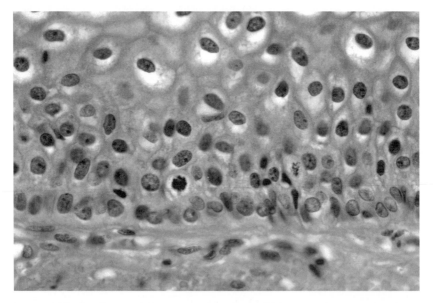

Figure 4. The basal zone of the squamous mucosa at high power demonstrating the transition from basal to the first parabasal cell and an occasional mitotic figure in the first cell above the basement membrane.

4 CARCINOGENESIS

While carcinogenesis is covered in other chapters in greater detail (see Chapters 3 and 4 in particular), a molecular model for HPV-induced carcinogenesis involving the interaction of HPV gene products with the tightly regulated network of cellular oncogenes and antioncogenes involved in the control of cell proliferation will be commented on here. This model is relevant to the schema of diagnostic classifications that follow, after which the relevant pathologic diagnoses will be defined in some detail (Stoler, 2000b).

Histogenetically, papillomaviruses must infect the "reserve, basal or stem" cell population of the cervical transformation zone: cells with the potential to differentiate along squamous, glandular, or neuroendocrine lines that are responsible for epithelial maintenance (Figure 5).

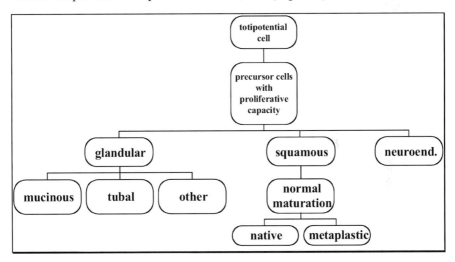

Figure 5. A schematic of normal histogenesis emphasizing that the reserve cells of the cervix can differentiate along squamous, glandular or neuroendocrine lines.

In cells committed to squamous differentiation there is an orderly program of maturation throughout the epithelial thickness both at the morphologic as well as the molecular level. As noted above, in normal squamous epithelia, the only cells capable of cell division are the basal or parabasal cells. In morphologically normal, but HPV-infected basal cells, papillomavirus gene expression is inhibited to near maintenance levels. Productive HPV gene expression is tightly regulated and permitted only in cells that have begun squamous maturation, with a concomitant loss of proliferative capacity (Figure 6). In the immediate suprabasal zone there is expression of the early regions of the viral genome, and as the cells differentiate, there is an induction of all viral genes as well as viral DNA synthesis, leading to assembly and production of virions in the cells just beneath the surface. In the cervix one recognizes such lesions as low-grade squamous intraepithelial lesions/mild dysplasia/CIN 1, most of which at some point, demonstrate koilocytotic atypia. Such lesions usually regress in 1-2 years, and rarely persist for extended periods. An explanation for some of the diagnostic criteria used by pathologists is implicit in this program of differentiation-linked expression. The nuclear enlargement and hyper-chromasia recognized as atypia is a direct result of E6/E7-mediated activation of host DNA synthesis. In a low-grade lesion this is regulated to occur in cells that can no longer divide (i.e., the intermediate squamous cells) and is primarily directed at the production of viral DNA (Figure 7). Given the small size of the viral genome, the several thousand copies of the virus present in a productively infected cell clearly cannot account for the two- to fourfold nuclear enlargement that is observed. It is a diagnostically fortunate coincidence that ineffective (in the sense of cell division) E6/E7 mediated host DNA synthesis produces the enlarged nuclei and increased N:C ratio recognized as abnormal. If the process is not fully developed, or is perhaps regressing, then the cells derived from the surface often have less nuclear abnormality (perhaps atypical squamous cells of uncertain significance, or ASCUS) than those seen in classical dysplasia. In the fully developed case, cells with well-developed koilocytotic atypia are classified as being derived from a mild dysplasia/LSIL. If the cells also have the correct amount and form of the cytokeratin binding protein HPV E4 expressed, then they appear as koilocytes. Koilocytotic atypia, while very often present, *does not have to be seen to recognize a low-grade lesion.* Every cytologist recognizes cells derived from the upper levels of a mild dysplasia that meet the diagnostic criteria for dysplasia yet do not have the characteristic perinuclear halo termed koilocytosis. Such lesions are just as HPV-associated as those that do have koilocytes and the differences undoubtedly represent temporal variation within the life cycle of a low-grade lesion.

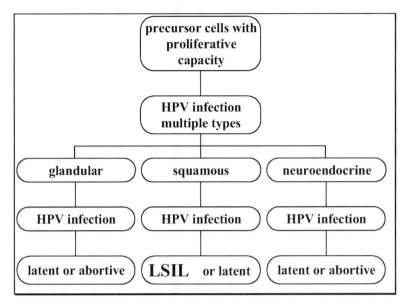

Figure 6. The pathogenesis of LSIL, emphasizing that only in a squamous milieu, will HPV infection be productive.

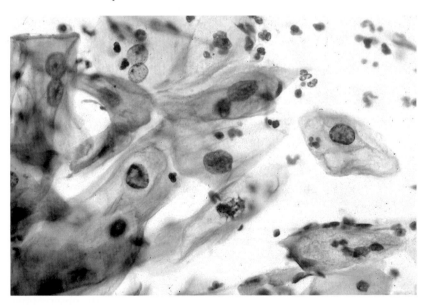

Figure 7. The cytology typical of a low-grade squamous intraepithelial lesion/mild dysplasia/CIN1.

If viral gene expression is so tightly regulated, how do high-grade lesions develop? The sine qua non of high-grade dysplasia is morphologic evidence of increased abnormal basal-like cell proliferation (Figure 8). In these cells, the coordinate link between differentiation and viral early gene expression is lost. How this occurs is unclear, although it certainly must be a rare event(s) given the high relative frequency of low versus high-grade lesions. Potential mechanisms might include viral integration or mutations in HPV E2; such that E2 mediated regulation of E6/E7 expression is lost. In such cases, the viral oncogenes E6 and E7 are *inappropriately expressed* in a population of cells that retain the capacity to divide, thereby *initiating* cell proliferation. As this population of cells proliferates, it overtakes the epithelium, producing lesions that are, by definition, characterized by less orderly squamous maturation and basal-like cell overgrowth with evident mitotic activity. Possible promoters of this process could be smoking, other viruses and infectious stimuli, inflammation or random mutation. The relative infrequency of these effects is biologically manifest by the latency and relative rarity of HSILs versus LSILs. Progression to the *proliferative phenotype* occurs most frequently, albeit not exclusively, with high-risk viral types, and results in the high grade squamous intraepithelial lesions also called moderate squamous dysplasia, severe squamous dysplasia, or squamous carcinoma in situ (CIN 2/3) (Figure 9). Thus, the Bethesda System's break between low-grade versus high-grade follows in part from the biologic changes manifest between these morphologies. Indeed, from the standpoint of epithelial biology, there is little rationale for separating moderate from severe dysplasia in that the critical break occurs between mild and moderate dysplasia with the switch to a *proliferative* as opposed to a differentiated and virally *productive* phenotype.

In high grade squamous intraepithelial lesions, the proliferating basaloid cells, driven by E6/E7 over expression, are at much greater risk for the acquisition of additional genetic errors, clonal selection, etc., perhaps under the influence of the same external mutagens and/or host genetic predisposition, which further *promotes* the development of the fully malignant phenotype, most often an invasive squamous cell carcinoma. The different subtypes of squamous cancer, e.g., keratinizing, etc., are probably related to the multi-step and somewhat random nature of the process. The proportion of different types may reflect the relative likelihood of different genetic pathways to a "successful" cancer, in part modulated by the microenvironment in which the lesion develops. Hence, early observations that keratinizing cancers are often more ectocervical than large cell nonkeratinizing or small cell malignancies, which tend to originate higher in the endocervical canal, have some contemporary validation.

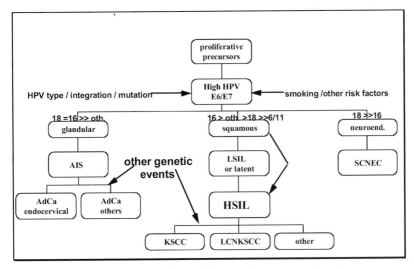

Figure 8. The possible pathogenesis of high-grade lesions and invasive cancer where inappropriate HPV oncogene expression drives the various types of epithelia to proliferate. Uncontrolled cell proliferation is the hallmark of true neoplasia. Abbreviations: AIS = adenocarcinoma in situ, AdCa = adenocarcinoma, KSCC = keratinizing squamous cell carcinoma, LCNKSCC = large cell non-keratinizing squamous cell carcinoma, LSIL/HSIL = low/high grade squamous intraepithelial lesion, SCNEC = small cell neuroendocrine carcinoma.

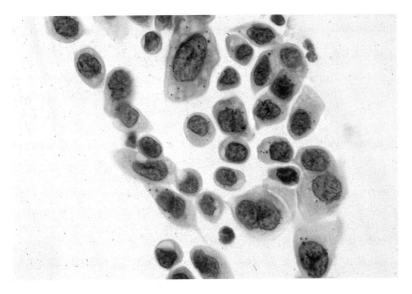

Figure 9. Cytology of a typical high-grade squamous intraepithelial lesion. The cells represented are consistent with the fact that the epithelium has been over run by proliferating cells such that they are close enough to the surface to be sampled with the usual Pap smear collection device.

Given this model for cervical squamous neoplasia, one still needs to account for the development of other epithelial tumors e.g., glandular and small cell neuroendocrine neoplasms. Reserve cells that are already committed to glandular differentiation are, because of a lack of an appropriate differentiation environment, not likely to be productive of virions. This is because the productive viral life cycle requires the cellular milieu of orderly squamous differentiation. If this is true, then viral infection in cells committed to glandular differentiation most often results (from the viral standpoint) in an abortive or latent infection of morphologically normal endocervical cells. Rarely, dysregulation of viral early gene expression occurs in these usually nonpermissive cells. This leads to hyperproliferative lesions of glandular cells, which pathologists recognize as severe endocervical dysplasia, better known as adenocarcinoma in situ (AIS). There is no established biologic correlate in this model of a low-grade glandular dysplasia. Hence, this nicely explains the inability of pathologists to reproducibly recognize, either cytologically or histologically, a clinically meaningful lesion less severe than what most call AIS. HPV 18 seems to be more successful at inducing neoplastic proliferation in glandular cells than HPV 16. Perhaps this is because HPV 18 has a greater disposition to integrate into the genome and perhaps because type 18 may have some preference for cells predisposed to other than squamous differentiation. Parenthetically, little if anything is known about the mechanisms of HPV type-specific cellular tropism. However, no HPV type can be exclusively trophic for non-squamous cells because, under the above model, that type of virus would be eliminated from the population. Depending upon the genetic switches that over time accompany virally induced glandular proliferations, the outcome may be an invasive adenocarcinoma, most often endocervical, but less frequently of another type, e.g., endometrioid or clear cell adenocarcinoma. The relative frequencies of the different types of cervical adenocarcinoma again may just reflect the relative frequency of the different populations committed towards various types of differentiation. Essentially identical arguments can be made for the development of small cell neuroendocrine carcinomas, tumors that are almost always associated with HPV 18 and whose low incidence probably reflects the relative abundance of a susceptible neuroendocrine-committed precursor cell population and the rarity of "successful" viral induction of cell proliferation in such cells.

5   CLASSIFICATION SYSTEMS AND HPV

Given the above background, the pathologic spectrum of HPV-associated neoplasia could be defined as those lesions in which HPV DNA is both present and expressed, so as to make the link between the presence of viral DNA and abnormal morphology pathogenetically feasible. Indeed this is exactly the case for the lesions that will now be defined and discussed. The WHO histologic classification of tumors of the uterine cervix and The Bethesda System (TBS) both recognize the importance of these concepts (Scully et al., 1994; Solomon et al., 2002) (Tables 1 and 2).

Table 1. WHO histologic classification of tumors and tumor-like lesions of the uterine cervix

	Epithelial Tumors and Related Lesions
1.1	Squamous lesions
1.1.1	Squamous papilloma
1.1.2	Condyloma acuminatum
1.1.3	Squamous metaplasia
1.1.4	Transitional metaplasia
1.1.5	Squamous atypia
1.1.6	Squamous intraepithelial lesions (dysplasia-carcinoma in situ; cervical intraepithelial neoplasia (CIN))
1.1.6.1	Mild dysplasia (CIN 1)
1.1.6.2	Moderate dysplasia (CIN 2)
1.1.6.3	Severe dysplasia (CIN 3)
1.1.6.4	Carcinoma in situ (CIN 3)
1.1.7	Squamous cell carcinoma
1.1.7.1	Keratinizing
1.1.7.2	Nonkeratinizing
1.1.7.3	Verrucous
1.1.7.4	Warty (condylomatous)
1.1.7.5	Papillary
1.1.7.6	Lymphoepithelioma-like carcinoma
1.2	Glandular Lesions
1.2.1	Endocervical polyp
1.2.2	Muellarian papilloma
1.2.3	Glandular atypia
1.2.4	Glandular dysplasia
1.2.5	Adenocarcinoma in situ
1.2.6	Adenocarcinoma
1.2.6.1	Mucinous adenocarcinoma
1.2.6.1.1	Endocervical type
1.2.6.1.2	Intestinal type
1.2.6.2	Endometrioid adenocarcinoma
1.2.6.3	Clear cell adenocarcinoma
1.2.6.4	Serous adenocarcinoma
1.2.6.5	Mesonephric adenocarcinoma

Table 1. WHO histologic classification of tumors and tumor-like lesions of the uterine cervix, *continued*

	Epithelial Tumors and Related Lesions
1.3	Other epithelial tumors
1.3.1	Adenosquamous carcinoma
1.3.2	Glassy cell carcinoma
1.3.3	Adenoid cystic carcinoma
1.3.4	Adenoid basal carcinoma
1.3.5	Carcinoid tumor
1.3.6	Small cell carcinoma
1.3.7	Undifferentiated carcinoma

Table 2. Bethesda System 2001

SPECIMEN TYPE: *Indicate conventional smear (Pap smear) vs. liquid-based vs. other*

SPECIMEN ADEQUACY
- ❑ Satisfactory for evaluation (*describe presence or absence of endocervical/transformation zone component and any other quality indicators, e.g., partially obscuring blood, inflammation, etc*)
- ❑ Unsatisfactory for evaluation ... (*specify reason*)
- ❑ Specimen rejected/not processed (*specify reason*)
- ❑ Specimen processed and examined, but unsatisfactory for evaluation of epithelial abnormality because of (*specify reason*)

GENERAL CATEGORIZATION (*optional*)
- ❑ Negative for Intraepithelial Lesion or Malignancy
- ❑ Epithelial Cell Abnormality: See Interpretation/Result (*specify 'squamous' or 'glandular' as appropriate*)
- ❑ Other: See Interpretation/Result (*e.g. endometrial cells in a woman > 40 years of age)*

AUTOMATED REVIEW
If case examined by automated device, specify device and result.

ANCILLARY TESTING
Provide a brief description of the test methods and report the result so that it is easily understood by the clinician.

INTERPRETATION/RESULT

Table 2. Bethesda System 2001, *continued*

NEGATIVE FOR INTRAEPITHELIAL LESION OR MALIGNANCY

(*when there is no cellular evidence of neoplasia, state this in the General Categorization above and/or in the Interpretation/Result section of the report, whether or not there are organisms or other non-neoplastic findings*)

ORGANISMS:
- ❑ *Trichomonas vaginalis*
- ❑ Fungal organisms morphologically consistent with *Candida* spp
- ❑ Shift in flora suggestive of bacterial vaginosis
- ❑ Bacteria morphologically consistent with *Actinomyces* spp.
- ❑ Cellular changes consistent with herpes simplex virus

OTHER NON-NEOPLASTIC FINDINGS (*Optional to report; list not inclusive*):
- ❑ Reactive cellular changes associated with:
  - o inflammation (includes typical repair)
  - o radiation
  - o intrauterine contraceptive device (IUD)
- ❑ Glandular cells status post hysterectomy
- ❑ Atrophy

OTHER
- ❑ Endometrial cells (*in a woman > 40 years of age*)
  (*Specify if 'negative for squamous intraepithelial lesion'*)

EPITHELIAL CELL ABNORMALITIES

SQUAMOUS CELL
- ❑ Atypical squamous cells
  - o of undetermined significance (ASC-US)
  - o cannot exclude HSIL (ASC-H)
- ❑ Low grade squamous intraepithelial lesion (LSIL) encompassing: HPV/mild dysplasia/CIN 1
- ❑ High grade squamous intraepithelial lesion (HSIL) encompassing: moderate and severe dysplasia, CIS/CIN 2 and CIN 3
  - o with features suspicious for invasion (*if invasion is suspected*)
- ❑ Squamous cell carcinoma

Table 2. Bethesda System 2001, *continued*
_____

GLANDULAR CELL
  ❑ Atypical:
      o   endocervical cells (NOS *or specify in comments*)
      o   endometrial cells (NOS *or specify in comments*)
      o   glandular cells (NOS *or specify in comments*)
  ❑ Atypical:
      o   endocervical cells, favor neoplastic
      o   glandular cells, favor neoplastic
  ❑ Endocervical adenocarcinoma *in situ*
  ❑ Adenocarcinoma:
      o   endocervical
      o   endometrial
      o   extrauterine
      o   not otherwise specified (NOS)
OTHER MALIGNANT NEOPLASMS: (*specify*)
EDUCATIONAL NOTES AND SUGGESTIONS: (*optional*)
     Suggestions should be concise and consistent with clinical follow-up
     guidelines published by professional organizations (references to
     relevant publications may be included).
_____

     The existing WHO formulation utilizes the cervical intraepithelial neoplasia
(CIN) terminology and can be easily translated into the traditional
dysplasia/carcinoma in situ (CIS) terminology or Bethesda terminology. Pap
smear terminology has progressively evolved as our concepts and knowledge
regarding pathogenesis have evolved (Table 3). Originally, the simple numeric
Papanicolaou classification while related to degree of severity soon became
problematic because the definition and clinical meaning varied widely amongst
laboratories (Kurman et al., 1991). The concept of cervical dysplasia most
widely promoted by Reagan and Patten sought to more formally relate the
spectrum of epithelial abnormality seen on Pap smear with the histologic
outcome on biopsy and conization (Patten, 1978; Reagan et al., 1961; Reagan
and Patten, 1962). The CIN classification introduced by Richart simplified the
number of categories and emphasized that there seemed to be a biologic
continuum of risk for the development of carcinoma (Richart, 1973; Richart
and Barron, 1969). It began the trend of realistically recognizing that some
pathologically defined categories were not very distinct or meaningful to the
patient or treating clinician. Specifically, it was argued that carcinoma in situ
and severe dysplasia were biologically the same and hence both were called
CIN III. Beginning in 1988 and now twice revised as recently as 2001, the
Bethesda System (TBS) was introduced to improve communication and
increase   reproducibility   between   pathologists   rendering   cytologic

interpretations (Kurman et al., 1991; Luff, 1992; Solomon et al., 2002). TBS is the first classification that takes into account recent knowledge of interobserver reproducibility, the distribution of HPV types and the clinical behavior and management of these lesions. The simplification and regrouping of lesions reflects many of the pathogenetic concepts raised in the just presented model. Low-grade lesions are the pathologic correlate of productive HPV infection. High-grade lesions are characterized by a proliferative phenotype and are generally not productive of virus. TBS classification of epithelial abnormalities presents a practical approach to cytologic diagnosis that is equally applicable to histologic interpretation. However, not all observers agree with that approach. Some compromise and use the CIN terminology for histology and the Bethesda terminology for cytology with either the CIN or dysplasia terminology in parentheses to provide translations for clinicians used to older terms.

Table 3. Comparison of Cytology Classifications For Squamous Lesions

PAP	PAP translation		Dysplasia/CIS	CIN	Bethesda
I	normal		normal	normal	normal
II	mild "atypia"		squamous atypia	atypical	ASC-US
III	suspicious		mild dysplasia	CIN I	LSIL
IV	probably malignant		moderate dysplasia	CIN II	HSIL
V	malignant		severe dysplasia	CIN III	HSIL
			carcinoma in situ	CIN III	HSIL
			cancer	cancer	cancer

6   SQUAMOUS CELL CYTOPATHOLOGY

6.1   Benign proliferative changes

Three different epithelial reactions have been classified as benign proliferative reactions in the uterine cervix (Bonfiglio and Patten, 1976; Geirsson et al., 1977; Patten, 1978). Included in this category are squamous metaplasia, hyperkeratosis and parakeratosis. While parakeratosis and hyperkeratosis are considered to be related processes, squamous metaplasia is quite dissimilar and is best considered separately and in somewhat more detail.

Squamous metaplasia in the cervix is the process whereby columnar glandular epithelium of the transformation zone is gradually replaced by a mature squamous epithelium (Figures 10 and 11). In the young female a portion of the face of the cervix is covered by a columnar endocervical-type of epithelium. Beginning at about the time of menarche and continuing throughout the reproductive years, this epithelium undergoes a trans-formation of variable extent into a squamous epithelium. This process occurs in virtually every female and is considered normal. Its etiology is uncertain, but is perhaps related to menarchal changes in bacterial flora and a lowering of vaginal pH. Adequate cellular samples which include material from the transformation zone in pre-menopausal women would therefore be expected to contain immature metaplastic cells as a normal finding.

Immature metaplastic cells in cytologic specimens have a round to oval configuration and relatively dense cytoplasm with nuclei that consistently average 50 square micrometers in total area. The nuclear:cytoplasmic ratio of the most immature metaplastic cells is quite high. As the epithelium undergoes maturation the cells acquire more cytoplasm and the nuclear-cytoplasmic ratio decreases.

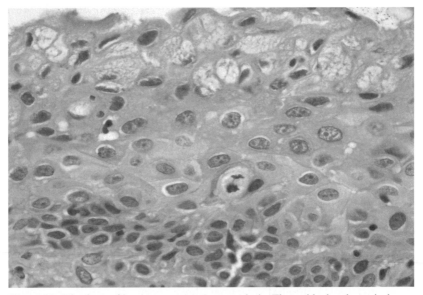

Figure 10. Histology of immature squamous metaplasia. The residual endocervical mucus-secreting epithelium can be seen on the surface as it is undermined by a proliferation of squamous cells that lack the features of dysplasia.

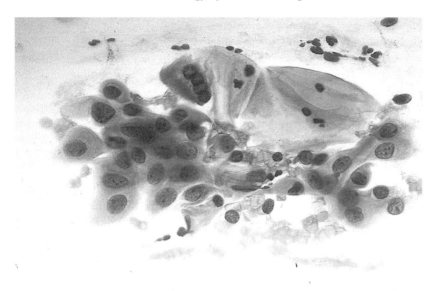

Figure 11. The cytology of immature squamous metaplasia. Note the cells of the lower part of the figure are a very good representation of the basal portion of the epithelium in Figure 10.

While squamous metaplasia is a normal physiologic process, an understanding of the process and its morphology is important to our understanding of carcinogenesis, for it is in the area of the transformation zone that the process of squamous metaplasia takes place, and where the precursor lesions to squamous cell carcinoma develop. The immature metaplastic epithelium of the squamous metaplastic process, more specifically the dividing basal cell population, seems to be that which is most susceptible to the suspected carcinogenic agent, namely human papillomavirus.

The normal squamous epithelium of the cervical mucosa does not contain a granular cell layer or a keratin layer (Rubio et al., 1976). Under some circumstances however, particularly in response to chronic irritation the epithelium undergoes hypermaturation and a granular cell layer with overlying keratinization develops. This occurrence is referred to as hyperkeratosis. A common situation associated with this process is uterine prolapse but any irritating stimulus, traumatic or inflammatory, may result in the development of hyperkeratosis.

Hyperkeratosis is diagnosed in cytologic samples by the identification of variable numbers of anucleate squamous cells that stain eosinophilic or orangeophilic with the Papanicolaou stain. The finding of hyperkeratosis alone does not appear to be associated with the presence or future development of any more significant epithelial lesion. While some intraepithelial processes and certain cases of invasive squamous carcinoma are marked by keratinization, these conditions almost always are identifiable cytologically by the concurrent presence of other cytologic abnormalities. Parakeratosis is a process that is similar to and may coexist with hyperkeratosis. It is characterized by multiple layers of miniature, keratinized cells with small pyknotic remnants of cell nuclei identifiable within their cytoplasm. The process occurs in squamous epithelium that is undergoing rapid turnover. While the underlying epithelium may otherwise appear normal, in some cases parakeratosis overlies an abnormal epithelium. Parakeratosis for example may be a feature associated with human papillomavirus related epithelial changes. Most typically, when the process is part of an intraepithelial lesion other cytologic abnormalities are present. Sometimes the presence of pleomorphic parakeratotic forms on a Pap smear is the only evidence that a significant lesion may be present. The presence of parakeratosis suggests that closer surveillance or further investigation of the patient may be indicated. The presence of pleomorphic parakeratosis where the parakeratotic cells have variability and atypia is an indication for further investigation such as colposcopy to exclude the possibility of a high-grade intraepithelial lesion.

6.2   Atypical Squamous Cells - ASC

One of the great virtues of TBS is the breaking up of the ambiguous diagnosis "atypical or Class II PAP" into specific diagnostic categories that correlate with either clinical or histologic diagnoses. Epithelial atypia is a term used to describe a spectrum of changes within the uterine cervix (Kurman and Solomon, 1994; Patten, 1978). Cells derived from this type of reaction, while not normal, do not have the characteristics of the more severe lesions classified as dysplasia or intraepithelial neoplasia. The cytologic changes in this category are related primarily to slight to moderate alterations in nuclear size and morphology. Etiologically, epithelial atypia of the uterine cervix can often be attributed to inflammation, repair/ regenerative processes, deficiency states, or perhaps the early manifestations of neoplasia.

A useful reference standard in cytologic material for evaluating size is the nucleus of the immature squamous metaplastic cell, which is a fairly constant 50 square micrometers in area. The nuclear size of the squamous cells classified as atypical is in the range of 75 to 125 square micrometers. This is in contrast to cells derived from dysplastic reactions that generally have nuclei in the range of 150 to 200 square micrometers. In general, the nuclear chromatin of "atypical nuclei" is finely granular, evenly distributed, and normochromatic as opposed to the hyperchromasia often associated with cells derived from dysplasia.

A number of different pathological processes can induce this type of nuclear alteration. In some instances the likely etiology of the atypia is evident from the examination of the cervical smear. Specific inflammatory processes, for example trichomoniasis, may be associated with the presence of atypical cells, which return to normal with the cessation of the inflammatory stimulus. In other cases the etiology and significance of the atypia may not be evident on the basis of the cytologic findings, thus they are of uncertain significance.

6.3   ASC-US

It is not uncommon to detect atypical squamous cells in cervical smears, which cannot be explained on the basis of any specific inflammatory process and which do not fit into the spectrum of intraepithelial lesions recognized as precursors to squamous carcinoma. This type of abnormality, which has also been referred to in the past as "benign" squamous atypia or borderline dyskaryosis, is characterized by a slight to moderate increase in nuclear size and mild nuclear hyperchromasia (Figure 12). The cells may have a mature-appearing cytoplasm resembling that of normal superficial or intermediate cells or an immature cytoplasm like that of immature squamous metaplastic cells. In recent years it has become clear that this borderline category is truly equivocal in that it correlates with true epithelial abnormality and HPV positivity approximately 50% of the time, compared to samples with unequivocal diagnostic SIL, which are HPV positive more than 90% of the time. Indeed it seems that this equivocal category is an important buffer for interpretive sensitivity and that it may well be defined in relation to the frequency of HPV positivity of cellular samples in the laboratory. Specifically a laboratory could calibrate its equivocal diagnoses to be between the low rates found in the normal population and the 85-95% high risk HPV positive rate expected in the SIL interpretive group (Solomon et al., 2001; Stoler, 2002).

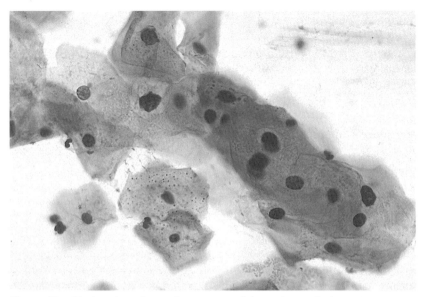

Figure 12.   Equivocal nuclear enlargement and hyperchromasia in mature squamous epithelial cells typical of ASC-US cytology.

6.4   ASC-H

An important minority of ASC diagnoses is the category of ASC-H. These are smears with cells that are worrisome but felt not to be diagnostic for HSIL (Figure 13). The cells of concern are immature metaplastic cells with a higher N:C ratio, some degree of hyperchromasia and perhaps mild nuclear contour irregularity compared to benign immature metaplasia. And yet by all criteria these cells fall short of those felt to be unequivocally diagnostic of HSIL. Often these cells are present in very small numbers on the slide contributing to the cytologist's tendency to equivocate. Yet their importance is clear as patients whose smears are interpreted as ASC-H have a higher frequency of ultimate HSIL compared to cases interpreted as ASC-US (Sherman et al., 2001; Sherman et al., 1999; Stoler, 1999).

ASC is primarily a cytologic interpretation. Histologically, equivocation tends to be minimized by pathologists, with a large number of resulting biopsies either interpreted as normal/inflammatory or diagnostic of SIL (Stoler and Schiffman, 2001). The concept that ASC interpretations are statements of equivocation and uncertainty rather than a linear progression state from normal to SIL is a recent conceptual advance.

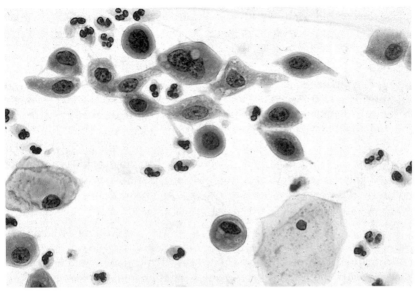

Figure 13. An image consistent with ASC-H. Metaplastic epithelial cells with mildly enlarged and hyperchromatic nuclei but not diagnostic of HSIL. Compare to Figure 9.

6.5 Cytology of SIL contrasted with ASC

The degree of severity of an intraepithelial neoplastic process is evaluated on a cytologic sample by a consideration of the morphologic characteristics of the constituent cells. Of less importance is the number of abnormal cells present. The morphologic features related to severity include those involving both the nucleus and the cytoplasm but the nuclear features are the most significant (Bonfiglio and Patten, 1976; Fu et al., 1981; Koss and Durfee, 1961; Meisels and Fortin, 1976; Patten, 1978; Purola and Savia, 1977; Reagan, 1965; Reagan, 1956, Reagan and Harmonic, 1962; Reagan et al., 1953).

The number of abnormal cells in the cytologic sample varies with the collection technique used. While counts of abnormal cells vary from one case to another, in general, lesser degrees of dysplasia are associated with fewer abnormal cells per slide while the more severe lesions are reflected by a markedly increased abnormal cell count. As reported in studies by Reagan and Patten and reemphasized in TBS, cells derived from dysplasia have nuclear areas in the size range of 150 to 200 square micrometers, i.e., about 4 times the nuclear area of the reference normal squamous cell nuclei. The nucleus of a normal intermediate squamous cell measures approximately 35 square micrometers and that of a cell derived from an immature squamous metaplasia approximately 50 square micrometers. The size varies somewhat with the differentiation of the dysplastic process. Nuclei from HSIL may range from 75 square micrometers up to 200 square micrometers, again depending on the subclass dysplasia.

In general, three chromatin patterns are associated with dysplasia. The nuclei of cells derived from dysplastic reactions may have a finely granular, evenly distributed chromatin; a finely granular, evenly distributed chromatin with some chromatin clumping; or, in keratinizing lesions, very dense, deeply staining, opaque chromatin. In some cases of HSIL, different chromatin patterns exist, consisting of evenly distributed, coarsely granular chromatin or evenly distributed, coarsely granular chromatin with interrupted nuclear membranes. Irregular chromatin distribution and so-called areas of nuclear clearing are generally not seen in the intraepithelial reactions but are characteristic of invasive processes.

With increasing severity of the lesion, there is decreasing cytoplasmic maturity. Mature, well-defined cytoplasm is characteristic of the superficial and intermediate cells of LSILs. Koilocytotic atypia (KA), the morphologic hallmark of what can be considered human papillomavirus cytopathic effect, is most commonly associated with these low-grade lesions. Other synonymous terms e.g., warty atypia, condylomatous atypia or koilocytosis have been used as cytologic diagnoses in cell samples characterized by these features. Microscopically, KA is defined as a cell with an atypical nucleus *and* a clearly defined, sharply delineated perinuclear halo. The atypical nuclei are characterized by hyperchromasia, nuclear enlargement and/or wrinkling of the nuclear envelope or more advanced degenerative changes including a smudging of the chromatin and pyknosis.

A perinuclear halo alone is not diagnostic. Cytoplasmic glycogen can sometimes give an appearance of a perinuclear clear zone particularly in tissue sections. Perinuclear halos, generally smaller and less well defined than those of koilocytes, are also seen as non-specific manifestations of inflammation and are particularly common with trichomonad infection. Smears with these characteristics should not be classified as dysplasia or SIL.

KA may be found in association with other cytologic features including "cherry-red amphophilia" of the cytoplasm of some cells and cell aggregates with dense, dyskeratotic cytoplasm and small, pyknotic nuclei. These latter features, while often associated with HPV infection, are not considered as pathognomonic of HPV infection. These so-called minor HPV changes, if present without koilocytosis or other evidence of dysplasia (SIL), are relatively non-specific. Hence, it is more appropriate to classify these cytologic changes as part of the ASC spectrum. Intraepithelial lesions demonstrating koilocytotic features but having nuclei smaller than those described above for dysplasia, that is, only mild nuclear enlargement on the order of 70 to 100 μm², may also be considered of undetermined significance.

Today, most consider mild dysplasia and koilocytotic atypia identical for purposes of patient management, treatment and follow up (Table 4). The latter concept is reinforced by studies demonstrating the inability of experienced pathologists to reproducibly separate the two lesions on the basis of morphology alone.

Table 4. Common features of koilocytotic atypia,mild dysplasia, and LGSIL

Same biologic potential	Require similar clinical management
Same heterogeneous HPV profile	Overlapping morphologic criteria

7   SURGICAL PATHOLOGY OF SQUAMOUS LESIONS

7.1   Squamous Papilloma

A squamous papilloma is defined as a benign papillary lesion covered by squamous epithelium without true koilocytosis (Kazal and Long, 1958; Kurman et al., 1992). Usually these have a more simple architecture than a condyloma. They are much more rare than true condylomata. Synonyms include fibroepithelial polyp, ectocervical polyp and fibroepithelioma, all of which may be preferable, since in other sites (e.g., larynx), squamous papillomas are equivalent to condylomata. As defined, these lesions are not HPV associated but are mentioned here because they are in the differential diagnosis of condylomata.

7.2   Condyloma acuminatum

Condylomata are papillary exophytic benign neoplasms caused by HPV. Tumors with this morphologic appearance are much more frequent on the external genitalia and compared to flat LSIL, these are relatively uncommon on the cervix. Condylomata frequently coexist at multiple anogenital sites (Isacson et al., 1996; Meisels and Fortin, 1976; Mittal and Chan, 1990; Purola and Savia, 1977).

While any HPV type can induce condylomatous histology, HPV types 6 and 11 are relatively more frequent in such lesions. Many researchers feel that the lesions with well-developed koilocytosis are the HPV-associated neoplasms that most frequently are the source of vegetative viral production, a feature that is probably best correlated with cytologic KA as defined above.

Grossly and colposcopically these lesions have an exophytic cauliflower (acuminate) appearance and a characteristic vascularity reflecting the richly vascular cores of the papillary fronds (Figure 14). Histologically, the epithelium is characterized by acanthosis, papillomatosis, and although less frequent in cervical than vulvar lesions, hyperkeratosis. Koilocytotic atypia as strictly defined above, is pathognomonic but may not be present depending on sectioning and the temporal evolution of the lesion. A useful clue, in the absence of koilocytes, is the presence of nuclear enlargement (cytologic atypia) inappropriate for the level of the epithelium, i.e., abnormally enlarged nuclei in the superficial layers. Parabasal hyperplasia is usually minimal and mitotic activity if present is usually confined to the basal zone. Moderate to marked parabasal hyperplasia, marked nuclear atypia, upper level mitoses or abnormal mitotic figures imply higher grade and a mixed terminology, e.g., condyloma with focal dysplasia/HSIL may be appropriate. Frequently this is not a problem as lesions with HSIL that still maintain their exophytic morphology are quite rare in the cervix, but similar concepts apply to the external genital lesions.

A recognized shortcoming, albeit not serious in cytologic screening, is the inability to distinguish condyloma acuminatum from LSIL. As presented, such distinctions are not really relevant as biologically these are very similar lesions. Most condylomata, as with LSIL, spontaneously regress or persist and are easily removed. Recurrence is quite common.

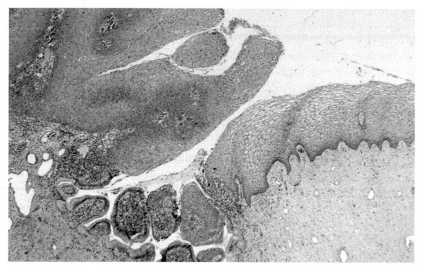

Figure 14. The cervical condyloma is evident in the left half of the field in which there is papillary hyperplasia of the epithelium, which at high power (see Figure 15) is cytologically consistent with a low-grade squamous intraepithelial lesion. In the right half of the figure normal ectocervical mucosa is evident consistent with the fact that the condyloma has arisen in the transformation zone.

7.3   Squamous Intraepithelial Lesions

The intraepithelial phase of the neoplastic process is characterized by a disordered development of the squamous epithelium, which is histologically manifest by a proliferation of primitive cells beginning in the lower portions of the epithelial layer (Ambros et al., 1990; Fu, 2002; Fu et al., 1981; Patten, 1978; Richart, 1973). This is accompanied by nuclear abnormalities including hyperchromasia, increased nuclear size, increased numbers of mitoses, and the presence of abnormal mitotic forms. In general, the more severe the process, the more the appearance of the epithelium deviates in appearance from the normal patterns of cervical epithelium. In the classical nomenclature, the term mild dysplasia (CIN 1/LSIL) is applied when the proliferating parabasal-like cells are confined to the lower one-third of the epithelium (Figure 15). While many such lesions have KA some do not. Moderate dysplasia (CIN 2) refers to those lesions in which the proliferating cells involve the middle one-third of the epithelium, and as the upper one-third of the epithelium becomes involved by these cells the dysplasia is considered to be severe (CIN 3) (Figures 16 and 17). If the entire thickness of the epithelium is replaced by the proliferation, the lesion has been termed carcinoma in situ (CIN 3). The spectrum of CIN 2-3 is thus characterized by cellular proliferation overtaking the epithelium and all are considered HSILs. HSILs increasingly have mitoses found at higher and higher levels in the epithelium and increased numbers of abnormal mitoses are identified. Fu et al. (1981) have shown that the presence of abnormal mitoses correlates with the presence of an aneuploid cell population and that this is predictive of those lesions that are most likely to progress. It is of interest that the presence of abnormal mitoses also correlates with identification of high-risk type papillomavirus DNA in these lesions.

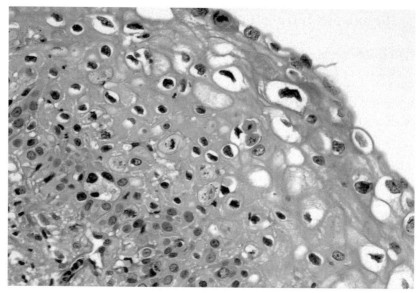

Figure 15. The histology of a typical low-grade squamous intraepithelial lesion. The proliferating zone is confined to the lower one-third of the epithelium. The superficial cells demonstrate koilocytotic atypia as defined.

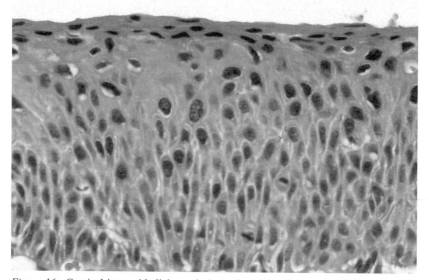

Figure 16. Cervical intraepithelial neoplasia grade 2. Note the parabasal-like cells extend into the middle third of the epithelium. Also, note the relative decrease in koilocytotic atypia.

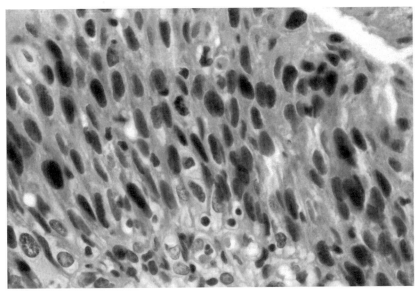

Figure 17. Cervical intraepithelial neoplasia grade 3. The proliferating cells replace the epithelium. Numerous mitotic figures and apoptotic figures are visible, indicative of the high rate of cell turnover.

In addition to subclassifying intraepithelial neoplasia by grade, one can also subdivide it on the basis of two basic morphologic patterns. The first and most common pattern is the one characteristic of lesions that usually arise in the transformation zone. This is referred to as the nonkeratinizing type, also called metaplastic dysplasia by Patten. The second type of lesion, termed keratinizing dysplasia because of the marked keratinization of many of the component cells, is much less common in the cervix although it is much more common in other genital sites like the vulva or penis where the epithelium normally has a stratum corneum (Figure 18). Marked cellular pleomorphism is also a characteristic of this lesion and this has led some to refer to the process as "pleomorphic dysplasia". With keratinizing dysplasia, no distinction is made between moderate, or severe dysplasia and carcinoma in situ, even in the traditional dysplasia/CIS system as the process by its nature always demonstrates evidence of cell differentiation and therefore does not fit into the accepted definition of classical carcinoma in situ. In TBS, keratinizing dysplasia is considered a HSIL.

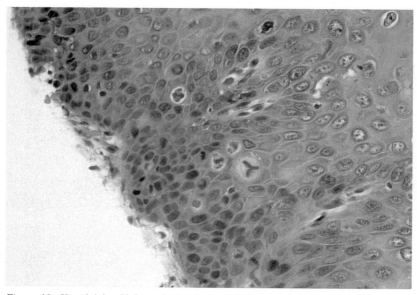

Figure 18. Keratinizing high-grade dysplasia. In this case similar to what often occurs on the vulva, the dysplastic epithelium is undergoing some degree of squamous maturation. But this is a high-grade proliferative lesion. Note the multiple mitotic figures including atypical (tripolar) forms.

It is important to emphasize that all SILs are full thickness abnormalities, even in mild cases. Although the proliferating cells do not involve the full thickness of the epithelium in lesions of less severity than carcinoma in situ, all cases of dysplasia demonstrate nuclear abnormalities, including increased size and hyperchromasia, even in the superficial portions of the reaction.

As described above, the cytologic manifestations of the squamous intraepithelial lesions reflect the morphologic appearance of these processes as seen in tissue samples. The pattern of the cellular sample derived from the various epithelial processes under consideration can be predicted from a study of the appearance of the cells in tissue biopsies taken from involved areas. The cells sampled by the cervical scrape and brush techniques are generally derived from the superficial cell layers of the epithelium and represent the cells seen in the more superficial portions of the epithelium of the proliferations.

7.3.1   Differential diagnosis of SIL

Many of the problems in biopsy differential diagnosis are related to specimen orientation, fixation, and processing. Immature metaplasia, atrophy, infection, and repair all enter the differential diagnosis. Usually there is no problem in proper grading of a biopsy but in some cases the distinction can be very difficult. Correlation with the available cytology is often of great help, and some adjunctive tests such as proliferation markers may be useful in selected cases (Keating et al., 2001; Klaes et al., 2002).

7.3.2 Natural history of SIL

There is still great controversy over whether CIN 1 is really precursor to CIN 2-3. The following rates are based on the meta-analysis of Ostor: For CIN 1, ~65% regress, ~15% progress to CIN 3 and relative risk (RR) for progression to CIN3 is 560 as compared to women without CIN. For CIN 2 there is still 50% regression, 35% progression and RR of 2000. For CIN 3 the risk of invasion depends upon length of follow-up, estimated to be at least 20% over 2 years (Ostor, 1993; Ostor and Mulvany, 1996). However, recent studies reflect the growing concept that there are two biologic states related to cervical HPV infection, LSIL and HSIL. LSIL, the manifestation of productive HPV infection mostly regresses. However the risk of concurrent HSIL or detectable HSIL in the near term is approximately 25% and is correlated with persistence of HPV positivity and high-risk type (Ho et al., 1998; Ho et al., 1995; Kiviat et al., 1992; Schiffman et al., 1993; Schiffman and Brinton, 1995). Given issues of diagnostic variability both colposcopic and pathologic, it is very difficult to document progression relative to misclassification. HSIL is a morphologic spectrum encompassing CIN2 and CIN 3 and is an epithelial state characterized by cell proliferation, and higher rates of persistent abnormality. HSILs are the most proximate precursors to invasive cancer and their eradication is the goal of cervical screening to prevent the development of invasive cancer. Remarkably, there is not broad agreement on the morphologic definition of HSIL (Scott et al., 2002). In some countries CIN2, because some fraction of it seems to "regress," is felt to be low grade. However, as defined above, CIN 2 can be viewed as important buffer or equivocal zone, which is more highly proliferative than LSIL. Defining it as high grade ensures patient safety. The management of CIN/SIL has recently been refined by a broad consensus process organized by the American Society of Colposcopy and Cervical Pathology (Wright et al., 2002).

7.4 Squamous Cell Carcinomas

The WHO classification of invasive squamous cell carcinoma of the uterine cervix is based on histologic morphology (Scully et al., 1994). It differs from the original Broders subclassification that was based on a nuclear grading system, additionally utilizing keratinization as the main index of differentiation (Broders, 1926). Wentz and Reagan first proposed the current WHO classification in 1959 (Wentz and Reagan, 1959). It divides squamous cell carcinoma into keratinizing, large cell non-keratinizing, and small cell types. This classification corresponds to the theories of histogenesis proposed by Reagan some of which over time have evolved with our knowledge base. Originally, the keratinizing type of cancer was felt to arise in the ectocervical area evolving from preexisting keratinizing dysplasia. In contrast, the nonkeratinizing variety was thought to arise in the transformation zone developing through the metaplastic dysplasia-carcinoma in situ pathway, and small cell carcinomas were felt to arise from small cell carcinoma in situ, which is preceded by atypical reserve cell hyperplasia usually high in the transformation zone within the canal. In the current WHO classification, the small cell tumors have been removed from the squamous category, as most of the small cell tumors that have an extremely poor prognosis have been demonstrated to have a neuroendocrine phenotype. The Reagan classification was originally adopted because of its correlation with tumor responsiveness to radiation therapy (Reagan and Fu, 1979). This correlation is controversial and currently with modern radiation therapy, histologic subtype and grading of the common carcinomas has little correlation to survival when adjusted for stage. For the surgical pathologist, the most important tumor descriptors are tumor size, depth of stromal invasion and presence of vascular space invasion and lymph node metastasis (Crissman et al., 1987; Lanciano et al., 1992; Roberts and Fu, 1990; Stoler, 2000a; Zaino et al., 1992).

Keratinizing carcinomas are composed of sheets and nests of infiltrating squamous epithelial cells characterized by the presence of well-formed keratin "pearls" formed by concentric rings of layered keratin (Figure 19). As defined, a single keratin pearl is sufficient for classification as a keratinizing cancer. Intercellular bridges are well formed between cells which usually have hyperchromatic often pyknotic nuclei. Mitoses are infrequent.

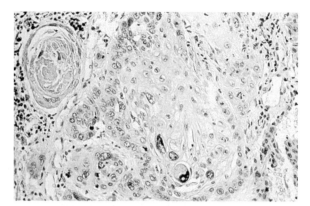

Figure 19. Keratinizing squamous cell carcinoma exhibiting keratin pearl formation. Because of the abundant cytoplasmic maturation and the relatively mild degree of nuclear pleomorphism, this tumor would also be considered to be well-differentiated or low grade.

Large cell non-keratinizing carcinomas are composed of polygonal cells usually arranged in sheets forming masses with pushing borders (Figure 20). Keratinization of single cells may be present but keratin "pearls" are not found. The nuclei are enlarged, variable in size and have prominent nucleoli and coarsely granular chromatin. Mitoses are more common than in the keratinizing tumors. These are the most common type of squamous cancer today accounting for ~75% of tumors.

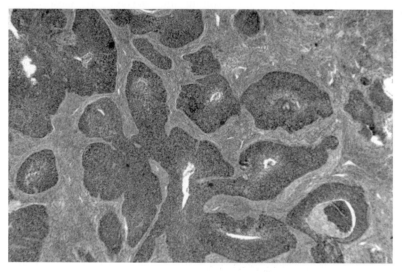

Figure 20. A low power view of large cell non-keratinizing squamous cell carcinoma demonstrating infiltrating nests of relatively undifferentiated epithelium. Depending upon the degree of nuclear pleomorphism at high power this tumor could be considered intermediate to high grade.

7.4.1   Squamous carcinoma variants

Verrucous carcinoma is a specific subtype of squamous carcinoma, which if strictly defined, is associated with a good prognosis (Masih et al., 1993; Okagaki et al., 1984; Roberts and Fu, 1990; Vayrynen et al., 1981). Diagnostic criteria are similar to those tumors at other sites, e.g., vulva where it is much more common. These are extremely well differentiated tumors characterized by exophytic and endophytic growth of markedly acanthotic epithelium with abundant hyperkeratosis. The deep portions of the tumor demonstrate bulbous masses of squamous cells with rounded/ pushing borders with minimal cytologic atypia. Invasion seems to occur as if by "pressure atrophy" rather than by infiltrative growth. Koilocytosis is often minimal or absent. The relationship of these tumors to HPV is less clear than for the usual type of squamous cancer. The confusion is in part because the so-called giant condyloma of Buschke-Lowenstein in the vulva is considered synonymous with verrucous carcinoma. Helpful differential features of condylomata are a rich fibrovascular network supporting the epithelium, prominent koilocytosis, and lack of downward growth, but obviously there can be overlap. Squamous cell carcinomas with a strikingly condylomatous appearance and architecture are termed condylomatous carcinoma. The deep margins are of the usual infiltrative type, compared to verrucous cancer.

Transitional cell-like tumors resemble papillary transitional cell carcinomas of the bladder. The papillae are covered by basaloid or transitional-like stratified epithelium. Complete excisional biopsies are necessary to distinguish invasive from noninvasive tumors. Some of these tumors have been associated with late recurrence, but the tumor is so rare that good data are not available.

Unlike the nasopharyngeal tumors as well as similar tumors throughout the GI tract, the rare lymphoepithelioma of the cervix have not been demonstrated to be EBV associated (Mills et al., 1985). We have seen three such tumors and two were HPV-associated. Depending upon the degree of inflammation, the differential diagnosis can include lymphoma, and immunohistochemistry may be quite helpful in resolving the nature of the process.

7.4.2   Microinvasive carcinoma

Microinvasive squamous cell carcinoma of the uterine cervix (Stage IA) is defined as a carcinoma which is no longer than 7mm. in linear extent, and that invades the stroma to a depth of no more than 5mm. More conservative definitions have been for a tumor that has invaded the cervical stroma to a depth no greater than 3 mm from the site of origin and does not demonstrate lymphatic or blood vessel invasion. This definition identifies a group of patients who are at extremely low risk for developing lymph node metastases or of dying as a result of their disease. Although some reports have indicated that lesions with up to 5 mm of invasion should be considered as microinvasive carcinomas and that the demonstration of lymphatic invasion has no association with metastases in these microinvasive tumors, other studies have shown that metastases, recurrences and deaths although uncommon, do occur in patients with greater than 3 mm of invasion or lymphatic involvement. Because of this controversy the current staging system stratifies tumors as those with invasion ≤3 (IA1) vs. those with >3 but ≤5 mm of invasion (IA2) (Burghardt et al., 1991; Christopherson et al., 1976; Ostor, 1995; Roche and Norris, 1975; Sevin et al., 1992; Tsukamoto et al., 1989b).

In the large majority of cases the invasive foci develop out of an overlying epithelium, which manifests CIN 3. The invasive foci usually appear as tongue-like projections into the underlying stroma (Figure 21). At the point of invasion the epithelium typically shows evidence of paradoxical cytoplasmic differentiation as compared to adjacent dysplasia/CIS. There is usually a dense plasma cell and lymphocytic infiltrate present in proximity to the invasive focus, which may represent a manifestation of host response to the tumor. The invasive foci tend to have an irregular margin as opposed to the smooth outline of endocervical glands involved by intraepithelial neoplasia. This is a helpful feature in distinguishing gland involvement from early invasion. The method of measurement is not well codified but most measure stromal invasion as perpendicular from the nearest basement membrane.

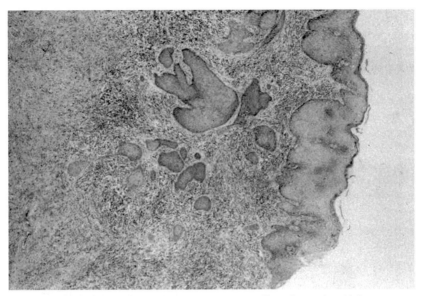

Figure 21. An example of microinvasive squamous cell carcinoma in which nests of infiltrating malignant epithelium are present less than three millimeters from the nearest basement membrane.

8　　GLANDULAR LESIONS

8.1　Adenocarcinoma in situ

Adenocarcinoma in situ of the cervix (AIS) is the recognized histogenetic precursor of most endocervical adenocarcinomas (Boon et al., 1981; Christopherson et al., 1979; Farnsworth et al., 1989; Gloor and Hurlimann, 1986; Gloor and Ruzicka, 1982; Jaworski, 1990; Jaworski et al., 1988; Weisbrot et al., 1972; Wells and Brown, 1986). In the 2001 Bethesda System revision, AIS is formally recognized as a specific diagnostic entity (Solomon et al., 2002). In that same system, lesions that are concerning for AIS, but are felt to be non-diagnostic are now referred to as atypical glandular cells (AGC), a reflection of diagnostic uncertainty. There is no recommendation for a specific cytologic category of glandular dysplasia/intraepithelial neoplasia less than AIS. Cases of endocervical adenocarcinoma as well as AIS are increasing in clinical frequency. Most of this is a relative increase due to effective screening for cervical squamous cell carcinoma and its precursors. Some authors do argue for an absolute increase as well, but these data seem less clear. Pap smears may detect AIS or AGC but their effectiveness for this class of lesions is clearly less than for squamous lesions. The reasons for this are complex and include the effectiveness of endocervical sampling, familiarity with diagnostic criteria, and the relative frequency of AIS/AGC in the population which, in most studies, is at least 10-fold less than the frequency of squamous abnormality. AIS is virtually always present in the transformation zone. AIS is associated with SIL, usually HSIL in roughly 40-70% of cases. As noted earlier, adeno-carcinomas of the cervix are also strongly associated with HPVs (Duggan et al., 1995; Farnsworth et al., 1989; Wilczynski et al., 1988). In several large multinational studies the frequency of HPV being associated with cervical adenocarcinoma is virtually the same as for squamous cancer, i.e., >90%, but with a different type distribution (Bosch and Sanjose, 2002a; Bosch et al., 2002b; Bosch et al., 1995; Munoz et al., 2003; Walboomers et al., 1999). HPV-18 and related viruses are relatively much more common in glandular lesions then the HPV-16 related group of viruses (16:18 group ratios of approximately 1:1 vs. about 5:1 for squamous lesions).

Histologically, AIS is localized to the squamocolumnar junction. AIS does not usually extend below the level of normal endocervical glands (3-5 mm.) unless it involves prominently dilated glands or tunnel clusters. AIS when present, has an associated SIL in 40-70% of cases. Conversely, AIS is quite rare relative to SIL and this frequency is highly dependent on the population under study. As noted above, AGC has a frequency of no more than 1/10 the SIL rate. In older studies the relative frequency of AIS/SIL was often cited at 1/200. In the NCI ALTS trial, which intensively studied 5000 women with equivocal or low grade Pap smear abnormality, the frequency was less than 1/1000 (unpublished data).

AIS is characterized by glandular structures lined by cells demonstrating hyperchromasia, altered, often coarse chromatin, nuclear pseudo-stratification, decreased mucin secretion, elevated N:C ratio, mitotic activity and apoptosis (Figures 22 and 23). The cell type is almost always of endocervical mucinous differentiation. Although rarely endometrial, ciliated and intestinal cell types may be present, causing issues in differential diagnosis. As described, the criteria for AIS are primarily cytologic, that is, they can be applied to individual cells or small groups of cells in histologic section. Mitoses and apoptotic bodies are probably the most specific criteria indicative of the proliferative phenotype characteristic of HPV-induced high-grade precursors (Biscotti and Hart, 1998). Essentially, any endocervical glandular abnormality with more than a rare mitosis, especially if it is associated with SIL, should be considered AIS for management purposes. Increased architectural complexity may also be present in the form of papillae and budding. However, gland fusion, true cribriform growth, very irregular gland out-pouching or stromal desmoplasia all suggest early invasive adenocarcinoma.

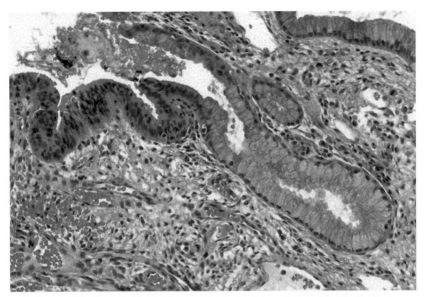

Figure 22. Adenocarcinoma in situ in which the hyperchromatic and stratified epithelial cells are seen to abruptly merge with the normal endocervical epithelium.

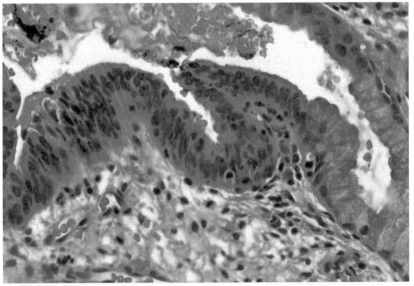

Figure 23. A high power view of adenocarcinoma in situ. One can appreciate the stratified hyperchromatic nuclei with both mitotic and apoptotic activity.

8.2   Endocervical glandular dysplasia (EGD)

WHO defined EGD as those lesions characterized by significant nuclear abnormalities more striking than those seen in glandular atypia but not sufficient for AIS (Casper et al., 1997; Farnsworth et al., 1989; Jaworski et al., 1988; Wells and Brown, 1986). In the AFIP cervix fascicle, Kurman suggested a quantitative criterion such that if only one gland profile or less is involved, than the diagnosis of EGD is preferred to that of AIS (Kurman et al., 1992). However, the criteria for EGD are really not well defined histologically, cytologically, biologically, or clinically in any of these publications. The concept that there must be a recognizable precursor of AIS stems from a misguided application of concepts of neoplastic development in squamous epithelia. Since there are morphologically, biologically, and clinically recognizable lesions of low- and high-grade squamous dysplasia, must there not also be the same for glandular lesions? In most series, attempts to separate lesion less than AIS into low grade or high-grade dysplasia are problematic (Jaworski, 1990; Jaworski et al., 1988). A review of the photographs and criteria invariably produces confusion in that the written or image based data for EGD, especially high grade EGD, are always remarkably similar to those used to make a diagnosis of AIS. This may represent the fact that the criteria for AIS are cytologic, applicable to a single cell. It seems improbable that one can reliably recognize a true neoplastic precursor, i.e., AIS, and also reliably distinguish at least two other intraepithelial neoplastic diagnoses in single glandular cells (e.g., low and high-grade dysplasia) and also reliably distinguish these three categories from all the other reactive processes that enter the differential diagnosis. Objective studies of diagnostic reproducibility strongly argue for lumping of intraepithelial neoplastic diagnoses, not splitting (Stoler and Schiffman, 2001). Furthermore, in series that have attempted to make these distinctions using molecular markers, high grade EGD looks very much like AIS (Farnsworth et al., 1989; Hurlimann and Gloor, 1984). This is true whether one uses HPV detection, HPV expression, cell proliferation markers, CEA expression or other immunohistochemical markers. Indeed, the HPV data are most persuasive assuming one believes that precursors of endocervical adenocarcinoma are HPV associated. Candidate cases of low-grade glandular dysplasia always have very low HPV detection rates. In contrast in LSIL, HPV is detectable in virtually 100% of accurately diagnosed cases. Ergo, low grade EGD is not EGD, that is, it (whatever *it* is) is not in the spectrum of intraepithelial neoplasia (Ioffe et al., 2003; Lee, 2003).

Finally, the implications of diagnoses "less than AIS" for clinicians should be seriously considered. Maintaining this distinction implies that biologically there is an entity that is less than AIS and by analogy, that entity might be safe to follow rather than to search out and destroy. Indeed, given the inability to colposcopically visualize AIS, the problems with sampling the endocervix cytologically and by curettage, the imprecision of our terminology and ability to clearly communicate the meaning of our diagnoses to clinicians, prudent management requires localization and ablation of these glandular abnormalities. In most of the literature as well as the ASCCP practice guidelines, the preferred method of treatment is cold knife conization to insure adequate margins, although the degree of reassurance is dependent upon the length of the margin. For patients that have completed child bearing, hysterectomy may still be part of the management of AIS.

The main differential diagnosis of AIS includes microglandular hyperplasia, a variety of inflammatory reactions or reparative changes, endometriosis and tubal metaplasia (Novotny et al., 1992). The most reliable single criterion for distinguishing AIS from its mimics is mitotic activity or other evidence of cell proliferation (Biscotti, 1997; Biscotti and Hart, 1998). The proliferative phenotype is highly correlated with the effect of HPV oncogenes on the cell cycle. Consequently, the judicious application of markers such as Ki-67, PCNA, cyclins, p16 and HPV may be quite useful in select problematic cases (Ronnett et al., 1999).

8.3   Adenocarcinoma

Adenocarcinomas of the cervix account for ~15% of all invasive carcinomas and are also associated with HPVs (Bosch et al., 1995; Duggan et al., 1995; Vesterinen et al., 1989; Wilczynski et al., 1988; Young and Scully, 1990). The WHO subclassification of glandular tumors, as for squamous lesions, is based on light microscopic appearance of routine H &E sections.

The usual well-differentiated endocervical adenocarcinoma typically forms gland-like spaces lined by columnar cells that may demonstrate some mucin production (Figure 24). Poorly differentiated tumors have a predominately solid growth pattern with only poorly formed glandular spaces evident (Figure 25). Moderately differentiated neoplasms demonstrate features that are intermediate between the two extremes. Subtypes of adenocarcinoma other than the usual, account for approximately 30% of glandular cancers. Besides the typical endocervical pattern primary cervical adenocarcinoma may have other patterns of differentiation. Mixed adenosquamous carcinomas make up about 5-15% of cervical carcinomas or roughly 30-50% of cervical carcinomas with a glandular component. In roughly decreasing frequency, endometrioid, clear cell, papillary villoglandular, papillary serous, and mesonephric types are also recognized as well as tumors having mixed patterns of differentiation.

8.3.1   Mucinous (endocervical, intestinal, and signet-ring cell types)

This type of tumor accounts for 70% of cervical adenocarcinomas. Epidemiologically it occurs 5-10 years later than AIS with a mean age of ~50. The grading schemes proposed for adenocarcinomas are analogous to the FIGO system used in endometrial tumors. CEA staining may be useful in differential diagnosis, as endocervical tumors are positive and most true endometrial tumors are not (Gilks et al., 1989; Steeper and Wick, 1986). Clinical outcome for adenocarcinoma is similar to or slightly worse than that for cervical squamous carcinoma, although in making such comparisons stage needs to be carefully controlled for (Ostor, 2000; Saigo et al., 1986; Sevin et al., 1992; Swan and Roddick, 1973). Because of location, these tumors are more difficult to screen for cytologically and hence they tend to present at a higher stage. Obviously metastatic gastrointestinal tract tumors enter the differential diagnosis of some mucinous cancers. When primary to the cervix, intestinal and signet ring cell patterns that mimic gastric cancer often coexist with other types of more usual adenocarcinoma.

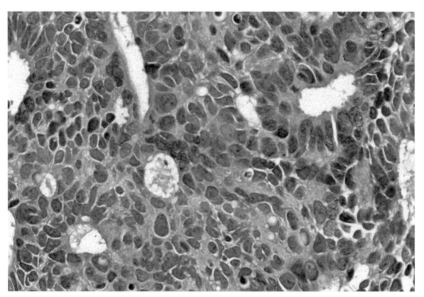

Figure 24.   Well differentiated endocervical adenocarcinoma in which glandular differentiation is readily evident. However, the glands are fused into irregular masses that infiltrate the stroma.

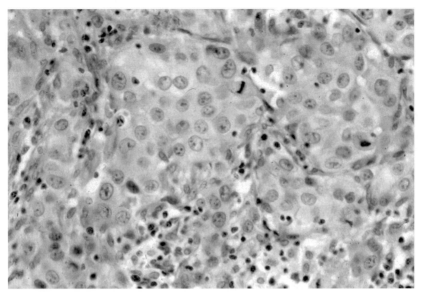

Figure 25. High power histology of a poorly differentiated adenocarcinoma. In this case there is little histologic evidence of glandular differentiation. Rather, the tumor grows as diffuse sheets and nests of markedly pleomorphic and cytologically atypical cells.

8.3.2   Endometrioid

This type of tumor mimics the appearance of primary endometrial adenocarcinoma both histologically and cytologically. In some cases both endocervical and endometrial types of differentiation are present. Differentiation from an endometrial adenocarcinoma arising in the lower uterine segment can be very difficult, and accurate gross description can be critical. Most tumors arising at the level of the transformation zone with endometrioid morphology are primary cervical. Other differential diagnostic considerations include endometriosis. There is no clear difference in clinical behavior between endometrioid and endocervical adenocarcinoma once stage and grade are accounted for.

8.3.3   Clear cell

These tumors account for about 5% of cervical neoplasms. Increasingly these tumors are unrelated to diethylstilbesterol exposure compared to the situation 1-2 decades ago (Hanselaar et al., 1991; Roth, 1974). This distinctive neoplasm may arise in any of the areas containing Muellarian derived epithelium and therefore may be seen in the vagina, cervix, endometrium or ovary. In all sites it is histologically and cytologically similar. The tumors may be solid, tubulo-cystic, papillary or some combination of these three patterns in their growth. In the tubulo-cystic and papillary areas typical "hobnail cells", in which the nuclei protrude into the gland lumen may be seen. The cells have a clear appearing cytoplasm in tissue sections due to the dissolution of the cytoplasmic glycogen in processing. In cytologic preparations the clear cytoplasm may not be as evident and the cells may demonstrate a granular pale eosinophilic or amphophilic cytoplasmic appearance. Cytologically, the abnormal cells may occur singly, in rounded clusters or in sheets. The cytoplasm has ill defined boundaries and varies in amount from abundant to scant. The nuclei are large, generally round or oval and tend to be centrally located. Nucleoli are prominent and the nuclear chromatin varies from finely to coarsely granular. Hyperchromasia is not a prominent feature. The differential diagnosis includes Arias-Stella reaction, microglandular hyperplasia, and mesonephric remnants.

8.3.4 Minimal deviation (adenoma malignum)

Much has been written about this very rare variant of mucinous carcinoma (Clement and Young, 1989; Gilks et al., 1989; Silverberg and Hurt, 1975; Steeper and Wick, 1986). It is associated with the Peutz-Jeghers syndrome as well as ovarian mucinous neoplasms. Hence its pathogenesis may not be HPV-associated. The tumor is characterized by deceptively benign epithelium resembling normal endocervix. The glands are inappropriate in their distribution being present too deep and varying greatly in size and shape. A desmoplastic stromal response is a helpful diagnostic feature. Extensive sampling is required and will usually demonstrate some glands with increased atypia and mitotic figures. Hence small biopsy or Pap smear diagnosis is treacherously unreliable. Because of this, these tumors often present at a late stage and it is uncertain as to whether the prognosis is different when adjusted for stage.

8.3.5 Well-differentiated (papillary) villoglandular

Recently described, this tumor tends to present in younger patients and is associated with a good prognosis probably because it tends to present at an early stage (Young and Scully, 1989). Stratified columnar epithelial cells, usually with low-grade nuclei, line the papillae. The stroma tends to be fibrous and thicker than in serous cancers and may also have a considerable inflammatory response. Superficial biopsy may miss the invasive component of the tumor.

8.3.6 Serous

This type of cervical adenocarcinoma is very rare (Gilks and Clement, 1992). It is histologically and cytologically similar to the same tumor in its more common location in the ovary and the endometrium. It has to be distinguished from the other two papillary neoplasms, clear cell carcinoma and the papillary variant of endometrioid adenocarcinoma. The serous lesions are characterized by arborizing thin fibrous stalks lined by cuboidal to or polygonal cells without evidence of a prominent clear cell pattern. The nuclear abnormalities are usually intermediate or high grade.

8.3.7 Mesonephric

These tumors are thought to arise from mesonephric remnants from which they have to be distinguished (Ferry and Scully, 1990). An infiltrative growth pattern is most helpful in differential diagnosis, as is a location in the lateral cervix and the absence of surface involvement in the overlying endocervical glands.

9 OTHER EPITHELIAL TUMORS

9.1 Adenosquamous carcinoma

Mixed adenosquamous carcinomas make up 8 to 10 percent of the malignancies of the cervix; that is, roughly half of glandular cervical cancers have a squamous component (Bethwaite et al., 1992; Christopherson et al., 1979; Gallup et al., 1985; Gordon et al., 1989). These tumors are composed of mixtures of squamous epithelial and glandular elements. In the poorly differentiated varieties, mucus containing tumor cells may be intermingled singly and in small groups with poorly differentiated squamous cells.

9.2 Glassy cell carcinoma

Glassy cell carcinoma is a poorly differentiated variant first described by Glucksman and Cherry (Littman et al., 1976; Pak et al., 1983; Tamimi et al., 1988). It is made up of large cells with amphophilic cytoplasm, which often has a ground glass appearance, and large nuclei with prominent nucleoli. The cells have distinct borders and form sheets. It is probably best considered a poorly differentiated high-grade adenosquamous carcinoma and it is associated with a poor prognosis.

9.3 Adenoid cystic carcinoma and adenoid basal carcinoma

These are rare neoplasms of the cervix, which were only recently clearly differentiated from each other (Brainard and Hart, 1998; Ferry and Scully, 1988; Fowler et al., 1978; Hart, 2002; Ramzy et al., 1975; Shingleton et al., 1977). Both tend to occur in older patients. The adenoid cystic tumor of the cervix resembles adenoid cystic carcinoma of the salivary gland in its histologic appearance and aggressive biologic behavior. The tumor is composed of small basaloid cells arranged in sheets and nests often having a cribriform pattern or small cyst-like formations, which contain a hyaline like material. These tumors frequently coexist with squamous cell carcinoma.

Adenoid cystic carcinoma must be distinguished from adenoid basal cell carcinoma, which represents a distinct morphologic and biologic entity. This tumor is composed of small oval to round nests of basaloid cells with uniform nuclei arranged in a pallisading fashion at the periphery of the nests. Small gland-like spaces or frank squamous differentiation may be present in the center of some nests. About half of the tumors are associated with a coexisting squamous carcinoma, either in situ or invasive. The prognosis for adenoid basal cell carcinoma is favorable. In the Ferry and Scully series, only 1 of 14 patients died of tumor.

9.4 Carcinoid tumor

Carcinoid tumors of the uterine cervix are rare, but are now well recognized as a form of low-grade neuroendocrine carcinoma (Albores-Saavedra et al., 1976; Tsukamoto et al., 1989a). Some consider them variants of adenocarcinoma or tumors with biphasic glandular and neuroendocrine differentiation, but this also occurs at other sites. The tumor is histologically similar to carcinoid tumors at other body sites consisting of small, relatively uniform cells growing in an insular or trabecular pattern with or without rosette formation. The presence of argyrophilic cytoplasmic granules is confirmatory evidence for this diagnosis. Neurosecretory granules can also be demonstrated by electron microscopy and immunocytochemical techniques can be used to demonstrate neuroendocrine markers such as neuron specific enolase, chromogranin or synaptophysin.

9.5   Small cell carcinoma

This neoplasm was originally classified as a subtype of squamous carcinoma. It is now recognized, however, that this is a poorly differentiated variant of neuroendocrine carcinoma resembling small cell carcinoma of the lung (Abeler et al., 1994; Ambros et al., 1991; Boruta et al., 2001; Clement, 1990; Stoler et al., 1991). This highly aggressive neoplasm is composed of diffusely infiltrating aggregates of small polygonal to irregular cells with little visible cytoplasm and small, rounded to irregularly shaped nuclei which are hyperchromatic and which contain small nucleoli (Figure 26). Mitoses are common and necrosis is frequently evident. Electron microscopy or immunocytochemical staining can demonstrate the presence of neurosecretory granules. This neoplasm should be distinguished from nonkeratinizing squamous cell carcinoma composed of relatively small cells as small cell carcinoma has an exceedingly poor prognosis. This tumor is almost exclusively HPV 18-associated.

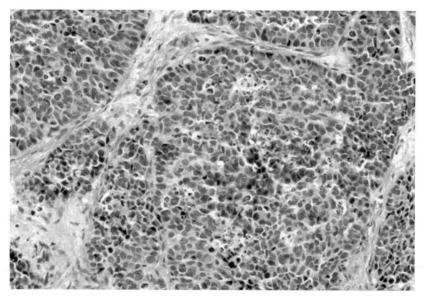

Figure 26. Small cell neuroendocrine carcinoma. Irregular masses of small cells with a very high nuclear to cytoplasmic ratio diffusely infiltrate the cervical stroma. Centrally in most masses there is degeneration and necrosis indicative of the high growth fraction of this aggressive neoplasm.

10 STAGING AND PROGNOSIS OF CERVICAL CARCINOMAS

Reviewing the literature on established prognostic markers is problematic. Case series vary from as few as 30 cases to more than 17,000 (Crissman et al., 1987; Crissman et al., 1985; Fuller et al., 1989; Hopkins and Morley, 1991; Rubens et al., 1988; Zaino et al., 1992). The methods of staging, lymph node sampling, pathologic criteria used and treatment approaches are rarely comparable. A most important problem is the fact that International Federation of Gynecology & Obstetrics (FIGO) staging which is in many series clinically based, does not take into account the patient's lymph node status, whereas the TNM stage grouping does. Hence the details regarding the staging system used and whether patients are classified by surgical or clinical criteria is critical. As frustrating as these problems may be, it seems there is reasonable consensus regarding the pathologic features that are essential aids to proper staging and have prognostic impact. For cancers of the cervix, stage is still the most important prognostic factor. When it is possible to assign a surgical stage and proper TNM stage grouping, prognostication is greatly enhanced by correcting the 20-50% of patients who are under-staged by the clinical staging system. Factors intimately related to FIGO stage and lymph node status, for example, estimates of tumor size, depth of invasion relative to overall wall thickness, lymphovascular space invasion, parametria and other margin status are all useful (Gerdin et al., 1994; Goodman et al., 1989; Hopkins and Morley, 1991; Hopkins and Morley, 1993; Inoue, 1984a; Inoue and Okumura, 1984b; Kosary, 1994). In a recent series of 377 stage I/II cervical cancer patients treated with radical hysterectomy and lymph node dissection and from which small cell carcinoma and microinvasive carcinoma patients were excluded, depth of invasion, lymphovascular space invasion, lymph node status and age were found to be significantly prognostic in a multivariate analysis that used a new statistical survival tree analysis (Sevin et al., 1996). The latter procedure may be superior to the more usual Cox proportional hazards model in that the analysis determines cut points rather than having them predetermined before the analysis. In many series, grade and histologic type still have some effect. Histologic type is usually more significant for nonsquamous histologies such as some of the poorly differentiated adenocarcinomas and small cell neuroendocrine carcinomas. Grading is controversial with unclear significance because there is widespread lack of consensus on which grading system to use and how they should be applied.

In summary, the TNM stage, which incorporates the FIGO staging estimate of tumor extent with the best available evaluation of the patient's lymph node status, is the most powerful prognostic factor. Within stages, accurate measurements of tumor size and/or the depth of invasion normalized for cervical thickness if possible, evaluation of vascular space invasion, evaluation

Chapter 1

of margins particularly the parametrium and enumeration of the number of positive nodes help to stratify patients. The factors that are available to the pathologist in the above list should be documented in the surgical pathology report and a synoptic type of report form facilitates this. Histologic typing and some attempt at grading should still be part of the rigor brought to diagnosis (Stoler, 2000a).

REFERENCES

Abeler VM, Holm R, Nesland JM, et al. Small cell carcinoma of the cervix. A clinicopathologic study of 26 patients. Cancer 1994;73:672-7.

Albores-Saavedra J, Larraza O, Poucell S, et al. Carcinoid of the uterine cervix: additional observations on a new tumor entity. Cancer 1976;38:2328-42.

Ambros RA, Kurman RJ. Current concepts in the relationship of human papillomavirus infection to the pathogenesis and classification of precancerous squamous lesions of the uterine cervix. Semin Diagn Pathol 1990;7:158-72.

Ambros RA, Park JS, Shah KV, et al. Evaluation of histologic, morphometric, and immunohistochemical criteria in the differential diagnosis of small cell carcinomas of the cervix with particular reference to human papillomavirus types 16 and 18 [published erratum appears in Mod Pathol 1992;5:40]. Modern Pathology 1991;4:586-93.

Bethwaite P, Yeong ML, Holloway L, et al. The prognosis of adenosquamous carcinomas of the uterine cervix. Br J Obstet Gynaecol 1992;99:745-50.

Biscotti CV, Gero MA, Toddy SM, et al. Endocervical adenocarcinoma in situ: an analysis of cellular features. Diagn Cytopathol 1997;17:326-32.

Biscotti CV, Hart WR. Apoptotic bodies: a consistent morphologic feature of endocervical adenocarcinoma in situ. Am J Surg Pathol 1998;22:434-9.

Bonfiglio TA, Patten SF. The histopathology of benign proliferative lesions and preinvasive neoplasia of the uterine cervix. J Reprod Med 1976;16:253-262.

Boon ME, Baak JP, Kurver PJ, et al. Adenocarcinoma in situ of the cervix: an underdiagnosed lesion. Cancer 1981;48:768-73.

Boruta DM, 2nd, Schorge JO, Duska LA, et al. Multimodality therapy in early-stage neuroendocrine carcinoma of the uterine cervix. Gynecol Oncol 2001;81:82-7.

Bosch FX, de Sanjose S. Human papillomavirus in cervical cancer. Curr Oncol Rep 2002a;4:175-83.

Bosch FX, Lorincz A, Munoz N, et al. The causal relation between human papillomavirus and cervical cancer. J Clin Pathol 2002b;55:244-65.

Bosch FX, Manos MM, Munoz N, et al. Prevalence of human papillomavirus in cervical cancer: a worldwide perspective. International biological study on cervical cancer (IBSCC) Study Group. J Natl Cancer Inst 1995;87:796-802.

Brainard JA, Hart WR. Adenoid basal epitheliomas of the uterine cervix: a reevaluation of distinctive cervical basaloid lesions currently classified as adenoid basal carcinoma and adenoid basal hyperplasia. Am J Surg Pathol 1998;22:965-75.

Broders AC. Carcinoma grading and practical application. Arch Pathol 1926;2:376-438.

Burghardt E, Girardi F, Lahousen M, et al. Microinvasive carcinoma of the uterine cervix (International Federation of Gynecology and Obstetrics Stage IA). Cancer 1991;67:1037-45.

Casper GR, Ostor AG, Quinn MA. A clinicopathologic study of glandular dysplasia of the cervix. Gynecol Oncol 1997;64:166-70.

Christopherson WM, Gray LA, Parker JE. Microinvasive carcinoma of the uterine cervix: A long-term followup study of eighty cases. Cancer 1976;38:629-32.

Christopherson WM, Nealon N, Gray LA, Sr. Noninvasive precursor lesions of adenocarcinoma and mixed adenosquamous carcinoma of the cervix uteri. Cancer 1979;44:975-83.

Cinel A, Oselladore M, Insacco E, et al. The accuracy of colposcopically directed biopsy in the diagnosis of cervical intraepithelial neoplasia. Eur J Gynaecol Oncol 1990;11:433-7.

Clement PB. Miscellaneous primary tumors and metastatic tumors of the uterine cervix. Semin Diagn Pathol 1990;7:228-48.

Clement PB, Young RH. Deep nabothian cysts of the uterine cervix. A possible source of confusion with minimal-deviation adenocarcinoma (adenoma malignum). Int J Gynecol Pathol 1989;8:340-8.

Crissman JD, Budhraja M, Aron BS, et al. Histopathologic prognostic factors in stage II and III squamous cell carcinoma of the uterine cervix. An evaluation of 91 patients treated primarily with radiation therapy. Int J Gynecol Pathol 1987;6:97-103.

Crissman JD, Makuch R, Budhraja M. Histopathologic grading of squamous cell carcinoma of the uterine cervix. An evaluation of 70 stage Ib patients. Cancer 1985;55:1590-6.

Duggan MA, McGregor SE, Benoit JL, et al. The human papillomavirus status of invasive cervical adenocarcinoma: a clinicopathological and outcome analysis. Human Pathology 1995;26:319-25.

Farnsworth A, Laverty C, Stoler MH. Human papillomavirus messenger RNA expression in adenocarcinoma in situ of the uterine cervix. Int J Gynecol Pathol 1989;8:321-30.

Ferry JA, Scully RE. "Adenoid cystic" carcinoma and adenoid basal carcinoma of the uterine cervix. A study of 28 cases. Am J Surg Pathol 1988;12:134-44.

Ferry JA, Scully RE. Mesonephric remnants, hyperplasia, and neoplasia in the uterine cervix. A study of 49 cases. Am J Surg Pathol 1990;14:1100-11.

Fowler WC, Jr., Miles PA, Surwit EA, et al. Adenoid cystic carcinoma of the Cervix. Report of 9 cases and a reappraisal. Obstet Gynecol 1978;52:337-42.

Fu YS. Pathology of the Uterine Cervix, Vagina, and Vulva. 2nd ed. Philadelpha: Saunders; 2002.

Fu YS, Reagan JW, Richart RM. Definition of precursors. Gynecol Oncol 1981;12:S220-31.

Fuller AF, Jr., Elliott N, Kosloff C, et al. Determinants of increased risk for recurrence in patients undergoing radical hysterectomy for stage IB and IIA carcinoma of the cervix. Gynecol Oncol 1989;33:34-9.

Gallup DG, Harper RH, Stock RJ. Poor prognosis in patients with adenosquamous cell carcinoma of the cervix. Obstet Gynecol 1985;65:416-22.

Geirsson G, Woodworth FE, Patten SF, Jr., et al. Epithelial repair and regeneration in the uterine cervix. I. An analysis of the cells. Acta Cytol 1977;21:371-8.

Gerdin E, Cnattingius S, Johnson P, et al. Prognostic factors and relapse patterns in early-stage cervical carcinoma after brachytherapy and radical hysterectomy. Gynecol Oncol 1994;53:314-9.

Gilks CB, Clement PB. Papillary serous adenocarcinoma of the uterine cervix: a report of three cases. Mod Pathol 1992;5:426-31.

Gilks CB, Young RH, Aguirre P, et al. Adenoma malignum (minimal deviation adenocarcinoma) of the uterine cervix. A clinicopathological and immunohistochemical analysis of 26 cases. Am J Surg Pathol 1989;13:717-29.

Gloor E, Hurlimann J. Cervical intraepithelial glandular neoplasia (adenocarcinoma in situ and glandular dysplasia). A correlative study of 23 cases with histologic grading, histochemical analysis of mucins, and immunohistochemical determination of the affinity for four lectins. Cancer 1986;58:1272-80.

Gloor E, Ruzicka J. Morphology of adenocarcinoma in situ of the uterine cervix: a study of 14 cases. Cancer 1982;49:294-302.

Goodman HM, Buttlar CA, Niloff JM, et al. Adenocarcinoma of the uterine cervix: prognostic factors and patterns of recurrence. Gynecol Oncol 1989;33:241-7.

Gordon AN, Bornstein J, Kaufman RH, et al. Human papillomavirus associated with adenocarcinoma and adenosquamous carcinoma of the cervix: analysis by in situ hybridization. Gynecol Oncol 1989;35:345-8.

Hanselaar AG, Van Leusen ND, De Wilde PC, et al. Clear cell adenocarcinoma of the vagina and cervix. A report of the Central Netherlands Registry with emphasis on early detection and prognosis. Cancer 1991;67:1971-8.

Hart WR. Symposium part II: special types of adenocarcinoma of the uterine cervix. Int J Gynecol Pathol 2002;21:327-46.

Ho GY, Bierman R, Beardsley L, et al. Natural history of cervicovaginal papillomavirus infection in young women. N Engl J Med 1998;338:423-8.

Ho GY, Burk RD, Klein S, et al. Persistent genital human papillomavirus infection as a risk factor for persistent cervical dysplasia [see comments]. J Natl Cancer Inst 1995;87:1365-71.

Hopkins MP, Morley GW. Stage IB squamous cell cancer of the cervix: clinicopathologic features related to survival. Am J Obstet Gynecol 1991;164:1520-7; discussion 1527-9.

Hopkins MP, Morley GW. Prognostic factors in advanced stage squamous cell cancer of the cervix. Cancer 1993;72:2389-93.

Howe DT, Vincenti AC. Is large loop excision of the transformation zone (LLETZ) more accurate than colposcopically directed punch biopsy in the diagnosis of cervical intraepithelial neoplasia? Br J Obstet Gynaecol 1991;98:588-91.

Hurlimann J, Gloor E. Adenocarcinoma in situ and invasive adenocarcinoma of the uterine cervix. An immuno-histologic study with antibodies specific for several epithelial markers. Cancer 1984;54:103-9.

Hutchinson M, Fertitta L, Goldbaum B, et al. Comparison of their ability to sample abnormal cells for cervical smears. J Reprod Med 1991;36:581-6.

Inoue T. Prognostic significance of the depth of invasion relating to nodal metastases, parametrial extension, and cell types. A study of 628 cases with Stage IB, IIA, and IIB cervical carcinoma. Cancer 1984a;54:3035-42.

Inoue T, Okumura M. Prognostic significance of parametrial extension in patients with cervical carcinoma Stages IB, IIA, and IIB. A study of 628 cases treated by radical hysterectomy and lymphadenectomy with or without postoperative irradiation. Cancer 1984b;54:1714-9.

Ioffe OB, Sagae S, Moritani S, Symposium part 3: should pathologists diagnose endocervical preneoplastic lesions "Less Than" adenocarcinoma in situ?: Point. Int J Gynecol Pathol 2003;22:18-21.

Irvin WP, Jr., Andersen WA, Taylor PT, Jr., et al. "See-and-treat" loop electrosurgical excision. Has the time come for a reassessment? J Reprod Med 2002;47:569-74.

Isacson C, Kessis TD, Hedrick L, et al. Both cell proliferation and apoptosis increase with lesion grade in cervical neoplasia but do not correlate with human papillomavirus type. Cancer Research 1996;56:669-74.

Jaworski RC. Endocervical glandular dysplasia, adenocarcinoma in situ, and early invasive (microinvasive) adenocarcinoma of the uterine cervix. Semin Diagn Pathol 1990;7:190-204.

Jaworski RC, Pacey NF, Greenberg ML, et al. The histologic diagnosis of adenocarcinoma in situ and related lesions of the cervix uteri. Adenocarcinoma in situ. Cancer 1988;61:1171-81.

Kazal H, Long J. Squamous cell papillomas of the uterine cervix. A report of 20 cases. Cancer 1958;11:1049-1059.

Keating JT, Cviko A, Riethdorf S, et al. Ki-67, cyclin E, and p16INK4 are complimentary surrogate biomarkers for human papilloma virus-related cervical neoplasia. Am J Surg Pathol 2001;25:884-91.

Kiviat NB, Critchlow CW, Kurman RJ. Reassessment of the morphological continuum of cervical intraepithelial lesions: does it reflect different stages in the progression to cervical carcinoma? IARC Sci Publ 1992:59-66.

Klaes R, Benner A, Friedrich T, et al. p16INK4a immunohistochemistry improves interobserver agreement in the diagnosis of cervical intraepithelial neoplasia. Am J Surg Pathol 2002;26:1389-99.

Kosary CL. FIGO stage, histology, histologic grade, age and race as prognostic factors in determining survival for cancers of the female gynecological system: an analysis of 1973-87 SEER cases of cancers of the endometrium, cervix, ovary, vulva, and vagina. Semin Surg Oncol 1994;10:31-46.

Koss LG, Durfee GR. Unusual patterns of squamous epithelium of the uterine cervix: cytologic and pathology study of koilocytotic atypia. Ann NY Acad Sci 1961;63:1245-1261.

Kurman R. Blaustein's Pathology of the Female Genital Tract. 5th ed. New York: Springer; 2002.

Kurman R, Norris H, Wilkinson E. Tumors of the Cervix, Vagina, and Vulva. 3rd ed; 1992.

Kurman RJ, Malkasian GD Jr, Sedlis A, et al. From Papanicolaou to Bethesda: the rationale for a new cervical cytologic classification. Obstet Gynecol 1991;77:779-82.

Kurman RJ, Solomon D. The Bethesda System for reporting cervical/vaginal cytologic diagnoses: Definitions, criteria, and explanatory notes for terminology and specimen adequacy. New York: Springer-Verlag; 1994.

Lanciano RM, Won M, Hanks GE. A reappraisal of the International Federation of Gynecology and Obstetrics staging system for cervical cancer. A study of patterns of care. Cancer 1992;69:482-7.

Lee KR. Symposium part 4: Should pathologists diagnose endocervical preneoplastic lesions "Less Than" adenocarcinoma in situ?: Counterpoint. Int J Gynecol Pathol 2003;22:22-4.

Littman P, Clement PB, Henriksen B, et al. Glassy cell carcinoma of the cervix. Cancer 1976;37:2238-46.

Luff RD. The Bethesda System for reporting cervical/vaginal cytologic diagnoses. Report of the 1991 Bethesda workshop. Am J Clin Pathol 1992;98:152-4.

Masih AS, Stoler MH, Farrow GM, et al. Human papillomavirus in penile squamous cell lesions. A comparison of an isotopic RNA and two commercial nonisotopic DNA in situ hybridization methods. Arch Pathol Lab Med 1993;117:302-7.

Meisels A, Fortin R. Condylomatous lesions of the cervix and vagina. I. Cytologic patterns. Acta Cytol 1976;20:505-9.

Mills SE, Austin MB, Randall ME. Lymphoepithelioma-like carcinoma of the uterine cervix. A distinctive, undifferentiated carcinoma with inflammatory stroma. Am J Surg Pathol 1985; 9:883-9.

Mittal KR, Chan W, Demopoulos RI. Sensitivity and specificity of various morphological features of cervical condylomas. An in situ hybridization study. Arch Pathol Lab Med 1990;114:1038-41.

Munoz N, Bosch FX, de Sanjose S, et al. Epidemiologic classification of human papillomavirus types associated with cervical cancer. N Engl J Med 2003;348:518-27.

Novotny DB, Maygarden SJ, Johnson DE, et al. Tubal metaplasia. A frequent potential pitfall in the cytologic diagnosis of endocervical glandular dysplasia on cervical smears. Acta Cytol 1992;36:1-10.

Okagaki T, Clark BA, Zachow KR, et al. Presence of human papillomavirus in verrucous carcinoma (Ackerman) of the vagina. Immunocytochemical, ultrastructural, and DNA hybridization studies. Arch Pathol Lab Med 1984;108:567-70.

Ostor AG. Natural history of cervical intraepithelial neoplasia: a critical review. Int J Gynecol Pathol 1993;12:186-92.

Ostor AG. Pandora's box or Ariadne's thread? Definition and prognostic significance of microinvasion in the uterine cervix. Squamous lesions. Pathol Annu 1995;30 Pt 2:103-36.

Ostor AG. Early invasive adenocarcinoma of the uterine cervix. Int J Gynecol Pathol 2000;19:29-38.

Ostor AG, Mulvany N. The pathology of cervical neoplasia. Curr Opin Obstet Gynecol 1996;8:69-73.

Pak HY, Yokota SB, Paladugu RR, et al. Glassy cell carcinoma of the cervix. Cytologic and clinicopathologic analysis. Cancer 1983;52:307-12.

Patten SF. Diagnostic Cytopathology of the Uterine Cervix. 2nd ed. Basel: Karger; 1978.

Peyton CL, Schiffman M, Lorincz AT, et al. Comparison of PCR- and hybrid capture-based human papillomavirus detection systems using multiple cervical specimen collection strategies [published erratum appears in J Clin Microbiol 1999;37:478]. J Clin Microbiol 1998;36:3248-54.

Pfenninger JL. Cervex-Brush and Cytobrush: comparison of their ability to sample abnormal cells for cervical smears. J Reprod Med 1992;37:A32.

Purola E, Savia E. Cytology of gynecologic condyloma acuminatum. Acta Cytol 1977;21:26-31.

Ramzy I, Yuzpe AA, Hendelman J. Adenoid cystic carcinoma of uterine cervix. Obstet Gynecol 1975;45:679-83.

Reagan JW. Dysplasia of the uterine cervix. In: Gray LA, editor. Dysplasia, Carcinoma in Situ and Microinvasive Carcinoma. Springfield: Thomas; 1965.

Reagan JW, Bell BA, Neuman JL, et al. Dysplasia in the uterine cervix during pregnancy: an analytic study of the cells. Acta Cytol 1961;5:17-29.

Reagan JW, Fu YS. Histologic types and prognosis of cancers of the uterine cervix. Int J Radiat Oncol Biol Phys 1979;5:1015-20.

Reagan JW, Harmonic MJ. Dysplasia of the uterine cervix. Ann NY Acad Sci 1956;63:1236-1241.

Reagan JW, Patten SF. Dysplasia: A basic reaction to injury in the uterine cervix. Ann NY Acad Sci 1962;97:662-683.

Reagan JW, Seideman IL, Saracusa Y. The cellular morphology of carcinoma in situ and dysplasia or atypical hyperplasia of the uterine cervix. Cancer 1953;6:224-235.

Richart RM. Cervical intraepithelial neoplasia. Pathol Annu 1973;8:301-28.

Richart RM, Barron BA. A follow-up study of patients with cervical dysplasia. Am J Obstet Gynecol 1969;105:386-93.

Roberts ME, Fu YS. Squamous cell carcinoma of the uterine cervix--a review with emphasis on prognostic factors and unusual variants. Semin Diagn Pathol 1990;7:173-89.

Roche WD, Norris HJ. Microinvasive carcinoma of the cervix. The significance of lymphatic invasion and confluent patterns of stromal growth. Cancer 1975;36:180-6.

Ronnett BM, Manos MM, Ransley JE, et al. Atypical glandular cells of undetermined significance (AGUS): cytopathologic features, histopathologic results, and human papillomavirus DNA detection. Hum Pathol 1999;30:816-25.

Roth LM. Clear-cell adenocarcinoma of the female genital tract. A light and electron microscopic study. Cancer 1974;33:990-1001.

Rubens D, Thornbury JR, Angel C, et al. Stage IB cervical carcinoma: comparison of clinical, MR, and pathologic staging. Am J Roentgenol1988;150:135-8.

Rubio CA, Soderberg G, Grant CA, et al. The normal squamous epithelium of the human uterine cervix: a histological study. Pathol Eur 1976;11:157-62.

Saigo PE, Cain JM, Kim WS, et al. Prognostic factors in adenocarcinoma of the uterine cervix. Cancer 1986;57:1584-93.

Schiffman MH, Bauer HM, Hoover RN, et al. Epidemiologic evidence showing that human papillomavirus infection causes most cervical intraepithelial neoplasia [see comments]. J Natl Cancer Inst 1993;85:958-64.

Schiffman MH, Brinton LA. The epidemiology of cervical carcinogenesis. Cancer 1995;76(Suppl):1888-901.

Scott DR, Hagmar B, Maddox P, et al. Use of human papillomavirus DNA testing to compare equivocal cervical cytologic interpretations in the United States, Scandinavia, and the United Kingdom. Cancer 2002;96:14-20.

Scully RE, Bonfiglio TA, Kurman RJ, et al. Histological Typing of Female Genital Tract Tumours. 2nd ed. Berlin: Springer-Verlag; 1994.

Sevin B-U, Lu Y, Bloch DA, et al. Surgically defined prognostic parameters in patients with early cervical carcinoma: A multivariate survival tree analysis. Cancer 1996;78:1438-46.

Sevin BU, Nadji M, Averette HE, et al. Microinvasive carcinoma of the cervix. Cancer 1992;70:2121-8.

Sherman ME, Mendoza M, Lee KR, et al. Performance of liquid-based, thin-layer cervical cytology: correlation with reference diagnoses and human papillomavirus testing. Mod Pathol 1998;11:837-43.

Sherman ME, Solomon D, Schiffman M. Qualification of ASCUS. A comparison of equivocal LSIL and equivocal HSIL cervical cytology in the ASCUS LSIL Triage Study. Am J Clin Pathol 2001;116:386-94.

Sherman ME, Tabbara SO, Scott DR, et al. "ASCUS, rule out HSIL": cytologic features, histologic correlates, and human papillomavirus detection. Mod Pathol 1999;12:335-42.

Shingleton HM, Lawrence WD, Gore H. Cervical carcinoma with adenoid cystic pattern: a light and electron microscopic study. Cancer 1977;40:1112-21.

Silverberg SG, Hurt WG. Minimal deviation adenocarcinoma ("adenoma malignum") of the cervix: a reappraisal. Am J Obstet Gynecol 1975;121:971-5.

Solomon D, Davey D, Kurman R, et al. The 2001 Bethesda System: terminology for reporting results of cervical cytology. JAMA 2002;287:2114-9.

Solomon D, Schiffman M, Tarone R. Comparison of three management strategies for patients with atypical squamous cells of undetermined significance: baseline results from a randomized trial. J Natl Cancer Inst 2001;93:293-9.

Steeper TA, Wick MR. Minimal deviation adenocarcinoma of the uterine cervix ("adenoma malignum"). An immunohistochemical comparison with microglandular endocervical hyperplasia and conventional endocervical adenocarcinoma. Cancer 1986;58:1131-8.

Stoler MH. The biology of papillomaviruses. Pathology Case Reviews 1997;2:1-13.

Stoler MH. Does every little cell count? Don't "ASCUS". Cancer 1999;87:45-7.

Stoler MH. Advances in cervical screening technology. Mod Pathol 2000a;13:275-84.

Stoler MH. Human papillomaviruses and cervical neoplasia: a model for carcinogenesis. Int J Gynecol Pathol 2000b;19:16-28.

Stoler MH. Toward objective quality assurance: the eyes don't have it. Am J Clin Pathol 2002;117:520-2.

Stoler MH, Mills SE, Gersell DJ, et al. Small-cell neuroendocrine carcinoma of the cervix. A human papillomavirus type 18-associated cancer. Am J Surg Pathol 1991;15:28-32.

Stoler MH, Schiffman M. Interobserver reproducibility of cervical cytologic and histologic interpretations: realistic estimates from the ASCUS-LSIL Triage Study. JAMA 2001; 285:1500-5.

Swan DS, Roddick JW. A clinical-pathological correlation of cell type classification for cervical cancer. Am J Obstet Gynecol 1973;116:666-70.

Tamimi HK, Ek M, Hesla J, et al. Glassy cell carcinoma of the cervix redefined. Obstet Gynecol 1988;71:837-41.

Tsukamoto N, Hirakawa T, Matsukuma K, et al. Carcinoma of the uterine cervix with variegated histological patterns and calcitonin production. Gynecol Oncol 1989a;33:395-9.

Tsukamoto N, Kaku T, Matsukuma K, et al. The problem of stage Ia (FIGO, 1985) carcinoma of the uterine cervix. Gynecol Oncol 1989b;34:1-6.

Vayrynen M, Romppanen T, Koskela E, et al. Verrucous squamous cell carcinoma of the female genital tract. Report of three cases and survey of the literature. Intl J Gynaecol Obstet 1981;19:351-6.

Vesterinen E, Forss M, Nieminen U. Increase of cervical adenocarcinoma: a report of 520 cases of cervical carcinoma including 112 tumors with glandular elements. Gynecol Oncol 1989;33:49-53.

Walboomers JM, Jacobs MV, Manos MM, et al. Human papillomavirus is a necessary cause of invasive cervical cancer worldwide. J Pathol 1999;189:12-19.

Weisbrot IM, Stabinsky C, Davis AM. Adenocarcinoma in situ of the uterine cervix. Cancer 1972;29:1179-87.

Wells M, Brown LJ. Glandular lesions of the uterine cervix: the present state of our knowledge. Histopathology 1986;10:777-92.

Wentz WB, Reagan JW. Survival in cervical cancer with respect to cell type. Cancer 1959;12:384-388.

Wilczynski SP, Bergen S, Walker J, et al. Human papillomaviruses and cervical cancer: analysis of histopathologic features associated with different viral types. Hum Pathol 1988;19:697-704.

Wright TC, Jr., Cox JT, Massad LS, et al. 2001 Consensus Guidelines for the management of women with cervical cytological abnormalities. JAMA 2002;287:2120-9.

Young RH, Scully RE. Villoglandular papillary adenocarcinoma of the uterine cervix. A clinicopathologic analysis of 13 cases. Cancer 1989;63:1773-9.

Young RH, Scully RE. Invasive adenocarcinoma and related tumors of the uterine cervix. Semin Diagn Pathol 1990;7:205-27.

Zaino RJ, Ward S, Delgado G, et al. Histopathologic predictors of the behavior of surgically treated stage IB squamous cell carcinoma of the cervix. A Gynecologic Oncology Group study. Cancer 1992;69:1750-8.

Chapter 2

The Natural History of Cervical Cancer

Anthony B. Miller, M.B., F.R.C.P.
Division of Clinical Epidemiology, Deutsches Krebsforschungszentrum

INTRODUCTION

Interest in the natural history of cancer of the cervix began with the recognition that for effective and efficient application of screening, "the natural history of the disease should be known" (Wilson and Junger, 1968). This is because screening is based on the expectation that the early detection of cancer, in what has been called the Detectable Preclinical Phase (DPCP) (Cole and Morrison, 1980), will result in a reduction in mortality from the disease. If effective screening is directed primarily to the detection of precursors, the development of invasive cancer will be prevented. Therefore, an effective program for screening for cancer of the cervix will result in a reduction in cancer incidence as well as a reduction in cancer mortality. Knowledge of the natural history of the disease will facilitate decisions on the appropriate ages to initiate and cease screening, and the optimal frequency of re-screening in those who test negative.

It is intuitively obvious that in order to gain knowledge of the natural history of the lesions discovered by screening, screening has to be performed and the detected abnormalities identified. However, as screening is a clinical activity performed in order to benefit the individual, it is rarely possible to avoid applying the currently best-known therapy for the condition. For "early" lesions this almost invariably involves surgical excision, which often, at least in the period before colposcopy management became routine for cervix screening, resulted in complete, or almost complete ablation of the cervical epithelium. Therefore, except in very unusual circumstances (Kinlen and Spriggs, 1978), it is not possible to determine the natural history of the detected lesions by observing them. Yet when cervical cancer screening programs based on cervical cytology were being introduced, it was appreciated that the number of cases of presumed precursors was too large compared to the numbers of invasive cancers that occurred in the same population (Burns et al., 1968; Fidler et al., 1968; Coppleson and Brown, 1975). This led to a series of studies that began to clarify the natural history of the disease as identified by the abnormalities detected by cytology. However, because of the impossibility of directly observing the outcome of lesions treated surgically, their natural history has to be inferred by statistical techniques, usually by applying models of the presumed natural history, that are valid only to the extent that the assumptions that led to the model are valid.

It is only fairly recently, when the natural history of cervical infection with human papillomaviruses (HPV) has been studied by specially designed investigations, that studies of the natural history of cervix cancer have been put on a new footing. Even here, however, ethical concerns over a process of observation that might unwittingly allow an invasive cancer to develop has resulted in the endpoints of studies being restricted to lesions which the earlier cytology-based studies showed were early in the process of progression to invasive cancer. This has resulted in considerable room for disagreement over the implications of the findings of these studies as will be shown in this chapter. However, the implication of the basis for both types of studies is that it is impossible to discuss the natural history of cancer of the cervix without considering screening for the disease. As implied above, the implications of such studies apply to policy issues such as the age at which to start screening, the age to stop, and the frequency of re-screening, as well the type of test used and how it is examined in the laboratory. These issues have been discussed elsewhere (Miller, 1999; Miller, 2002), and for the most part they will not be referred to in this chapter.

Because it seems not to be possible to understand the studies of the natural history of HPV in relation to the development of cancer of the cervix without understanding the knowledge gained by the earlier cytology-based studies, the first part of this chapter is devoted to a review of such studies. In the second part of the chapter, the discussion focuses on our emerging understanding of the natural history of the lesions identified by HPV DNA testing. A final section attempts to bring both types of information together in an integrated whole.

1   FINDINGS FROM CYTOLOGY-BASED STUDIES

1.1   A note on terminology

In the original WHO classification (Riotten et al., 1973) the precursors of cancer of the cervix were considered in two groups, carcinoma-in-situ, a full thickness change in the squamous epithelium of the cervix with malignant appearing nuclei but without invasion of the basement membrane, and various degrees of dysplasia, which involved lesser degrees of involvement of the epithelium without full thickness change. The degrees of dysplasia were identified as mild, moderate and severe. In the hands of experienced observers, the distinction between carcinoma-in-situ and severe dysplasia was usually made consistently. Subsequently, Richart (1980) proposed the cervical intraepithelial neoplasia (CIN) terminology, categorizing mild dysplasia as CIN 1, moderate dysplasia as CIN 2, and severe dysplasia and carcinoma-in-situ combined as CIN 3. However, in 1989 the "Bethesda" system was promulgated in the United States, with CIN 1 together with cellular evidence of HPV effects combined as Low Grade Squamous Intraepithelial lesions (LSIL) and CIN 2 and 3 combined as High Grade Squamous Intraepithelial lesions (HSIL) (National Cancer Institute Workshop, 1989) (Table 1).

Table 1. Classification of preinvasive lesions of the uterine cervix

Descriptive (WHO) classification	Cervical Intraepithelial Neoplasia (CIN) classification	Bethesda classification
Unclassified	Unclassified	ASCUS/AGUS
Unclassified	HPV effects	LSIL
Mild dysplasia	CIN 1	LSIL
Moderate dysplasia	CIN 2	HSIL
Severe dysplasia	CIN 3	HSIL
Carcinoma-in-situ	CIN 3	HSIL

More recently, the Bethesda system has been modified further in an attempt to remove some of the ambiguities associated with the ASCUS designation (Solomon et al., 2002). Although the intent of the Bethesda system was to simplify reporting and facilitate clinical management, while avoiding some of the observer variation inseparable from a multigrade system, the impact of the spread of this system on understanding of the natural history of the precursors has been adverse, as will be discussed further below. Nevertheless, it will be impossible to avoid using the terminology adopted by the authors, though the equivalence of some (and the grouping of other) abnormalities should be kept in mind.

1.2   The natural history of carcinoma-in-situ of the cervix

As indicated earlier, when data began to become available from the early screening programs for cancer of the cervix, it was noticed that the number of cases of carcinoma-in-situ of the cervix was far greater than was "required" to account for the incidence of invasive cancer of the cervix in the absence of screening. The difference between the cumulative incidence of carcinoma in situ (CIS) by age less the prevalent (non-progressed) cases of carcinoma-in-situ and the cumulative incidence of invasive cancer in data from the British Columbia screening program was named the "yawning gap" (Boyes et al., 1982) (Figure 1). The expectation, if all cases of carcinoma-in-situ progress to invasive cancer, was that these two curves should overlap.

However, there were several other potential explanations for the gap. The first was false negative error. If a case of carcinoma-in-situ was missed at the first or subsequent screens in error, but was diagnosed subsequently at a later screen, the cumulative incidence of carcinoma in situ would be increased artefactually, and the prevalence of carcinoma in situ would be reduced, thus contributing to the yawning gap. The second potential explanation was denominator error. If women who returned for re-screening did so after a change of name as a result of marriage, or if the initial records were so deficient that the initial and subsequent screens could not be linked in the laboratory's file, then the prevalence would be reduced artifactually by inclusion in the denominator of the same women screened a second or third time, with lower resultant risk of disease.

The effect on the cumulative incidence of carcinoma-in-situ would be less, as their true risk is similar to those already correctly included in the computations for incidence, and so again the yawning gap would be increased. A third potential explanation was that there was a cohort effect. If more recent birth cohorts had a greater lifetime risk of disease than older cohorts, then a gap would be created, as the younger cohorts in a cross sectional study would largely comprise those at risk for carcinoma-in-situ, whereas the older cohorts would be at risk for invasive carcinoma. The remaining explanation was regression of carcinoma-in-situ. If all the other explanations were discounted, then the excess of carcinoma-in-situ would be caused by the fact that not all cases are destined to progress to invasive cancer, nor even remain unchanged in a woman; rather, some would regress to lesser degrees of abnormality or even to normal epithelium.

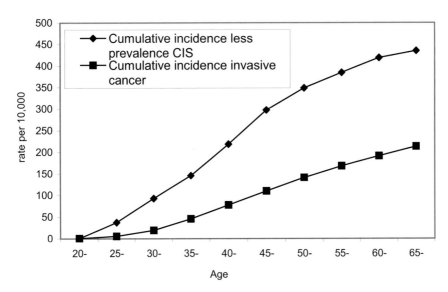

Figure 1. The "yawning" gap

The British Columbia cohort study was set up to evaluate these different explanations for the yawning gap. The study utilized the records in the central cytology laboratory, the only one in the province. Records on all women born in 1914-18 and 1929-33 with follow-up to 1969 were extracted, and related to population data on invasive cancer, deaths, marriage and hysterectomies. The major concentration in the analysis was on corrected rates of prevalence and incidence of carcinoma-in-situ and of invasive cervical cancer. It was found that the gap persisted in spite of corrections for the false negative error and denominator error, and that the two cohorts 15 years of age apart had almost identical risks of carcinoma-in-situ at comparable ages (Boyes et al., 1982). Thus the only remaining explanation for the gap was regression, which probably occurred in 40-60% of the detectable cases, especially at younger ages. An extension of this study, with follow-up to 1985, including a younger cohort born in 1944-48, confirmed these conclusions, and showed even more regression at younger ages than had been computed for the older cohorts (Miller et al., 1991).

1.3   The natural history of dysplasia of the cervix

In the British Columbia Cohort Study, the inclusion of identified cases of dysplasia did not increase the proportion of those with preclinical abnormalities that developed progressive disease. Indeed, the majority of these cases appeared to regress, confirming that only among those few cases that progressed to carcinoma-in-situ was there a risk of invasive carcinoma (Boyes et al., 1982). However, the British Columbia data did not distinguish between separate degrees of dysplasia. Therefore, to address this deficiency, a large cohort of women identified through one pathology laboratory in Toronto and whose records of cytological examinations spanned many years was studied (Holowaty et al., 1999). The pathologists serving this laboratory had made a consistent attempt to identify the different degrees of dysplasia by cytology, and only referred women for further assessment if there was cytological evidence of progression. By linking the records extracted from the laboratory with those of the Ontario Cancer Registry, women who were subsequently diagnosed with carcinoma-in-situ or invasive carcinoma of the cervix were identified (Holowaty et al., 1999). Once again there was evidence of regression. The maximum extent of regression occurred in those with cytological evidence of mild dysplasia, but in addition, over 50% of those with cytological evidence of moderate dysplasia showed regression. Progression to severe dysplasia or worse within 10 years occurred in only 10% of those with mild dysplasia and in 32% of those with moderate dysplasia. Most of these progressions occurred within 5 years. There was even less progression, even within ten years, when invasive cancer was used as the endpoint (Table 2). Equally as important, a category identified in the laboratory as minimal dysplasia, a grouping that encompasses those that in the Bethesda system would be labelled as ASCUS, hardly showed any evidence of progression at all. Therefore, the results of the study supported the conclusions of a Canadian workshop (Miller et al., 1991), which proposed that there is prognostic value in the classification of moderate dysplasia separately from severe dysplasia, and that cytologic surveillance rather than immediate referral to colposcopy should be recommended for those with a cytologic diagnosis of mild dysplasia.

Table 2. Estimates of progression in the Toronto Dysplasia Study
(Holowaty et al, 1999)

Progression within 10 years to carcinoma-in-situ or worse:

	Probability	RR
Controls	0.006	
Mild dysplasia	0.03	4.7
Moderate dysplasia	0.10	17.0
Severe dysplasia	0.21	35.1

Progression within 10 years to invasive cancer of the cervix:

	Probability	RR
Controls	0.0006	
Mild dysplasia	0.003	5.7
Moderate dysplasia	0.009	16.3
Severe dysplasia	0.029	52.8

Although the study of Holowaty et al. (1999) was one of the largest studies of the natural history of dysplasia, and one of the few to obtain data on invasive cervical cancer as an endpoint, a number of other studies also considered this issue. These earlier studies were reviewed by Ostor (1993) who also concluded that a high proportion of cases of dysplasia regressed.

1.4   Implications of mathematical models of the natural history of cancer of the cervix for screening frequency

An early evaluation of the British Columbia data using a Markov-Chain model supported a prolonged natural history of carcinoma-in-situ (an average sojourn time of at least 9 years) (Yu et al., 1982). It also suggested that cytologically negative women should be rescreened every five years (Yu et al., 1982).

However, a critical study which increased our understanding of the appropriate approach to re-screening was coordinated by the IARC Working Group on Cervical Cancer Screening (1986). This study largely provided the basis for international recommendations for three yearly or even less frequent repeat screening and underlined the importance of concentrating screening between the ages of 35 and 64 (Miller, 1992). However, an underlying difficulty with these recommendations is that probably the most successful screening program in the world is the organized program in Finland, which utilized only five-yearly screening and achieved the levels of success that the IARC model suggested would require three-yearly screening. A re-evaluation of the British Columbia data using the Miscan model developed in Rotterdam (van Oortmarssen and Habbema, 1995) showed that although the median duration for progression from carcinoma in situ to invasive cancer in the IARC study was of the order of 5-8 years, this was calculated by including screen-detected cancers, whose prognosis is extremely good and who are affected by the lead time gained by screening. Correcting for such screen-detected cancers resulted in a median duration from carcinoma in situ to invasive cancer of 15 years. The implication of this is that screening every 5, not 3 years, will give a 90% reduction in invasive cancer incidence and mortality.

Table 3 shows the results from these models in terms of the expected impact on the cumulative incidence of invasive cancer of the cervix in optimally screened populations. It is important to recognize that in these optimal circumstances, based on highly efficient cytology screening programs from many countries, no realistic screening schedule results in abolition of the occurrence of invasive cancer.

Table 3. IARC study - modified, low incidence country

Age and schedule of screening	Cumulative rate per 100,000	Reduction in incidence*	Number of tests in a lifetime
None	1575		
20-64:			
3 yrly	47	97%	15
5 yrly	158	90%	9
26-64:			
3 yrly	63	96%	13
5 yrly	189	88%	8

*In women with at least one prior negative screen, assuming 100% compliance with screening schedule

In many countries, including the US, the outcome will be less impressive. Part of the reason for this is failure of an essential component of the program, which can occur at the level of the woman, her physician, or the laboratory examining her smears (Miller, 1995), but another reason is likely to be the natural variability of the natural history in different women. The models are based on averages of transition probabilities, each with a different distribution or range of time periods during which some lesions progress from one state to the next, while others regress to normal, and still others remain stable for long periods of time. Some lesions may progress so rapidly that they cannot be found in a curable stage even with annual screening, and it seems unlikely that the majority of such lesions would be detected by more frequent screening. This does not mean there are different types of cancers of the cervix, as suggested many years ago (Ashley, 1966), just that the fast-growing lesions represent one extreme of the distribution of progression (sojourn) times. However, the fact they occur is what has tended to drive the search for more sensitive tests, and particularly the current enthusiasm for HPV testing.

2 THE NATURAL HISTORY OF CERVICAL INTRAEPITHELIAL NEOPLASIA AS IDENTIFIED BY HPV TESTING

Human papillomavirus infection of young women is frequent, and in the large majority of women transient. Infection with HPV would be of little concern if it had not been conclusively demonstrated that cervix uteri cancer was caused by this virus, or rather certain types of HPV virus (16,18, 31,33,35,39, 45, 51, 52,56,58,59, 68). Of these, HPV type 16 is by far the most frequent world wide, though countries vary in the prevalence of HPV types in their population. Thus, oncogenic types of human papillomaviruses (HPV) can be found in nearly all cancers of the cervix (Walboomers et al., 1999). The evidence that certain types of HPV cause cancer of the cervix has been categorized as *sufficient* by the International Agency for Research on Cancer (1995).

As discussed in the first section of this chapter, much is known about the natural history of the abnormalities identified by cytology screening. Many are likely to regress without treatment. However, it is not clear that this is also true for the lesions identified by HPV testing. Melkert et al. (1993) found a higher prevalence of HPV infection using the polymerase chain reaction (PCR) for testing in women under the age of 35 than in older women, and concluded that most such infections were transient. This was confirmed by Jacobs et al. (2000) who also found a decreasing HPV prevalence with increasing age in cytologically negative women. They suggested that each year at least 70% of HPV infections cleared spontaneously. In a further study from the same group of investigators in the Netherlands, involving women who had CIN 3, Remmink et al. (1995) suggested that only women who were infected with high risk HPV types were likely to have progressive disease, and only in women with persistent infection was their disease likely to progress. Further, Zielenski et al. (2001) suggested that infection with HPV precedes the development of a cytologic abnormality. However, cross-sectional surveys (conducted across ages at one point in time), such as those just described, do not provide much information on natural history. It is necessary to follow groups of women for some time, and conduct repeated tests, to obtain such information, but to date, relatively few studies of this type have been performed.

Ho et al. (1998) followed 608 college students for 6 months to 2 years. They estimated that after 3 years, 43% of such women would have acquired an HPV infection. Increased risk was associated with young age, being black, having many sexual partners, and with alcohol and tobacco use. The median duration of infection was 8 months. Of those who acquired HR HPV infection, 37% had an abnormal smear. Similar risks were also reported by other US investigators. Koutsky et al. (1992) reported that after 2 years of follow-up, those initially HPV positive had a cumulative risk of CIN 2 or 3 of 28% compared to a cumulative risk of 3% for those initially HPV negative. Risk was highest for those women infected with HPV 16 or 18, the relative risk for those infected with type 16 being 11 (95% CI 4.6-26) for the development of a squamous intraepithelial lesion (SIL) compared to those without an HPV 16 infection. Gaarenstroom et al. (1994) also showed that low-grade SIL progressed to high-grade disease only if it contained high-risk HPV types.

In the UK, Woodman et al. (2001) reported the results of a study designed to determine the natural history of human papillomavirus (HPV) infections. They recruited a cohort of 1075 young women who agreed to undergo intensive cytology and HPV screening, and who on average had repeat tests every 7 months. This enabled Woodman et al. to determine accurately the timing of HPV infections, and the development of CIN that followed some of these infections. Somewhat surprisingly, of the 240 women who developed abnormal smears whose HPV status was known, 41% tested negative for HPV and another 34% only tested HPV positive at the same visit as that in which their abnormal smear was detected. Thus, for only 25% was a positive HPV test predictive of abnormal cytology, though this translated into a cumulative risk of 33% at 3 years. However, as anticipated, the risk of a moderate or severe dyskariosis (cellular evidence of dysplasia, in the UK terminology) was substantially greater in those who tested HPV positive, and of the 28 women who developed high grade CIN during follow-up, 82% had become HPV positive after a median follow-up of 26 months. Nevertheless, compared to those who were HPV negative during follow-up, the risk of moderate or severe dyskariosis was maximal at 6 months after the first HPV positive test (RR 25.3, 95% CI 8.8-72.8), and declined rapidly thereafter (RR >12 months 6.3, 95% CI 2.1-19.6). So in this study, maximal risk was not demonstrated in those with evidence of persistent HPV infection. This finding is different from that from the cohort study of Ho et al. (1998), where persistence of HPV infection was associated with increased risk of squamous intraepithelial lesions. However the US study was smaller, and the number of lesions less than in the study of Woodman et al. (2001), and the intensity of observation of the cohort was less in the US compared to the UK. Woodman et al. (2001) thus confirmed the transitory nature of most HPV infections, identified the variability in HPV types that may accompany such infections, but also showed that cytology may identify abnormalities after a remarkably short latent period from the first evidence of HPV infection. Their data suggest that if women are screened with HPV tests, whether or not they test positive and are then found to have CIN is subject to far more of the vagaries of chance than most have assumed until now.

Other data suggest that the intensity of an HPV infection (i.e., the viral load) is relevant as to whether detectable disease develops. Thus, Cuzick et al. (1994) showed that in women with cytological abnormalities, a high viral load detected by a semi-quantitative PCR was strongly related to high grade CIN. Ho et al. (1995) also suggested that women with SIL with a high viral load are more likely to have persistent SIL than those with a low level of DNA. They conducted a study of 70 subjects with histopathologically confirmed cervical dysplasia, followed at 3-month intervals for 15 months. Those with HPV type-specific infection and with a high viral load had the highest risk of persistent SIL compared to those with a low-level of type-specific persistent infection or no type-specific infection (OR 4.97, 95% CI 1.45-17.02).

Liaw et al. (1999) followed a cohort of 17654 cytologically-negative women using the records of Kaiser Permanente in California. Enrollment in the cohort commenced in 1989, and women were followed to the end of 1994. On average, each woman had 0.6 smears a year, and 20% had no repeats. A total of 380 incident cases of cytologic abnormality were identified, 154 with ASCUS, 179 with LSIL and 47 with HSIL. Cervix lavages had been collected and stored at enrollment, and on diagnosis, another lavage specimen was collected. Similarly specimens were collected from up to 3 matched controls without abnormality, and all specimens were tested for HPV DNA using PCR. The data were analyzed as a nested case-control study. Compared with women who were HPV DNA negative on enrollment, those who were positive at enrolment had an OR of 3.8 (95% CI 2.6-5.5) for being diagnosed with LSIL, and an OR of 12.7 (6.2-25.9) for HSIL. Infection with HPV type 16 was most likely to predict the development of SIL. The associations were much stronger for HPV positivity detected at diagnosis.

Josefsson et al. (2000) and Ylitalo et al. (2000) in case-control studies nested within a cohort of screened women in Sweden, and using a sensitive PCR assay, demonstrated that cervical carcinoma-in-situ associated with

HPV 16 occurred mainly in HPV type 16-positive women who had consistently high viral loads long-term. These studies, based on tests of archived specimens, confirmed the long natural history of carcinoma-in-situ, as previously inferred from cytology. Thus Ylitalo et al. (2000) computed that the mean time from a first confirmed HPV infection under age 25 to a diagnosis of carcinoma-in-situ in women with high and intermediate viral loads was 17 years and 19 years, respectively. Approximately 22% of women with evidence of a high viral load of type 16 HPV infection were eventually diagnosed with carcinoma-in-situ. Further, Josephson et al. (2000) found that women in the highest 20% of the HPV 16 DNA viral load distribution were at a 60-fold higher risk of being diagnosed with carcinoma-in-situ than women negative to HPV 16. Subsequently, van Duin et al. (2002) found, in a cohort study that in women with normal cytology, as well as those with abnormal cytology, an increased HPV 16 viral load conferred an increased risk of developing a cervical lesion.

The potential role of HPV DNA testing for cervical screening has been evaluated in several studies, such as in South Africa (Wright et al., 2000) and Costa Rica (Schiffman et al., 2000). Both these studies compared the sensitivity and specificity of HPV DNA testing and cytology in detecting presumed cervical cancer precursors, but in neither study was sufficient information given to allow assessment of the sensitivity and specificity of HPV testing for detection of CIN 3. Both studies confused the issue by adding cases of invasive cancer to the high-grade lesions. However, a greater difficulty is the utilization in these studies of the High Grade SIL designation, encompassing both cytologically diagnosed CIN 2 as well as CIN 3. In this context, we are not interested in CIN 2, as the majority of such lesions will regress spontaneously, and it is the sensitivity with regard to CIN 3, which is critical. Unfortunately, Clavel et al. (2001) in France also used the same endpoint in a cross-sectional study. They studied 7932 women enrolled in a screening program with a commercial HPV detection test (Hybrid-Capture-II) together with cytology for primary screening. Of 7339 women cytologically negative, 773 (11.9%) had evidence of an HPV infection. The same group later reported results of follow-up of a subsample of 3091 women with normal smears at first entry, among whom 659 (21%) had evidence of HPV infection (Bory et al., 2002). Of these 659, 241 (3% of the total studied) had a persistent HPV infection at 2 to 4 examinations, with a final diagnosis of high grade SIL in 51 (0.7% of the total studied) within 4 to 36 months. The women who developed high grade SIL had a higher viral load than those with transitory infections. All these women developed cytological abnormalities prior to or at the time of the colposcopy that led to the diagnosis. In contrast, of 2432 women who were negative for HPV and followed for a similar period as for the HPV positive women, only two developed a high grade SIL. In contrast to the findings of Roozendaal et al.

(1996), these authors did not find a higher positive predictive value of a persistent high-risk HPV infection for detection of a high-grade SIL in women older than 30 than in those younger, perhaps because they dichotomized age at too low a value for this French population.

It is difficult to assess the implications of such results, given that the majority of the high grade SIL cases of these authors would probably have been classified as moderate dysplasia by Holowaty et al. (1999), and would have eventually regressed. However, Nobbenhuis et al. (1999) concentrated on CIN 3 as their end point. They used cytology and HPV testing by PCR to monitor for an average of 33 months 353 women who had been referred to gynaecologists with mild to moderate or severe dysplasia. Thirty-three women reached clinical progression, defined as CIN 3 covering three or more cervical quadrants, or a smear result of suspected cervical cancer. All had persistent infection with a high risk HPV type. The cumulative 6-year incidence of clinical progression among these women was 40% (95% CI 21%-59%).

3   DISCUSSION

The lessons from the HPV studies seem clear. Infection with HPV, including oncogenic HPV types, is predictive of the subsequent development of SIL, but such infection occurs far too frequently compared to the amount of cervical cancer expected in these populations. A cumulative incidence of invasive cervical cancer of 1.5 % is unusual, and as high as 5% exceptional. Thus the large majority of infections in young women are not only transient, but even the majority of those that appear persistent, are of no concern. This conclusion has also been reached concerning many of the abnormalities identified by cytology (Holowaty et al., 1999; Miller et al., 2000).

In all countries, the incidence of invasive cancer of the cervix peaks at around age 55, and invasive cases are rare before age 30. However, carcinoma in situ and the dysplastic lesions that comprise the DPCP are detectable in some women even from the age of 15, while in women who become sexually active at a younger age HPV tests may be positive from the age of 11 or 12. However, the large majority of such detectable precursor lesions in young women will not have progressed, and the majority will have regressed, by age 35. Nevertheless, it appears to be established that testing by both cytology and for HR HPV identifies women with CIN 3, the proximate precursor for cervix cancer. Further, although the early cytology-based studies showed that at least 50% of women with detectable carcinoma-in-situ will not progress, the HPV-based studies support the view that only cases of CIN 3 with high risk HPV infection are at risk for progressive disease, while the proportion that regresses is of a similar order to the proportion that progresses.

There is, however, at least one other missing piece of information concerning the natural history of high-risk HPV infections. It is important to know what causes persistence of infection with oncogenic HPV viruses, and what causes precursors to progress and not regress. Is there a single co-carcinogen or two or more? It is unlikely to be a feature of the virus, given the high prevalence of non-persistent infection in young women, so that a refined test for HPV infection will not provide the answer. It may be a feature of the host, or it may be something else, as yet unenvisaged.

Ideally, we require a test that indicates that an oncogenic HPV has already enhanced genetic instability and rendered infected cells susceptible to transformation, thereby facilitating the development of cancer. The ideal test in this respect should have the ability to detect those progressive cytological abnormalities that are caused by high risk HPV infections and to discriminate them from transient low grade lesions and those that only mimic morphologic criteria of the onset of dysplasia or harbor HPV as an independent, but simultaneous event. Such an HPV-based test should have greater true biologic sensitivity and specificity than cytology and could possibly solve two problems inherent to conventional cytology. It could be the solution to the ASCUS/LSIL dilemma since, as already pointed out, these categories represent mostly transient infections or in the case of ASCUS mainly diagnostic uncertainty. The other problem that contributes to low sensitivity of conventional cytology is overlooking and/or misinterpreting abnormal cells, a problem that also ideally should be overcome by a test that fulfills the criteria specified above.

A new test that can be applied to both standard Pap smears and Thin Prep™ specimens which may have these desirable characteristics is CINtec™. This test identifies a cellular protein marker (cell cycle associated cyclin inhibitor p16INK4a) that is upregulated in potentially harmful HPV-associated CIN 2/3 lesions and a subset of CIN 1 lesions. The basis of this approach is that continuous expression of the viral oncogenes E6 and E7 interferes with normal cell cycle control by targeting p53 and pRB, respectively. This phenomenon is a general event in persistent high-risk HPV infections but seems not to be induced by low risk types. The functional loss of pRB by binding of E7 protein in turn leads to an increase in cell cycle regulating p16INK4a, possibly as a negative feedback loop. Therefore, it should be possible to use the detection of overexpression of this cell cycle regulatory protein as a surrogate marker for essential steps in early cervical carcinogenesis (Klaes et al., 2001). Klaes et al. (2001) studied more than 200 histology slides and demonstrated overexpression of p16INK4a in all CIN 2/3 lesions and in virtually all cervical cancers. Results from the same study show that the marker is not expressed in normal epithelium or in normal proliferating cells. Except for a faint and focal staining in a small percentage of inflammatory or metaplastic lesions, these entities and low grade CIN lesions not infected with high risk HPV were negative by

CINtec™ staining. Since the clinical specimens in this study were derived from cervical cone biopsies it is possible that weak staining in the case of inflammation or metaplasia is a remnant of a lesion that had already regressed. A study has been designed to evaluate this test in comparison with conventionally stained cytology smears in terms of biologically relevant endpoints. It is hoped that such a study will be initiated within the next 12 months in centers in developed and developing countries.

In the meantime, it seems clear that although the HPV studies are clarifying our understanding of the natural history of preclinical abnormalities of the cervix originally obtained from cytology. Figure 2 attempts to encapsulate this diagrammatically. It is important to recognize that although precise numbers cannot be given, as one moves from left to

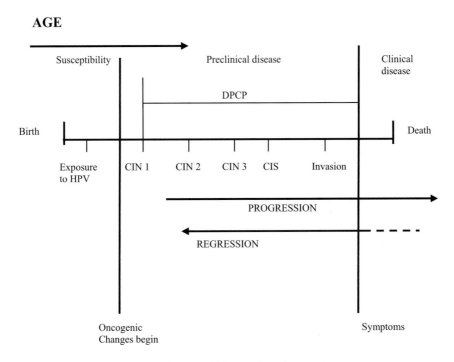

Figure 2. The natural history of cervix cancer

right across this figure, the probability of progression becomes less, and as one moves in the opposite direction, the probability of regression grows more. At present, in terms of application, our knowledge has not yet reached the stage when we can abandon cytology and substitute HPV testing. Research continues, however, and we can expect much more understanding in the years to come.

REFERENCES

Ashley, DJB. Evidence for the existence of two forms of cervical carcinoma. J Obstet Gynaecol Br Comm 1966; 73:382-9.

Bory JP, Cucherousset J, Lorenzato M, et al. Recurrent human papillomavirus infection detected by hybrid capture II selects women with normal smears at risk for developing high grade cervical lesions: a longitudinal study of 3091 women. Int J Cancer 2002; 102:519-25.

Boyes DA, Morrison B, Knox EG, et al. A cohort study of cervical cancer screening in British Columbia. Clinical Investigative Medicine 1982; 5:1-29.

Burns EL, Hammond EC, Percy C, et al. Detection of uterine cancer. Results of a community program of 10 years. Cancer 1968; 22:1108-19

Clavel C, Masure M, Bory JP, et al. Human papillomavirus testing in primary screening for the detection of high-grade cervical lesions: a study of 7932 women. Br J Cancer 2001; 84: 1616-23.

Cole P, Morrison AS. Basic issues in population screening for cancer. J Natl Cancer Inst 1980; 64:1263-72.

Coppleson LW, Brown B. Observations on a model of the biology of the cervix: a poor fit between observation and practice. Am J Obstet Gynecol 1975; 122: 127-36.

Cuzick J, Beverley E, Terry G, et al. HPV testing in primary screening of older women. Br J Cancer 1999; 81: 554–8.

Fidler HK, Boyes DA, Worth AJ. Cervical cancer detection in British Colombia. J Obstet Gynaec Br Comm 1968; 75: 392-404.

Gaarenstroom KN, Melkert P, Walboomers JMM, et al. Human papillomavirus DNA genotypes: prognostic factors for progression of cervical intraepithelial neoplasia. Int J Gynecol Cancer 1994; 4:73-8.

Ho GYF, Burk RD, Klein S, et al. Persistent genital human papillomavirus infection as a risk factor for persistent cervival dysplasia. J Natl Cancer Inst 1995; 87: 1365-71.

Ho GY, Bierman R, Beardsley L, Chang CC, Burk RD. Natural history of cervicovaginal papillomavirus infection in young women. N Engl J Med 1998; 338: 423–8.

Holowaty P, Miller AB, Rohan T, To T. The natural history of dysplasia of the uterine cervix. J Natl Cancer Inst 1999; 91: 252–8.

IARC Monographs on the evaluation of carcinogenic risks to humans. Volume 64 Human Papillomaviruses. Lyon, International Agency for Research on Cancer, 1995.

IARC Working Group on Cervical Cancer Screening. Summary Chapter. In: Hakama M, Miller AB, Day NE, (eds). Screening for Cancer of the Uterine Cervix. IARC Scientific Publications No. 76. Lyon, International Agency for Research on Cancer, 1986, 133–42.

Jacobs MV, Walboomers JMM, Snijders PJF, et al. Distribution of 37 mucosotropic HPV types in women with cytologically normal cervical smears: the age-related patterns for high-risk and low- risk types. Int J Cancer 2000; 87:221-7.

Josefsson AM, Magnusson PK, Ylitalo N, et al. Viral load of human papillomavirus 16 as a determinant for development of cervical carcinoma in situ: a nested case-control study. Lancet 2000; 355: 2189-93.

Kinlen LJ, Spriggs AI. Women with positive cervical smears but without surgical intervention. Lancet 1978; ii 463-5.

Klaes R, Friedrich T, Spitkovsky D, et al. Overexpression of p16INK4a as specific marker for dysplastic and neoplastic epithelial cells of the cervix uteri. Int J Cancer 2001; 92:276-84.

Koutsky LA, Holmes KK, Critchlow CW, et al. A cohort study of the risk of cervical intraepithelial neoplasia grade 2 or 3 in relation to papillomavirus infection. New Eng J Med 1992, 327: 1272-8.

Liaw K, Glass G, Manos M, et al. Detection of human papillomavirus DNA in cytologically normal women and subsequent cervical squamous intraepithelial lesions. J Natl Cancer Inst 1999; 91: 954–60.

Melkert PJW, Hopman E, van den Brule AJC, et al. Prevalence of HPV in cytomorphologically normal cervical smears as determined by the polymerase chain reaction is age-dependent. Int J Cancer 1993, 53:919-23.

Miller AB. Cervical cancer screening programmes. Managerial Guidelines. Geneva, World Health Organization, 1992.

Miller AB. Editorial: Failures of Cervical Cancer Screening. Am J Pub Hlth 1995; 85:761-2.

Miller AB. Cervix cancer. In: Kramer BS, Gohagan JK, Prorok PC, (eds) Cancer Screening, Theory and practice. New York, Marcel Dekker, Inc; 1999, 195-217.

Miller AB. Screening. In: Franco EL, Rohan, TE (eds). Cancer precursors. Epidemiology, detection and prevention. New York Berlin Heidelberg Springer-Verlag, 2002, 365-73.

Miller AB, Anderson G, Brisson J, et al. Report of a National Workshop on Screening for Cancer of the Cervix. Can Med Ass J 1991; 145:1301-25.

Miller AB, Knight J, Narod S. The Natural History of Cancer of the Cervix, and the implications for screening policy. In Cancer Screening, Miller AB et al (eds). Cambridge, Cambridge University Press, 1991, 144-52.

Miller AB, Nazeer S, Fonn S, Brandup-Lukanow A, et al. Report on consensus conference on cervical cancer screening and management. Int J Cancer 2000; 86: 440–7.

National Cancer Institute Workshop. The 1998 Bethesda System for reporting cervical/ vaginal cytological diagnoses. JAMA 1989; 262:931-4.

Nobbenhuis MAE, Walboomers JMM, Helmerhorst TJM, et al. Relation of human papilloma-virus status to cervical lesions and consequences for cervical-cancer screening: a prospective study. Lancet 1999, 354: 20-5.

Ostor AG. Natural history of cervical intraepithelial neoplasia: a critical review. Int J Gynecol Pathol 1993; 12: 186–92.

Remmink AJ, Walboomers JMM, Helmerhorst TJM, et al. The presence of persistent high-risk HPV types in dysplastic cervical lesions is associated with progressive disease: natural history up to 36 months. Int J Cancer 1995; 61:306-11.

Richart RM. The patient with an abnormal Pap smear: screening techniques and management. N Eng J Med 1980; 302:332-4.

Riotten G, Christopherson WM, Lunt R. Cytology of the female genital tract. International Histological Classification of Tumours No. 8. Geneva, World health Organization, 1973.

Rozendaal L, Walboomers LMM, van der Linden, JC et al. PCR-based high risk HPV test in cervical cancer screening gives objective risk assessment of women with cytomorphologically normal cervical smears. Int J Cancer 1996; 68:766-9.

Schiffman M, Herrero R, Hildesheim A, et al. HPV DNA testing in cervical cancer screening. Results from women in a high risk province of Costa Rica. JAMA 2000; 283:87-93.

Solomon D, Davey D, Kurman R, et al. The 2001 Bethesda System. Terminology for Reporting Results of Cervical Cytology. JAMA 2002; 287: 2114-9.

van Duin M, Snijders PJ, Schrijnemakers HF, et al. Human papillomavirus 16 load in normal and abnormal cervical scrapes: an indicator of CIN II/III and viral clearance. Int J Cancer 2002; 98: 590-5.

van Oortmarssen GJ, Habbema, JDF. Duration of preclinical cervical cancer and reduction in incidence of invasive cancer following negative Pap smears. Int J Epidemiol 1995; 24: 300-7.

Walboomers JM, Jacobs MV, Manos MM, et al. Human papillomavirus is a necessary cause of invasive cervical cancer worldwide. J Pathol 1999; 189: 12–9.

Wilson JMG, Junger G. Principles and practice of screening for disease. Public Health Paper (No. 34). Geneva. World Health Organization, 1968: 26.

Woodman CBJ, Collins S, Winter H, et al. The natural history of cervical human papillomavirus infection and its relationship to the occurrence of cervical intraepithelial neoplasia in young women. Lancet 2001; 357:1831-6.

Wright TC, Denny L, Kuhn L, et al. HPV DNA testing of self-collected vaginal samples compared with cytologic screening to detect cervical cancer. JAMA 2000; 283:81-6.

Ylitalo N, Sorensen P, Josefsson AM, et al. Consistent high viral load of human papillomavirus 16 and risk of cervical carcinoma in situ: a nested case-control study. Lancet 2000; 355: 2194-8.

Yu SZ, Miller AB, Sherman GJ. Optimising the age, number of tests, and test interval for cervical screening in Canada. J Epidemiol Community Health 1982; 36:1-10.

Zielinski GD, Snijders PJF, Rozendaal L et al. HPV precedes abnormal cytology in women developing cancer and signals false negative smears. Br J Cancer, 2001, 85: 398-404.

Section 2

HUMAN PAPILLOMAVIRUS

Chapter 3

The Biology of Human Papillomavirus Infections

Patti E. Gravitt, M.S., Ph.D.[1] and Keerti V. Shah, M.D., Dr.P.H.[2]
Departments of [1]Epidemiology and [2]Molecular Microbiology and Immunology, Johns Hopkins Bloomberg School of Public Health

INTRODUCTION

HPV infections are ubiquitous, and while they are etiologically linked to cervical cancer, the progression of an HPV infection to invasive cancer is a rare event and occurs over a period of many years. In this chapter, the properties of human papillomaviruses, the characteristics of HPV infections, and the potential mechanisms by which an HPV infection can progress to invasive cancer are described.

1   INFECTIOUS AGENT

1.1   Virion Structure

Papillomaviruses were formerly included in the broader virus family termed papovaviridae, which was subdivided into papillomavirus and polyomavirus subfamilies. However, more extensive molecular and biological characterization of these viruses has led to a reclassification into two distinct DNA virus families: the papillomaviruses and polyomaviruses.

Papillomaviruses are small, double stranded DNA viruses with a genome size of approximately 8000 base pairs. The circular DNA genome (episome) is encapsulated in a non-enveloped icosahedral capsid measuring ~ 55nm in diameter. Papillomaviruses (PVs) are highly species specific, and are widely distributed among vertebrate animals. There is remarkable similarity of the virus structure and genome organization between the PVs of various host species.

1.2   Genome Organization

The HPV genome is organized into 8-9 open reading frames (ORFs) and a non-coding region that has variably been referred to as the upstream regulatory region (URR) and the long control region (LCR). The coding regions for the viral proteins all lie on the same strand of the DNA, and transcription is initiated from one of several viral promoters. The coding regions are subdivided into 'early (E)' and 'late (L)' regions, based on the timing of expression following viral entry into the host cell. The organization of the genome is well-conserved across the spectrum of papillomaviruses. The functions of each of the early and late viral-encoded proteins are summarized in Table 1 (Stanley, 2001a), and discussed in more detail in Chapter 4.

Table 1. Function of HPV proteins

HPV ORF	Putative function
E1	Plasmid replication
E2	Regulation of viral DNA transcription and replication
E4	Disruption of cytokeratin matrix
E5	Localized to membrane components; possible interaction with growth factor signaling pathways
E6	Transformation and immortalization; p53 binding
E7	Transformation and transcriptional regulation; pRB, p107, and p130 binding
L1	Codes for major capsid protein
L2	Codes for minor capsid protein
LCR/URR	Contains regulatory motifs and origin of replication

2   HPV CLASSIFICATION

2.1   HPV diversity

Historically, serologic assays for detection of exposure to HPV infection have been insensitive. As a result, in contrast to many other viral infections, HPV types are not defined by seroreactivity, but by DNA sequence relatedness. The DNA sequence-based definition has engendered a 'genotype'-based nomenclature of human papillomaviruses. To date, over 100 HPVs have been identified. Genotypes are defined as having <90% nucleotide sequence identity with other HPV types in the L1 open reading frame, which is the most conserved ORF in the papillomavirus genome (de Villiers, 1994). Subtypes have between 90 and 98% sequence identity to a prototype sequence, and variants of a genotype have <2% sequence difference in the coding regions (Chan et al., 1995).

Phylogenetic analyses of the L1 sequences have identified clear groupings of the PV types based on their relative genetic relatedness (Figure 1) (Chan et al., 1995). Groupings based on E6 sequences are similar to the L1-based groupings in Figure 1. These groupings are remarkably consistent with observable PV phenotypes, including species of origin, tissue tropism, and association with benign versus malignant lesions.

The tissue tropism of the HPVs is reflected in the division of the genotypes into two large supergroups: A & B. Supergroup A includes HPVs that have been predominantly isolated from the genital mucosa. HPVs belonging to Supergroup B have been most frequently isolated from cutaneous epithelium, particularly among patients affected with a rare inherited disorder termed epidermodysplasia verruciformis (EV); therefore, Supergroup B viruses are also known as EV-associated viruses. Two other cutaneous HPV genotypes are found in Supergroup E (HPV 1 and HPV 41). While it is apparent that the Supergroups evolved by adapting to particular tissue types and locations, the predilection for site of infection is not absolute. For example, HPV 16 is found predominantly in the genital mucosal epithelium of the cervix, and is the type most commonly found in cervical cancers. However, HPV 16 has also been found both in non-genital mucosa (e.g., oropharynx) (Naghashfar et al., 1985) and cutaneous genital epithelium (e.g., penile foreskin) (Chow et al., 1991).

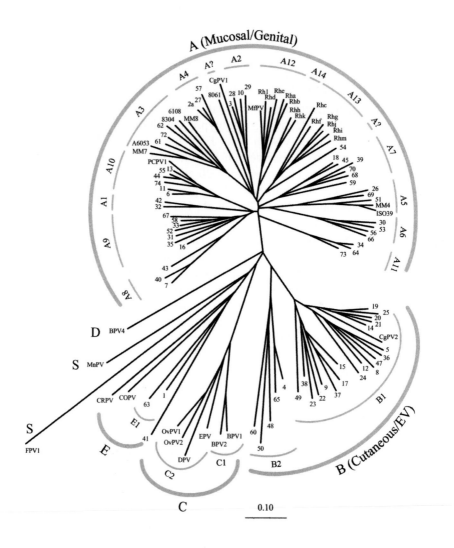

Figure 1. Phylogenetic tree based on L1 sequences from the NCI-Los Alamos National Labs HPV compendium (http://hpvweb.lanl.gov/stdgen/virus/hpv/ compendium/htdocs/ COMPENDIUM_PDF/97PDF/1/Intro97.pdf)

The non-human PVs cluster phylogenetically into Supergroups C, D and E, the latter of which also contains some human papillomaviruses. Supergroup C unites ungulate PVs which manifest typically as fibropapillomas. Included in this group are bovine PV (BPV 1 and 2), deer PV (DPV), European elk (EPV), and ovine (sheep) PV (OvPV). Supergroup D contains another set of BPV types (BPV 3, 4, and 6) that are distinct from BPV 1 and 2 in Supergroup C in that they manifest as true papillomas, rather than fibropapillomas. Supergroup E contains the canine oral PV (COPV) and cottontail rabbit PV (CRPV), as well as three cutaneous HPV types (HPV 1, 41 and 63).

2.2   Oncogenic and non-oncogenic HPV genotypes

The genital HPV genotypes comprising Supergroup A are further stratified into evolutionarily related subgroups, or clades. Chan defines a clade as having been 'formed by all species with shared derived ancestral characters and their most recent common ancestor' (Chan et al., 1995). The genital HPV types are divided into eleven separate clades, with CP8061, LVX82, and HPV 54 remaining unassigned due to poor resolution with the other lineages. The clade assignment for 48 genital HPV types is summarized in Table 2.

Table 2. Genital HPV categorization by phylygenetic clade assignment. Genotypes considered to be carcinogenic in bold (Munoz et al., 2003).

Clade	HPV types
A1	13, 42
A2	3, 10, 28, 29
A3	61, 62, 72, 84, 89, CP8304
A4	2, 27, 57
A5	**26, 51**, 69, **82**
A6	30, **53, 56, 66**
A7	**18, 39, 45, 59, 68**, 70
A8	7, 40, 43
A9	**16, 31, 33, 35, 52, 58**, 67
A10	6, 11, 13, 44, 55
A11	34, 64, **73**

The sequence-based categorization of the HPV genotypes felicitously groups the HPV types with known cancer association at the clade level. The HPV types most convincingly demonstrated epidemiologically to be linked to cervical cancer, HPV types 16, 18, 31, 33, 35, 45, 51, 52, 58, and 59, group to just three clades – A5, A7, and A9. Known low risk types, such as HPV 6 and 11, group to a single clade (A10). The evolutionary clustering of the HPV types determined observationally to be associated with cancer is consistent with molecular and epidemiologic evidence for causality. For example, large epidemiologic studies consistently show that genotypes in clades A7 and A9 have similar strengths of association with invasive cervical cancer (OR > 50), whereas types in clade A10 have almost no association with invasive cancer (Munoz, 2000). As discussed in detail in Chapter 4 there are also important molecular distinctions between the high risk HPVs in clades A7 and A9 and the low risk HPVs in clade A10. For example, high-risk types bind p53 and pRB with higher affinity than low risk HPVs (Crook et al., 1991; Li and Coffino, 1996; Heck et al., 1992), and differ in viral oncogene transcription (Hummel et al., 1992; Di Lorenzo et al., 1995). The remaining clades contain types that are unlikely to be associated with cancer. One interesting group is the A6 group. HPVs 53, 56, and 66 are all quite commonly found in the population (Peyton et al., 2001; Lazcano-Ponce et al., 2001; Herrero et al., 2000), but have only very rarely been found in invasive cervical cancers (Bosch et al., 1995). The grouping of these types with equally ambiguous cancer association further substantiates the clinical relevance of the phylogenetic clustering.

3   INFECTIOUS CYCLE

3.1   Normal infectious cycle

The HPVs infect the basal layers of stratified epithelium, presumably accessing this lower cell stratum through local microtrauma. An epithelial receptor mediating viral entry has not been clearly defined, although the $\alpha6\beta4$ integrin is a promising candidate (Evander et al., 1997). This complex is expressed on epithelial cells, and anti-$\alpha6$ antibodies can block HPV virus-like particle (VLP) uptake (Yoon et al., 2001). Completion of the viral life cycle is tightly linked to the differentiation program of the epithelial tissue. Non-vegetative replication occurs within the primarily infected basal cells following expression of the viral immediate early (IE) proteins E1, E2, and possibly E5; expression of HPV E6 and E7 proteins is quite low in the dividing basal cells (Iftner et al., 1992). However, E6 and E7 gene expression is upregulated in the differentiating suprabasal cells. The high level of E6/E7 expression is instrumental in the induction of the host DNA replication machinery, thereby allowing for vegetative viral DNA replication in a differentiated, non-dividing cell (reviewed in Stanley, 2001a). To this end, E6 and E7 proteins exhibit pleiotropic effects in the infected keratinocytes, including interaction with two important cell cycle regulatory proteins, p53 and pRB (reviewed in zur Hausen, 2002). The E7-pRB interaction results in functional inactivation of pRB, allowing for activation of the host replication machinery in the absence of external signaling. The E6-mediated degradation of p53 interferes with normal stress response in the infected cells, and is an important factor in HPV induced carcinogenesis. These interactions are stronger for high-risk HPVs. The viral DNA undergoes a vegetative DNA replication cycle in the differentiated cells, amplifying viral episomes to approximately 1000 copies per cell. The expression of late viral capsid proteins, L1 and L2, and viral assembly occur in the upper spinous layers of the differentiated epithelium. Therefore complete virions are found only in the most superficial layers of the epithelium. Viral exit does not appear to utilize cytolytic pathways, and is generally thought to be shed via normal exfoliation of the stratum corneum of the squamous epithelium.

4 PROGRESSION TO MALIGNANCY

HPV plays a necessary role in the etiology of cervical cancer by increasing the life span of the infected keratinocytes, followed by induction and maintenance of genetic instability. This ultimately leads to the accumulation of genetic damage responsible for the cellular changes underlying cancer development. A conceptual model of the natural history of cervical cancer is represented in Figure 2. The determinants for acquisition of HPV are described in detail in Chapter 6. This section will focus on virus and host-specific factors that have been associated with neoplastic progression. Many of these factors represent promising biomarkers for identification of infected individuals at high risk for cancer progression.

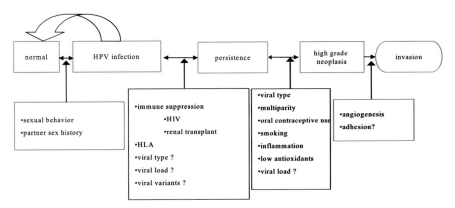

Figure 2. Natural history model of HPV associated cervical carcinogenesis

4.1 Viral factors in progression to malignancy

The HPVs are a heterogeneous group of viruses, and intertypic differences in transmissibility, immune evasion, and cellular interactions likely contribute to the pathogenesis of cervical cancer.

4.1.1 Viral genotype

As described in Section 2.2, of the >50 HPV genotypes known to infect the genital tract, only ~18 are thought to confer a substantial risk for invasive cancer (Table 2) (Munoz et al., 2003). The expression of the E6 and E7 oncoproteins from these types results in cellular changes that lead to loss of cell cycle control and increased genomic instability. For example, E7-mediated inactivation of pRB results in disruption of an important G1-S cell cycle regulatory pathway. A by-product of this interaction is loss of a negative feedback loop regulating expression of a cyclin-dependent kinase inhibitor, p16^{INK4a}. Studies have shown that overexpression of p16 (as determined by immunohistochemical staining) correlates with expression of high risk HPV E7; therefore p16 overexpression is being evaluated as a potential generic biomarker of high risk HPV infection (Klaes et al., 2001). High risk HPV E7 also induces centrosome-related mitotic disturbances, which may directly increase the genomic instability in high risk, HPV E7-expressing cells (reviewed in Duensing and Munger, 2002). The resulting loss of spindle integrity may increase the risk for chromosome mis-segregation and aneuploidy, where loss of tumor suppressors or gain of oncogenes can result in a cell population with a selective survival advantage. In cervical cancer, frequent abnormalities have been detected in chromosome 3, including the loss of 3p which contains the putative fragile histidine triad (FHIT) tumor suppressor (Wistuba et al., 1997) and gain of 3q which contains the RNA component of the human telomerase gene (Heselmeyer et al., 1997).

4.1.2 Viral persistence

Most studies confirm that persistent HPV detection is associated with an increased risk of progression to HSIL and cancer (Schlecht et al., 2001; Liaw et al., 1999; Wallin et al., 1999; Ho et al., 1998a). Winer and Koutsky summarize the epidemiology of HPV persistence in Chapter 6. A putative etiologic role of persistence in increasing cancer risk is recognized when examining the conceptual model presented in Figure 2 as a multi-stage carcinogenesis model. Persistent HPV infection may represent an early 'hit' through inactivation of p53 and pRB as a result of continued expression of E6 and E7. This creates a window of opportunity for subsequent 'hits' leading to increasing cellular dysregulation and genetic instability. Differences in the host immune response to HPV infection are clearly an important determinant for risk of persistence. The role of genetic susceptibilities to and protection from HPV infection are discussed in the next section.

4.1.3   Viral integration

The viral genome is always integrated in HPV 18 related cancers and is integrated in a majority of HPV 16-related cancers. Viral integration may potentially contribute to the progression to cervical cancer. HPV appears to integrate relatively indiscriminately at fragile sites in the host genome, but uniformly results in disruption of the HPV episome within the E1/E2 ORFs (Kalantari et al., 2001; Thorland et al., 2000). Integration thus releases E6/E7 expression from viral gene regulatory elements due to loss of the major repressor protein E2, resulting in constitutive expression of E6/E7 (Park et al., 1997). It is not clear whether malignant progression results from the unregulated expression of the viral oncoproteins following integration, or occurs as a result of genomic instability in cell populations already expressing transformed phenotypes. Preliminary evidence suggests that integrated transcripts are rarely detected in high-grade lesions (Klaes et al., 2001), indicating that it may represent a relatively late event in the carcinogenic pathway.

4.1.4.   Viral load

No single gold standard method for HPV quantitation has been described, and studies estimating the association of HPV viral load with neoplasia and cancer have used a variety of strategies for viral quantitation. An additional impediment to the interpretation of an HPV viral load measurement is the difficulty in obtaining a true random sample of infected cells from the cervix. Despite these methodologic and sampling limitations, some consistent observations have emerged. Generally, prevalent squamous intraepithelial lesions (SIL) have significantly higher viral load relative to HPV infected but cytologically normal controls (Schiffman et al., 2000; Swan et al., 1999; Sun et al., 2001; Healey et al., 2001; Sherman et al., 2002). A few studies have also demonstrated that high HPV 16 viral load (measured by TaqMan PCR) predicts risk of incident high grade SIL and carcinoma *in situ* (van Duin et al., 2002; Ylitalo et al., 2000; Josefsson et al., 2000). Other studies examining baseline viral load as measured by Hybrid Capture 2 (a cumulative measure of viral burden from 13 HPV types) did not show a significant difference in risk of incident HSIL between women with high and low viral load at baseline (Lorincz et al., 2002; Bory et al., 2002). Some of the discrepancies in the association between HPV viral load and cervical SIL prevalence and incidence may be explained by differences in the assays used to quantitate HPV and may be resolved as standardized quantitative assays become available (Gravitt et al., 2003).

4.1.5   HPV type-specific variants

HPVs of certain types, specifically HPVs 16 and 18, have been shown to have sufficient nucleic acid heterogeneity to form phylogenetically distinct subgroups within the same viral type. Sequencing of one or more ORFs from E6, E7, and L1, as well as the long control region (LCR) has identified multiple variants of HPV 16 and HPV 18 that can broadly be categorized as European (E) and non-European (NE) variants (Ho et al., 1991; Yamada et al., 1995; Ong et al., 1993; Chan et al., 1992). Multiple studies have shown an increased risk of cervical cancer and SIL among women infected with the HPV 16 or 18 NE variant relative to the E variant (Villa et al., 2000; Berumen et al., 2001; Hildesheim et al., 2001a; Burk et al., 2001). Functional differences between these variants in terms of viral oncogenicity or immune recognition have not been fully determined, but are under investigation (Kammer et al., 2000; Veress et al., 1999).

4.2   Host factors in progression to malignancy

As stated at the beginning of this chapter, HPV infections – even with high-risk genotypes – are common among sexually active individuals. Therefore, interindividual differences among infected women must figure predominantly in the constellation of sufficient causes for cervical cancer, a comparatively rare outcome of infection. Epidemiologic studies have identified a variety of behavioral and environmental factors associated with cervical cancer, as well as a clear genetic heritability of cervical cancer. A study using the Swedish Cancer Register and the National Family Register examined the relative contribution of shared environment and genetic effects in cervical cancer development and concluded that 27% of the variation in liability to cervical tumors was due to a heritable genetic effect, compared to only 2% due to shared environment between sisters (Magnusson et al., 1999; Magnusson et al., 2000).

4.2.1   Immune response

Multiple studies have examined the association of HLA class I and II alleles with cervical cancer. Specific HLA class II alleles are reported to confer either protection (e.g., DRB1*1301) or susceptibility (e.g., B*07 plus DQB1*0302) to cervical cancer (Apple et al., 1995; Wang et al., 2001; Lin et al., 2001). One study identified protection via DRB1*1301 for both LSIL and HSIL/cancer, suggesting that the effect modifies risk of persistent infection and therefore plays a role in the early stages of cancer progression (Wang et al., 2001). Limited data suggest a protective role of the DQ*0202 class I allele (Wang et al., 2002). These HLA susceptibilities may explain some of the genetic heritability of cervical cancer.

4.2.2   Environmental and behavioral exposures

Reproductive hormones such as estrogens and progestins have been shown to alter HPV gene expression *in vitro*, to varying degrees and effects (Chan et al., 1989; Chen et al., 1996). These *in vitro* observations, coupled with the epidemiologic evidence that multiparity (Munoz et al., 2002; Hildesheim et al., 2001b; Kjellberg et al., 2000; Schiff et al., 2000) and long duration oral contraceptive use (Moreno et al., 2002) appear to increase the risk of HPV associated cervical cancer (see Chapter 7). As epidemiologic methods and HPV exposure assessment have improved, a consistent increased risk of cervical cancer among cigarette smokers has been observed (Castle et al., 2002; Hildesheim et al., 2001b; Santos et al., 2001; Deacon et al., 2000; Kjellberg et al., 2000). Again, data showing carcinogenic metabolites in the cervical mucus of female smokers provide a biologically plausible mechanism supporting the observed epidemiologic association (Prokopczyk et al., 1997). Cigarette smoke is regarded as one of the strongest inducers of oxidant stress, and changes in the redox state of HPV infected keratinocytes may well affect the normal differentiation signaling program, leading to deregulation of the typical HPV and host protein interactions. In addition, the high potential for mutagenesis as a result of the tobacco carcinogen exposure can contribute a second 'hit', in a cell whose primary hit was the HPV induced inactivation of pRB and p53. Epidemiologic studies have also found other associations that are consistent with redox changes in the local microenvironment. In a few studies, chronic inflammation is associated with a slightly increased risk of HPV associated cervical cancer (Yang et al., 2001; Castle et al., 2001), and high levels of dietary antioxidants (e.g., tocopherol and reduced ascorbic acid) (Ho et al., 1998b) have been shown to have a protective association.

4.3   Host response to HPV infection

4.3.1   Innate immunity

Generally, the human response to viral infection relies both on non-specific innate responses as well as antigen-specific adaptive immunity. Innate immunity is important for controlling infection while the adaptive response is initiated. It is becoming increasingly clear that the innate response plays an important role in directing the nature of the adaptive response (reviewed in Woodworth, 2002). In the case of HPV infection, one of the most general immunoevasive characteristics is related to the nature and site of HPV infection. HPV establishes a local infection that does not result in either lysis of infected cells or in a systemic phase of the infection, which together limit the opportunity for the virus to encounter professional antigen presenting cells (reviewed in Tindle, 2002). Similarly, the highly antigenic repetitive elements of the viral capsid are expressed only in the more superficial layers of the epithelium, away from the sub-basal localization of dendritic cells involved in epithelial immune surveillance. In addition, high risk HPVs appear to quickly act to subvert the innate, immediate early response to viral infection by downregulating type-1 interferon-responsive signaling that is traditionally stimulated upon intracellular viral infection (Nees et al., 2001; Barnard et al., 2000; Park et al., 2000; Chang et al., 2000). Because of this IFN non-responsiveness, HPV infections are characteristically non-inflammatory infections. This results in substantial delay in recruitment of important immune cells to the site of HPV infection. These immunoevasive mechanisms work in concert to keep HPV relatively hidden from the human immune system so the immune system does not have a sufficient opportunity to 'see' the virus in the early stages of infection. This possibly explains the relatively long time to clearance of a typical HPV infection.

4.3.2   Adaptive immunity

Relatively little is known about the natural course of the adaptive immune response to HPV. However, much can be inferred from studies in animal PV infections, observational cross-sectional studies of immune characteristics in humans, and experimental results from participants in the early HPV VLP vaccine trials. What is clear from these studies is that both antibody and cellular immune response can be stimulated by infection with HPV. Evidence for induction of humoral immunity comes from the demonstration that seroconversion occurs in ~60% of women with incident HPV 6, 16, or 18 infections within 18 months of infection (Carter et al., 2000). It is not clear whether the seronegative women with detectable HPV

DNA fail to develop an antibody response, or do so at titers below the limit of the detection of the serologic assays. The median time to seroconversion is estimated at ~10-12 months, again suggestive that the virus remains hidden from immune recognition during the early phases of infection. These data reflect antibody responses to the L1 capsid protein in serologic assays which use the L1 VLP as capture antigen. Antibody responses to early proteins are variable, and may be related to disease stage (Sun et al., 1994; Meschede et al., 1998; Silins et al., 2002).

While the development of an antibody response may be critical to prevent lateral spread of the infection and to protect against reinfection, efficient viral clearance is predicated on an effective cellular immune response (reviewed in Stanley, 2001b). The cellular immune response is a complicated interplay between professional antigen presenting cells (APCs), CD4+ T-helper cells, CD8+ cytolytic T cells (CTLs), and the infected keratinocyte. The role of co-stimulation from cytokine signaling is of critical importance, as the nature of the cytokine response is paramount for appropriate activation of the APCs, CD4+ and CD8+ cells. These immune cells recognize HPV antigens presented on the cell surface via MHC class II antigens (on the APCs), or MHC class I antigens (on the infected keratinocytes). HPV infections have been shown to interfere with MHC class I antigen presentation, both by downregulating class I expression on infected keratinocytes (Brady et al., 2000), and by disruption of peptide transport to class I molecules by loss of expression of transporter-associated with antigen presentation-1 (TAP-1) (Evans et al., 2001).

Local cytokine milieu influences the expression of co-stimulatory surface antigens required for activation of the CTL (reviewed in Tindle, 2002). Recognition of HPV antigen via MHC class I presentation in the absence of co-stimulatory molecules can lead to tolerance or anergy, effectively disabling the CTL response. In addition, the type of response is usually balanced between a Th1 (CTL) and Th2 (humoral) response, but may be polarized to either arm based on dramatic changes in cytokine balance. Thus, an effective cellular immune response to HPV relies on a tightly cross-regulated system of autocrine and paracrine cytokine signals. Disruptions of this pathway likely contribute substantially to defects in immune responsiveness to HPV infections, and are of considerable interest in development of effective therapies against persistent HPV infections.

4.3.3 Clearance vs. latency

HPV clearance as discussed in the preceding sections is defined by the lack of detectable HPV DNA at the site of initial infection. It is not clear if this reflects complete viral clearance, or establishment of a latent phase where the virus is present, but is undetectable. Evidence from HIV-induced immunosuppressed populations suggest that latent HPV does exist, given the marked increase in HPV prevalence among HIV-positive versus HIV-negative women despite similar sexual histories (Benton et al., 1996). In addition, some population prevalence studies of HPV show an increase in HPV DNA prevalence among post-menopausal women (Herrero et al., 2000). This U-shaped curve in age-specific HPV prevalence could be explained as a cohort effect, wherein older women were more likely exposed to HPV infection, or it could represent activation of latent infections. A putative site of HPV latency is the basal epithelial cells; detection of HPV DNA, if existing solely in the basal epithelium, is unlikely to be detected because exfoliative procedures do not adequately sample basal cells.

CONCLUSION

The evidence supporting HPV as a necessary cause of cervical cancer rests on data derived from many approaches, ranging from basic molecular virology to population-based epidemiologic studies and clinical trials. However, the fundamental understanding of the biology of HPV serves as an anchor in the causal argument, providing strong evidence of biologic plausibility for HPV as a tumor virus.

REFERENCES

Apple RJ, Becker TM, Wheeler CM, et al. Comparison of human leukocyte antigen DR-DQ disease associations found with cervical dysplasia and invasive cervical carcinoma. J Natl Cancer Inst 1995; 87:427-36.

Barnard P, Payne E, McMillan NA. The human papillomavirus E7 protein is able to inhibit the antiviral and anti-growth functions of interferon-alpha. Virology 2000; 277:411-9.

Benton EC, Arends MJ. Human papillomavirus in the immunosuppressed. In: Lacey C (ed), Papillomavirus Reviews: Current Research on Papillomaviruses. Leeds University Press, 1996. pp. 271-279.

Berumen J, Ordonez RM, Lazcano E, et al. Asian-American variants of human papillomavirus 16 and risk for cervical cancer: a case-control study. J Natl Cancer Inst. 2001; 93:1325-30.

Bory JP, Cucherousset J, Lorenzato M, et al. Recurrent human papillomavirus infection detected with the hybrid capture II assay selects women with normal cervical smears at risk for developing high grade cervical lesions: a longitudinal study of 3,091 women. Int J Cancer 2002; 102:519-25.

Bosch FX, Manos MM, Munoz N et al. Prevalence of human papillomavirus in cervical cancer: a worldwide perspective. J Natl Cancer Inst 1995; 87:796-802.

Brady CS, Bartholomew JS, Burt DJ, et al. Multiple mechanisms underlie HLA dysregulation in cervical cancer. Tissue Antigens 2000; 55:401-11.

Burk R, Schiffman M, Herrero R, et al. HPV 18 variants are associated with decreased risk of CIN 2/3 and cervical cancer. 19th International Papillomavirus Conference. 2001. Florianopolis, Brazil.

Carter JJ, Koutsky LA, Hughes JP, et al. Comparison of human papillomavirus types 16, 18, and 6 capsid antibody responses following incident infection. J Infect Dis 2000; 181;1911-19.

Castle PE, Wacholder S, Lorincz AT, et al. A prospective study of high-grade cervical neoplasia risk among human papillomavirus-infected women. J Natl Cancer Inst 2002; 94: 1406-14.

Castle PE, Hillier SL, Rabe LK, et al. An association of cervical inflammation with high-grade cervical neoplasia in women infected with oncogenic human papillomavirus (HPV). Cancer Epidemiol Biomarkers Prev 2001; 10:1021-7.

Chan SY, Ho L, Ong CK, et al. Molecular variants of human papillomavirus type 16 from four continents suggest ancient pandemic spread of the virus and its coevolution with humankind. J Virol 1992; 66:2057-66.

Chan S-Y, Delius H, Halpern AL, et al. Analysis of genomic sequences of 95 papillomavirus types: Uniting typing, phylogeny, and taxonomy. J Virol 1995; 69:3074-83.

Chan WK, Klock G, Bernard HU. Progesterone and glucocorticoid response elements occur in the long control regions of several human papillomaviruses involved in anogenital neoplasia. J Virol 1989; 63:3261-9.

Chang YE, Laimins LA. Microarray analysis identifies interferon-inducible genes and Stat-1 as major transcriptional targets of human papillomavirus type 31. J Virol 2000; 74:4174-82.

Chen YH, Huang LH, Chen TM. Differential effects of progestins and estrogens on long control regions of human papillomavirus types 16 and 18. Biochem Biophys Res Commun 1996; 224:651-9.

Chow VT, Tay SK, Tham KM, et al. Subclinical human papillomavirus infection of the male lower genital tract: colposcopy, histology and DNA analysis. Int J STD AIDS 1991; 2:41-5.

Crook T, Fisher C, et al. Modulation of immortalizing properties of human papillomavirus type 16 E7 by p53 expression. J Virol 1991; 65: 505-10.

de Villiers EM. Human pathogenic papillomavirus types: an update. Curr Top Microbiol Immunol 1994; 186:1-12.

Deacon JM, Evans CD, Yule R, et al. Sexual behaviour and smoking as determinants of cervical HPV infection and of CIN3 among those infected: a case-control study nested within the Manchester cohort. Br J Cancer 2000; 83:1565-72.

DiLorenzo T, Steinberg B. Differential regulation of HPV type 6 and 11 early promoters in cultured cells derived from laryngeal papillomas. J Virol 1995; 69: 6865-72.

Duensing S, Munger K. Human papillomaviruses and centrosome duplication errors: modeling the origins of genomic instability. Oncogene 2002; 21:6241-8.

Evander M, Frazer IH, Payne E, et al. Identification of the α_6 integrin as a candidate receptor for papillomaviruses. J Virol 1997; 71:2449-56.

Evans M, Borysiewicz LK, Evans AS, et al. Antigen processing defects in cervical carcinomas limit the presentation of a CTL epitope from human papillomavirus 16 E6. J Immunol 2001; 167:5420-8.

Gravitt PE, Burk RD, Lorincz A, et al. A comparison between real-time PCR and hybrid capture 2 for HPV DNA quantitation. Cancer Epidemiol Biomarkers Prev 2003;12:477-84.

Healey SM, Aronson KJ, Mao Y, et al. Oncogenic human papillomavirus infection and cervical lesions in aboriginal women of Nunavut, Canada. Sex Trans Dis 2001; 28:694-700.

Heck DV, Yee CL, Howley PM, Munger K. Efficiency of binding the retinoblastoma protein correlates with the transforming capacity of the E7 oncoproteins of the human papillomaviruses. Proc Natl Acad Sci USA 1992; 89: 4442-6.

Herrero R, Hildesheim A, Bratti C, et al. Population-based study of human papillomavirus infection and cervical neoplasia in rural Costa Rica. J Natl Cancer Inst 2000; 92:464-74.

Heselmeyer K, Macville M, Schrock E, et al. Advanced-stage cervical carcinomas are defined by a recurrent pattern of chromosomal aberrations revealing high genetic instability and a consistent gain of chromosome are 3q. Genes Chromosomes Cancer 1997; 19:233-40.

Hildesheim A, Schiffman M, Bromley C, et al. Human papillomavirus type 16 variants and risk of cervical cancer. J Natl Cancer Inst 2001a; 93:315-8.

Hildesheim A, Herrero R, Castle PE, et al. HPV co-factors related to the development of cervical cancer: results from a population-based study in Costa Rica. Br J Cancer 2001b; 84:1219-26.

Ho G, Bierman R, Beardsley L, et al. Natural history of cervicovaginal papillomavirus infection in young women. N Engl J Med 1998a; 338:423-8.

Ho GY, Palan PR, Basu J, et al. Viral characteristics of human papillomavirus infection and antioxidant levels as risk factors for cervical dysplasia. Int J Cancer 1998b; 78:594-9.

Ho L, Chan SY, Chow V, et al. Sequence variants of human papillomavirus type 16 in clinical samples permit verification and extension of epidemiological studies and construction of a phylogenetic tree. J Clin Microbiol 1991; 29:1765-72.

Hummel M, Hudson JB, Laimins LA. Differentiation-induced and constitutive transcription of human papillomavirus type 31b in cell lines containing viral episomes. J Virol 1992; 66: 6070-80.

Iftner T, Oft M, Bohm S, et al. Transcription of the E6 and E7 genes of human papillomavirus type 6 in anogenital condylomata is restricted to undifferentiated cell layers of the epithelium. J Virol 1992; 66:4639-46.

Josefsson AM, Magnusson PK, Ylitalo N, et al. Viral load of human papilloma virus 16 as a determinant for development of cervical carcinoma in situ: a nested case-control study. Lancet 2000; 355:2189-93.

Kalantari M, Blennow E, Hagmar B, et al. Physical state of HPV16 and chromosomal mapping of the integrated form in cervical carcinomas. Diagn Mol Pathol 2001; 10:46-54.

Kammer C, Warthorst U, Torrez-Martinez N, et al. Sequence analysis of the long control region of human papillomavirus type 16 variants and functional consequences for P97 promoter activity. J Gen Virol 2000; 81:1975-81.

Kjellberg L, Hallmans G, Ahren A-M, et al. Smoking, diet, pregnancy, and oral contraceptive use as risk factors for cervical intra-epithelial neoplasia in relation to human papillomavirus infection. Br J Cancer 2000; 82:1332-8.

Klaes R, Friedrich T, Spitkovsky D, et al. Overexpression of p16(INK4A) as a specific marker for dysplastic and neoplastic epithelial cells of the cervix uteri. Int J Cancer 2001; 92:276-84.

Klaes R, Woerner SM, Ridder R, et al. Detection of high-risk cervical intraepithelial neoplasia and cervical cancer by amplification of transcripts derived from integrated papillomavirus oncogenes. Cancer Res 1999; 59:6132-6.

Lazcano-Ponce E, Herrero R, Munoz N, et al. Epidemiology of HPV infection among Mexican women with normal cervical cytology. Int J Cancer 2001; 91;412-20.

Li X, Coffino P. High-risk human papillomavirus E6 protein has two distinct binding sites within p53, of which only one determines degradation. J Virol 1996; 70: 4509-16.

Liaw K-L, Glass A, Manos M, et al. Detection of human papillomavirus DNA in cytologically normal women and subsequent cervical squamous intraepithelial lesions. J Natl Cancer Inst 1999; 91:954-60.

Lin P, Koutsky LA, Critchlow CW, et al. HLA class II DR-DQ and increased risk of cervical cancer among Senegalese women. Cancer Epidemiol Biomarkers Prev 2001; 10:1037-45.

Lorincz AT, Castle PE, Sherman ME, et al. Viral load of human papillomavirus and risk of CIN3 or cervical cancer. Lancet 2002; 360:228-9.

Magnusson PKE, Lichtenstein P, and Gyllensten UB. Heritability of cervical tumors. Int J Cancer 2000; 88:698-701.

Magnusson PKE, Sparen P, Gyllensten UB. Genetic link to cervical tumors. Nature 1999; 400:29-30.

Meschede W, Zumbach K, Braspenning J, et al. Antibodies against early proteins of human papillomaviruses as diagnostic markers for invasive cervical cancer. J Clin Microbiol 1998; 36:475-80.

Moreno V, Bosch FX, Munoz N, et al. Effect of oral contraceptives on risk of cervical cancer in women with human papillomavirus infection: the IARC multicentric case-control study. Lancet 2002; 359:1085-92.

Munoz N, Bosch FX, de Sanjose S, et al. Epidemiologic classification of human papilloma-virus types associated with cervical cancer. N Engl J Med 2003; 348:518-27.

Munoz N, Franceschi S, Bosetti C, et al. Role of parity and human papillomavirus in cervical cancer: the IARC multicentric case-control study. Lancet 2002; 359:1093-101.

Munoz N. Human papillomavirus and cancer: the epidemiological evidence. J Clin Virol 2000; 19:1-5.

Naghashfar Z, Sawada E, Kutcher MJ, et al. Identification of genital tract papillomaviruses HPV-6 and HPV-16 in warts of the oral cavity. J Med Virol. 1985; 17:313-24.

Nees M, Geoghegan JM, Hyman T, et al. Papillomavirus type 16 oncogenes downregulate expression of interferon-responsive genes and upregulated proliferation-associated and NF-kappaB-responsive genes in cervical keratinocytes. J Virol 2001; 75:4283-96

Ong CK, Chan SY, Campo MS, et al. Evolution of human papillomavirus type 18: an ancient phylogenetic root in Africa and intratype diversity reflect coevolution with human ethnic groups. J Virol 1993; 67:6424-31.

Park JS, Hwang ES, Park SN, et al. Physical status and expression of HPV genes in cervical cancers. Gynecol Oncol 1997; 65:121-9.

Park JS, Kim EJ, Kwon HJ, et al. Inactivation of interferon regulatory factor-1 tumor suppressor protein by HPV E7 oncoprotein. Implication for the E7-mediated immune evasion mechanism in cervical carcinogenesis. J Biol Chem 2000; 275:6764-9.

Peyton CL, Gravitt PE, Hunt WC, et al. Determinants of genital human papillomavirus detection in a US population. J Infect Dis 2001; 183:1554-64.

Prokopczyk B, Cox JE, Hoffmann D, et al. Identification of tobacco-specific carcinogen in the cervical mucus of smokers and nonsmokers. J Natl Cancer Inst 1997; 89: 868-73.

Santos C, Munoz N, Klug S, et al. HPV types and cofactors causing cervical cancer in Peru. Br J Cancer 2001; 85:966-71.

Schiff M, Miller J, Masuk M, et al. Contraceptive and reproductive risk factors for cervical intraepithelial neoplasia in American Indian women. Int J Epidemiol 2000; 29:983-90.

Schiffman M, Herrero R, Hildesheim A, et al. HPV DNA testing in cervical cancer screening: results from women in a high-risk province of Costa Rica. JAMA 2000; 283:87-93.

Schlecht NF, Kulaga S, Robitaille J, et al. Persistent human papillomavirus infection as a predictor of cervical intraepithelial neoplasia. JAMA 2001; 286:3106-14.

Sherman ME, Schiffman M, Cox JT. Effects of age and human papilloma viral load on colposcopy triage: data from the randomized atypical squamous cells of undetermined significance/low-grade squamous intraepithelial lesion triage study (ALTS). J Natl Cancer Inst 2002; 94:102-7.

Silins I, Avall-Lundqvist E, Tadesse A, et al. Evaluation of antibodies to human papilloma-virus as prognostic markers in cervical cancer patients. Gynecol Oncol 2002; 85:333-8.

Stanley M. Human papillomavirus and cervical cancer. Best Practice & Res Clin Obstet Gynecol 2001a; 15:663-76.

Stanley M. Immunobiology of papillomavirus infections. J Reproductive Immunol 2001b; 52:45-59.

Sun CA, Lai HC, Chang CC, et al. The significance of human papillomavirus viral load in prediction of histologic severity and size of squamous intraepithelial lesions of uterine cervix. Gynecol Oncol 2001; 83:95-9.

Sun Y, Eluf-Neto J, Bosch FX, et al. Human papillomavirus-related serological markers of invasive cervical carcinoma in Brazil. Cancer Epidemiol Biomarkers Prev 1994; 3:341-7.

Swan D, Tucker R, Tortolero-Luna G, et al. Human papillomavirus (HPV) DNA copy number is dependent on grade of cervical disease and HPV type. J Clin Microbiol 1999; 37:1030-4.

Thorland EC, Myers SL, Persing DH, et al. Human papillomavirus type 16 integrations in cervical tumors frequently occur in common fragile sites. Cancer Res 2000; 60:5916-21.

Tindle RW. Immune evasion in human papillomavirus-associated cervical cancer. Nature Reviews Cancer 2002; 2:59-65.

van Duin M, Snijders PJ, Schrijnemakers HF, et al. Human papillomavirus 16 load in normal and abnormal cervical scrapes: an indicator of CIN II/III and viral clearance. Int J Cancer 2002; 98:590-5.

Veress G, Szarka K, Dong XP, et al. Functional significance of sequence variation in the E2 gene and the long control region of human papillomavirus type 16. J Gen Virol 1999; 80: 1035-43.

Villa LL, Sichero L, Rahal P, et al. Molecular variants of human papillomavirus types 16 and 18 preferentially associated with cervical neoplasia. J Gen Virol 2000; 81:2959-2968.

Wallin KL, Wiklund F, Angstrom T, et al. Type-specific persistence of human papillomavirus DNA before the development of invasive cervical cancer. N Engl J Med 1999; 341:1633-8.

Wang SS, Wheeler CM, Hildesheim A, et al. Human leukocyte antigen class I and II alleles and risk of cervical neoplasia: results from a population-based study in Costa Rica. J Infect Dis 2001; 184:1310-4.

Wang SS, Hildesheim A, Gao X, et al. Comprehensive analysis of human leukocyte antigen class I alleles and cervical neoplasia in 3 epidemiologic studies. J Infect Dis 2002; 186:598-605.

Wistuba II, Montellano FD, Milchgrub S, et al. Deletions of chromosome 3p are frequent and early events in the pathogenesis of uterine cervical carcinoma. Cancer Res 1997; 57:3154-8.

Woodworth CD. HPV innate immunity. Front Biosci 2002; 7:d2058-71.

Yamada T, Wheeler CM, Halpern AL, et al. Human papillomavirus type 16 variant lineages in United States populations characterized by nucleotide sequence analysis of the E6, L2, and L1 coding segments. J Virol 1995; 69:7743-53.

Yang YC, Chang CL, Huang YW, et al. Possible cofactor in cervical carcinogenesis: proliferation index of the transformation zone in cervicitis. Chang Gung Med J 2001; 24:615-20.

Ylitalo N, Sorensen P, Josefsson AM, et al. Consistent high viral load of human papillomavirus 16 and risk of cervical carcinoma in situ: a nested case-control study. Lancet 2000; 355:2194-8.

Yoon C-S, Kim K-D, Park S-N, et al. α_6 integrin is the main receptor of human papillomavirus type 16 VLP. Biochem Biophys Res Commun 2001; 283:668-73.

zur Hausen H. Papillomaviruses and cancer: from basic studies to clinical application. Nat Rev Cancer 2002; 2:342-50.

Chapter 4

The Molecular Pathogenesis of Human Papillomavirus-Associated Cancer

Stephen T. Oh, Ph.D. and Laimonis A. Laimins, Ph.D.
Department of Microbiology – Immunology, Feinberg School of Medicine, Northwestern University

INTRODUCTION

Human papillomaviruses (HPVs) are small, non-enveloped, double-stranded DNA viruses that induce hyperproliferative lesions in epithelial tissues (Howley, 1996). More than 100 different types of HPV have been identified and each of these exhibits greater than 10% difference at the nucleotide level in the L1 capsid coding sequence (Meyers et al., 1996; zur Hausen, 2002). These HPV types infect a range of epithelial tissues. For instance, HPV 1 infects epithelial tissues on the soles of feet while HPV types 2, 4 and 7 infect cutaneous epithelia to induce common hand warts. The most well characterized HPV types, however, are those that infect genital epithelia, and these can be sub-grouped based on their association with cervical and other anogenital cancers. "High-risk" HPV types such as HPV 16, 18, 31, and 45 induce lesions that can lead to cancer, while "low-risk" types such as HPV 6 and 11 induce benign lesions that rarely progress (zur Hausen, 2002; Howley, 1996).

1   VIRAL LIFE CYCLE

The life cycle of all HPV types is closely linked to the differentiation state of the host epithelia (Figure 1) (Howley, 1996; Laimins, 1996). Initial infection occurs through small lesions that expose cells in the basal layer to viral entry. Following infection, the viral genome is established as episomes at approximately 50 to 100 copies per cell. These infected basal cells replicate viral DNA in synchrony with chromosomal DNA. Following cell division, infected daughter cells migrate away from the basal layer and begin to differentiate. In the highly differentiated suprabasal layers, viral late gene expression and amplification of the viral genome are induced. Productive viral replication is dependent on cellular enzymes, and one consequence of HPV infection is that cells remain active in the cell cycle as they undergo differentiation. In normal epithelia, cells immediately exit the cell cycle as they leave the basal layer and often nuclei are degraded in highly differentiated cells. In HPV infected epithelia, nuclei are present in all layers and production of virions occurs in the highly differentiated cells. Following viral amplification, genomes are packaged into capsids consisting of the L1 and L2 proteins and newly assembled virions are released.

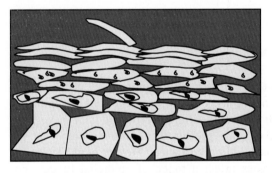

DNA synthesis	capsid synthesis
+	+++
+++	+
+/-	-
+/-	-

Figure 1: Cartoon of differentiating epithelia with basal and suprabasal layers. Sites of HPV viral DNA synthesis as well as capsid synthesis are indicated.

2   HPV GENOME ORGANIZATION AND REGULATION OF VIRAL GENE EXPRESSION

2.1   Genomes and transcripts

The HPV genomes consist of circular, double-stranded DNAs of approximately 8 kb in length (Figure 2). The genomes are organized into three regions: an early region containing six to eight open reading frames

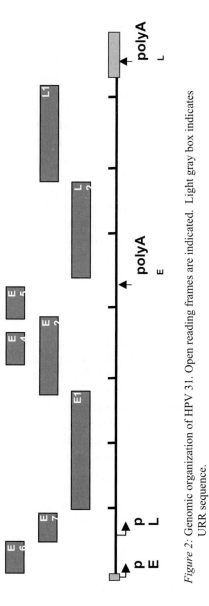

Figure 2: Genomic organization of HPV 31. Open reading frames are indicated. Light gray box indicates URR sequence.

(ORFs), a late region, and an upstream regulatory region (URR). This overall genomic organization is shared across all HPV types. Furthermore, all HPV gene products are expressed from polycistronic messages that are transcribed from multiple promoters (Howley, 1996). These promoters are coordinately regulated in concert with the differentiation status of the stratified epithelium. For example, the high-risk HPV 31 genome contains two major promoters, p97 and p742 (Hummel et al., 1992). Early genes are primarily expressed in undifferentiated cells from p97 located upstream of the E6 open reading frame, while late genes are expressed in differentiated cells from p742 which is located in the middle of the E7 gene. In contrast, the low-risk HPV 11 genome contains two early promoters that direct initiation of transcripts upstream of E6 and E7 respectively and a single late promoter is localized to a similar region as in HPV 31 (DiLorenzo et al., 1995; Chow et al., 1987). Post-transcriptional regulation of HPV gene expression plays an important role in the life cycle and involves alternative splicing mechanisms as well as differential usage of two tandemly arranged polyadenylation sites (del Mar Pena and Laimins, 2002).

2.2   Viral protein functions

E6 and E7 are the first two open reading frames in the HPV early region. The E6 proteins from both high and low risk types are approximately 150 amino acids in size and contain two zinc finger domains (Cys-X-X-Cys). The high risk E6 protein is found both in the nucleus as well as the cytoplasm and has been implicated in binding to over 12 different cellular proteins (zur Hausen, 2002). E7 is a small nuclear protein of approximately 100 amino acids in size that contains a single zinc binding motif (Howley, 1996). The presence of zinc binding regions in both E6 and E7 suggests that these genes may have evolved by gene duplication. The specific functions of these two viral proteins will be discussed in detail in subsequent sections.

The HPV E1 and E2 proteins are required for viral replication and regulation of early gene expression (Laimins, 1998). The HPV origin is located in the URR adjacent to the start sites for early transcripts. It consists of A/T-rich sequences flanked by multiple binding sites for the E2 protein. E1 can bind to these A/T-rich DNA sequences with low affinity, while E2 binds to its recognition sites with high affinity (Laimins, 1998). In addition to binding origin sequences independently, E1 and E2 can form a complex with each other, facilitating a stable interaction between E1 and the A/T-rich sequences (Mohr et al., 1990; Ustav and Stenlund, 1991). The E2 protein specifically binds to the palindromic sequence $ACCN_6GGT$, and it can either activate or repress early transcription, depending on the promoter context (Spalholz et al., 1985; Thierry et al., 1987).

The functions of E4 and E5 are not well understood at this time. E5 is a hydrophobic membrane protein that can modulate EGF receptor signaling. It has been suggested that E5 associates with the vacuolar ATPase and blocks endosomal acidification, thus inhibiting the downregulation of activated EGF receptors (Conrad et al., 1993; Straight et al., 1995). However, recent studies have examined the effects of mutating E5 in the context of the complete viral genome and have implicated it in modulation of late viral functions (Fehrman et al., 2002). In BPV 1, E5 has been shown to encode the major transforming activity of the virus and that this results from its association with the platelet derived growth factor receptor (Petti et al., 1992). No such activities have been demonstrated for the E5 proteins of HPVs.

Although designated as an early gene, E4 is primarily expressed upon differentiation along with the late genes, and its function is also unclear. Some studies have shown that E4 can induce the collapse of cytokeratin networks, while one recent study demonstrated that E4 associates with a putative RNA helicase, suggesting that E4 might be involved in the regulation of mRNA stability and translation (Doorbar et al., 1991; Doorbar et al., 2000; Roberts et al., 1993).

The L1 and L2 open reading frames encode the capsid proteins and these are synthesized following viral DNA amplification. L1 is the major capsid protein, representing approximately 80% of the total protein in the virion, while L2 is the minor capsid protein. Together, the two capsid proteins form an icosahedral capsid, composed of 72 pentameric capsomeres arranged on a T=7 surface lattice (Howley, 1996).

2.3 Regulation of viral expression and tissue specificity

The HPV early promoter from the high-risk viruses directs initiation of transcription at sites upstream of the E6 ORF and has been extensively studied. The transcription factors that regulate the early promoters bind to sequences located within the URR regions (del Mar Pena and Laimins, 2002). An analysis of URR regions of different human papillomavirus types has revealed a number of binding sites, which are common to all types as well as some which are unique. It is likely that the variation in the spectrum of binding factors contributes to the tissue tropism of papillomaviruses. Factor binding sites common among all HPV types include those for TFIID binding to canonical TATA boxes located approximately 30 base pairs upstream from the early start sites. Adjacent to these sequences and present in most HPV types are Sp-1 and AP-1 binding sites (del Mar Pena and Laimins, 2002). All URR sequences contain a series of AP-1 sites though the number and exact locations vary according to type. Other factor binding sites include those for NF-1, TEF-1, TEF-2, Oct-1, KRF-1, NF-1, AP-2, YY1 as well as glucocorticoid responsive elements (GRE) (Apt et al., 1993; Butz et al., 1993; Chang et al., 1990; Gloss et al., 1987; Ishiji et al., 1992; Kyo et al., 1997; O'Conner et al., 1995).

The search for determinants of the epithelial tropism of HPVs has largely relied on transient expression assays. In these assays, URR reporter constructs were found to be most active in cells of squamous epithelial origin and significantly less active in lines derived from other tissues (Gloss et al., 1987; Gius et al., 1988; Cripe et al., 1987; Gius et al., 1988). As a result, it has been postulated that keratinocyte-specific enhancers are present in the URR regions and that these contribute to tissue tropism. Chang et al. hypothesized that it is the particular combination of ubiquitous factors working in concert that determines the cell type specific expression (Chang et al., 1990). The majority of evidence indicates that this latter model is correct.

In addition to positive elements located in the HPV promoter, a negative or silencer element has been identified at the distal end of the HPV 6 URR. This element binds the transcriptional repressor, CCAAT displacement protein (CDP) and represses early gene expression (Pattison et al., 1997). Upon epithelial differentiation, the repressive activity of the CDP protein is reduced. Other negative regulators include those for C/EBPβ that has been shown to regulate HPV 11 expression (Wang et al., 1996).

Much less information is available concerning the factors that activate late gene expression. The tight linkage of viral late gene expression and epithelial differentiation suggests that differentiation-specific cellular factors control this process. Studies have demonstrated that viral DNA must be maintained as episomes for the activation of late expression (Frattini et al., 1996). It addition it has been shown that the rearrangement of chromatin occurs at the late promoter region upon epithelial differentiation (del Mar Pena and Laimins, 2001). With the availability of methods for genetic analysis of HPV functions during the viral life cycle, a detailed examination of the interplay of differentiation and amplification in the activation of the late promoter is now possible.

3   THE ROLE OF E6 AND E7 IN IMMORTALIZATION AND TRANSFORMATION

The major oncoproteins of high risk HPVs are encoded by the E6 and E7 genes (Howley, 1996). Although expression of E7 alone can lead to transformation of established rodent cell lines, studies from several laboratories have demonstrated that expression of both E6 and E7 from high-risk HPV types is necessary to induce immortalization of primary epithelial cells (Hawley-Nelson et al., Vousden et al., 1989; Munger et al., Phelps et al., 1989; Hudson et al., 1990). Not only are E6 and E7 required for the events that initiate immortalization, their continued expression is required to maintain the transformed state. One striking example of this is the Hela cell line which was derived from a biopsy of an HPV 18 positive cervical cancer over 50 years ago yet when expression of the E6 and E7 genes is abrogated, this cell line undergoes senescence (Hwang et al., 1996). Numerous studies have implicated p53 and Rb as the primary cellular targets of E6 and E7, respectively, though recent evidence suggests that there additional targets that play important roles in transformation (Dyson et al., 1989; Huibregtse et al., 1991; Scheffner et al., 1990).

3.1   E7 and Rb

The HPV E7 proteins (Figure 3) share sequence homology with the oncoproteins of other small DNA tumor viruses, including SV40 large T antigen (TAg) and adenovirus E1A. Like these other viral oncoproteins, E7 can bind to the retinoblastoma protein, Rb, and inhibit its functions (Dyson et al., 1989; Munger et al., 1989). The finding that Rb binding-deficient mutants of E7 cannot immortalize primary cells even in the presence of high-risk E6 demonstrates that this interaction is highly important for transformation (Jones et al., 1997). The low-risk E7 proteins also bind to Rb, but with a 10-fold lower affinity than the high-risk proteins (Heck et al., 1992).

3.2   E6 and p53

The high-risk E6 proteins, like SV40 TAg and adenovirus E1B, bind to p53, however only E6 is able to target p53 for degradation (Scheffner et al., 1990). This effect is mediated by complex formation with the cellular ubiquitin ligase E6-AP (Huibregtse et al., 1991). The structure of the E6 protein is shown in Figure 4. Degradation of p53 by E6 is specific to high-risk HPV types, although some evidence suggests that low-risk forms of E6 may be able to bind to p53 with a low affinity (Crook et al., 1991; Li and Coffino, 1996). Some mutants of E6 that can bind to p53 but do not target it for degradation, still retain the capability to block its effects on transcription, suggesting that binding of p53 by E6 alone has functional implications (Lechner et al., 1994).

In normal cells, the level of p53 is low, but upon exposure to a variety of DNA damaging agents, p53 levels are upregulated through post-translational mechanisms (Ko and Prives, 1996). p53 acts as a sequence-specific transcription factor that can activate or repress a number of downstream genes, including p21, bax, and MDM2.

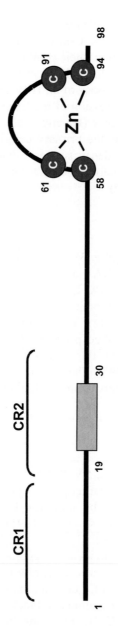

Figure 3: Structure of high-risk E7 proteins. CR1 and CR2 Rb interaction domains as well as zinc finger domain are indicated.

Furthermore, the low risk E7 proteins, even when expressed together with high risk E6, cannot immortalize cells. Recent evidence suggests that E7 binding to Rb also leads to its destabilization and subsequent degradation (Boyer et al., 1996; Jones et al., 1997). Rb is hypophosphorylated in early G1 and becomes progressively phosphorylated as the cells enter S-phase. Hypophosphorylated Rb binds to the E2F family of transcription factors and represses their ability to activate expression of S-phase-specific genes. Rb-mediated repression of E2F activity is relieved by phosphorylation resulting in progression of cells into S-phase. E7 binds to hypophosphorylated Rb and abrogates its repression of E2F family members leading to constitutive expression of S-phase specific genes (Lukas et al., 1996). In addition, it has been shown that expression of E7 leads to reactivation of DNA synthesis in the suprabasal layers of a stratified epithelium, suggesting that inactivation of Rb may be necessary to facilitate productive viral replication in differentiating epithelia (Woodworth et al., 1992; Cheng et al., 1995). Recent evidence suggests that other activities of E7 may also be important for transformation. Several mutants of E7 that can still bind to Rb and inhibit its function have been shown to be transformation-deficient (Banks et al., 1987; Edmonds and Vousden, 1989; Phelps et al., 1992). This notion is consistent with the finding that HPV 1 E7 binds to Rb with an affinity similar to that of the high-risk HPV types yet does not induce any malignancies in vivo (Schmitt et al., 1994). The elucidation of these additional targets of E7 is an area of high importance.

Depending on the context, activation of p53 can lead to either cell cycle arrest or apoptosis. Thus, the loss of p53 function in cells expressing E6 can have multiple consequences. For example, in response to DNA damage, p53 induces cell cycle arrest at the G1/S transition (Ko and Prives, 1996). In cells expressing E6, however, the lack of functional p53 results in a failure to arrest in G1/S (Foster et al., 1994; Kessis et al., 1993; Gu et al., 1994). Similarly, the role of p53 in modulating the mitotic spindle checkpoint at G2/M is affected by E6. In normal cells, treatment with spindle inhibitors induces a block at the G2/M transition. However, in cells lacking p53, this checkpoint is abrogated, resulting in the reduplication of DNA without cell division (Di Leonardo et al., 1997). This phenomenon is also seen in cells expressing E6 and can lead to the appearance of polyploid chromosomes that may promote the development of malignancy (Thomas et al., 1998; Thompson et al., 1997).

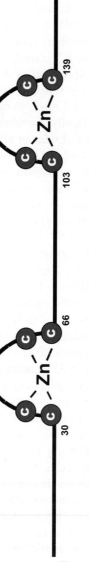

Figure 4: Structure of high-risk E6 proteins. Zinc finger domains are indicated.

In addition to initiating cell cycle arrest, p53 can also induce apoptosis. Cells expressing high risk E7 alone have high levels of p53 and are sensitized to apoptosis. However, co-expression of E6 in the presence of E7 decreases p53 levels and reduces the rate of apoptosis (Wang et al., 1996). This suggests that a primary role of E6 is to block the induction of p53-mediated apoptosis induced by E7 (Pan and Griep, 1994). Thus, the full effects of E6 and E7 are only seen when both proteins are co-expressed, allowing one to offset the negative effects of the other. E6 mutants that cannot degrade p53 are also unable to induce immortalization, suggesting that p53 is a key target of E6 (Huibregtse and Beaudenon, 1996; Jones et al., 1996). However, some mutants of E6 that retain the ability to target p53 for degradation nonetheless lose the ability to immortalize primary cells (Kiyono et al., 1998). This indicates that additional cellular targets may be important for E6 action.

3.2   Activation of telomerase by E6

In addition to targeting p53 for degradation, E6 proteins from high-risk HPV types have been shown to activate telomerase through the expression of the catalytic subunit, hTERT (Klingelhutz et al., 1996). Telomerase is responsible for synthesizing hexamer repeats at the ends of chromosomes. In normal cells, which lack telomerase, a gradual loss of telomere length is observed upon successive cell divisions in vitro. Eventually, telomere length reaches a critical size and cellular senescence is induced. Not surprisingly, telomerase activity is detected in virtually all tumors and is consistent with their immortalized phenotype in tissue culture. While fibroblasts can be readily immortalized by hTERT expression alone, immortalization of human foreskin keratinocytes (HFKs) requires both the activation hTERT expression as well as the inactivation of the Rb pathway (Kiyono et al., 1998). In infections by high-risk HPV types, these effects are mediated by the E6 and E7 proteins, respectively.

Interestingly, some studies suggest that immortalization of HFKs does not require p53 inactivation (Kiyono et al., 1998). Mutants of E6 have been described which retain the capability to target p53 for degradation but can no longer immortalize primary cells (Huibregtse and Beaudenon 1996; Kiyono et al., 1998). In addition, the finding that hTERT can substitute for E6 in immortalization of HFKs indicates that a critical function of E6 may be the activation of telomerase (Kiyono et al., 1998). More likely, both functions are relevant, with telomerase activation being important for the extension of lifespan and p53 degradation being critical for the development of secondary mutations and the progression to malignancy. The mechanism by which E6 activates hTERT expression remains unclear. Some studies have suggested that activation of myc expression by E6 is involved while others have suggested it is through its degradation or by myc-independent pathways (Oh et al., 2001; Gewin and Galloway, 2001). Clearly, more work needs to be done in this area.

3.3   A role for E6 and E7 in the HPV productive life cycle

Recent work has demonstrated that E6 and E7 also play an important role in the productive life cycle of human papillomaviruses (Flores et al., 2000; Thomas, 1999; Cheng et al., 1995). A tissue culture model has been developed that reproduces all aspects of a productive HPV infection (Frattini et al., 1996). In this system, cloned HPV sequences are transfected into normal human keratinocytes and cell lines established that maintain viral episomes. These cells mimic HPV infected basal cells in vivo. Upon differentiation of these cells in organotypic raft cultures, the activation of late viral functions along with the synthesis of virions is observed. These methods have been used to perform extensive genetic analyses of the HPV life cycle (Thomas et al., 1999; Stubenrauch et al., 1998; Frattini et al., 1996). It has been demonstrated that in the absence of E6 or E7 expression, high-risk HPV 31 genomes cannot be maintained as episomes (Thomas et al., 1999). Although genomes lacking E6 or E7 can be replicated in transient assays, they cannot be maintained in stable replication assays. Additional studies have implicated E7 in the activation of differentiation-dependent activities in the viral life cycle (Flores et al., 2000). Clearly, the primary role of E6 and E7 in the viral life cycle is not in oncogenesis but rather in some aspect related to replication. This is underscored by the fact that both proteins are expressed in low risk infections which rarely result in malignancy. Further elucidation of the roles of these proteins in the viral life cycle is an area of active research.

3.4   Other targets of E6 and E7

A number of other cellular factors are known to be modulated by E6 and/or E7. For example, E6 has been shown to bind to the putative calcium-binding protein E6-BP (Chen et al., 1995). In addition, type 16 E6 but not low-risk E6 binds to the focal adhesion protein paxillin. E6 proteins of the high risk HPV types but not of the low risk viruses contain PDZ binding domains at their C-termini. Mutation of these domains has been shown to abrogate the ability of these proteins to transform rodent fibroblasts and similar effects may occur in human keratinocytes. E6 has been shown to bind to several cellular proteins through the PDZ domain including hDLG, MUPP-1, MAGI-1, and hScrib (Gardiol et al., 1999). Furthermore, E6 induces the degradation of a number of these proteins and this may further contribute to transformation (Gardiol et al., 1999). Other properties associated with high-risk E6 proteins is its ability to inhibit transcriptional co-activation mediated by CBP and p300 (Patel et al., 1999; Zimmerman et al., 1999). Of course, it is not clear which of these activities are physiologically important and the genetic systems described above will provide useful insights. In addition to Rb, E7 interacts with other "pocket proteins" such as p107 and p130 proteins (Jones and Munger, 1996; Kubbutat and Vousden, 1996; Dyson et al., 1989). It has also been shown that E7 binds to other cell cycle regulators, such as the E2F/cyclin A complex, cyclin E, and p21 (Arroyo et al., 1993; McIntyre et al., 1996; Jones et al., 1997).

Several studies have linked E6 and E7 to the interferon-response pathway. For example, E7 has been shown to abrogate IFNα-signaling by blocking the nuclear translocation of p48 (Barnard et al., 1999). Furthermore, it has been reported that E7 impairs the activation of interferon regulatory factor 1 (IRF-1) (Perea et al., 2000). Similarly, E6 binds to IRF3 and blocks its activity (Ronco et al., 1998). Microarray analysis has shown that STAT-1 and several downstream interferon-response genes are repressed in cells containing episomal copies of the HPV 31 genome (Chang et al., 2000). Similar findings have been described for cells expressing HPV 16 E6 and E7 (Nees et al., 2001). Thus, multiple aspects of the interferon-response pathway appear to be targeted by E6 and E7.

It is likely that other targets of E6 and E7 have yet to be identified. Most effects attributed to E6 and E7 are specific to the high-risk types and this is not surprising given the association of high-risk HPV types with cancer. However, despite the lack of association with malignancy, low-risk HPV types are known to induce extensive hyperproliferative lesions. The cellular determinants of this phenotype have yet to be identified. Given the immortalizing functions of high-risk E6 and E7, it is likely that low-risk E6 and E7 are also important mediators of the hyperproliferation.

CONCLUSION

Significant advances in understanding the molecular pathogenesis of HPV infections and their links to cervical cancer have been achieved in the last few years. Despite this increased knowledge, little is known about the productive phase of the viral life cycle and the mechanisms by which cells progress from initial infection to malignancy. Understanding this last point is an important undertaking and will likely require an integration of molecular and epidemiological methodologies.

REFERENCES

Apt D, Chong T, Liu Y, et al. Nuclear factor I and epithelial specific transcription of HPV 16. J Virol 1993; 67: 4455-63.

Arroyo M, Bagchi S, Raychaudhuri P. Association of the human papillomavirus type 16 E7 protein with the S-phase-specific E2F-cyclin A complex. Mol Cell Biol 1993;13: 6537-46.

Banks L, Spence P, Vousden KH. Identification of human papillomavirus type 18 E6 polypeptide in cells derived from human cervical carcinoma. J Gen Virol 1987; 68: 1351-9.

Barnard P, McMillan NA. The human papillomavirus E7 oncoprotein abrogates signaling mediated by interferon-alpha. Virology 1999;259: 305-13.

Boyer SN, Wazer DE, Band V. E7 protein of human papillomavirus-16 induces degradation of retinoblastoma protein through the ubiquitin-proteosome pathway. Cancer Res 1996;56(20): 4620-4.

Butz K, Hoppe-Seyler F. Transcriptional control of HPV oncogene expression: composition of HPV 18 upstream regulatory region. J Virol 1993; 67: 6476-86.

Chang T, Chan W, Bernard H-U. Transcription of transforming genes of oncogenic HPV 16 is stimulated by tumor promoters through AP-1 sites. Nuc Acids Research 1990;18: 465-70.

Chang YE, Laimins LA. Microarray analysis identifies interferon-inducible genes and Stat-1 as major transcriptional targets of HPV 31. J Virol 2000;74: 4174-82.

Chen JJ, Reid CE, Band V, et al. Interaction of papillomavirus E6 oncoproteins with a putative calcium-binding protein. Science 1995;269: 529-30.

Cheng S, Schmidt-Grimminger DC, Murant T, et al. Differentiation-dependent up-regulation of the human papillomavirus E7 gene reactivates cellular DNA replication in suprabasal differentiated keratinocytes. Genes Dev 1995;9: 2335-49.

Chow LT, Nasseri S, Wolinsky S, et al. Human papillomavirus types 6 and 11 mRNAs from genital condyloma acuminata. J Virol 1987;61: 2581-88.

Conrad M, Bubb V, Schlegel R. The human papillomavirus 6 and 16 E5 proteins are membrane-associated proteins which associate the 16-kilodalton pore-forming protein. J Virol 1993;67: 6170-8.

Cripe T, Haugen T, Turk J, et al. Transcriptional regulation of the HPV 16 E6/E7 promoter by a keratinocyte-dependent enhancer and by the E2 transactivator and repressor gene products: implications for cervical cancer. EMBO J 1987;6: 3745-53.

Crook T, Fisher C, Vousden KH. Modulation of immortalizing properties of human papillomavirus type 16 E7 by p53 expression. J Virol 1991;65: 505-10.

del Mar Pena L, Laimins LA. Differentiation-dependent chromatin-rearrangement coincides with activation of HPV 31 late gene expression. J Virol 2001;75: 10005-13.

del Mar Pena L, Laimins LA. Regulation of HPV expression in the vegetative life cycle. In: McCance D, ed. Progress in Medical Virology. Amsterdam: Elsevier, 2002:31-52.

Di Leonardo A, Khan SH, Linke SP, et al. GM. DNA replication in the presence of mitotic spindle inhibitors in human and mouse fibroblasts lacking either p53 or pRb function. Cancer Res 1997;57: 1013-19.

DiLorenzo T, Steinberg B. Differential regulation of human papillomavirus type 6 and 11 early promoters in cultured cells derived from laryngeal papillomas. J Virol 1995;69:6865-72.

Doorbar J, Ely S, Sterling J, et al. Specific interaction between HPV 16 E1-E4 and cytokeratins results in collapse of the epithelial cell intermediate filament network. Nature 1991; 352: 824-7.

Doorbar J, Elston RC, Napthine K, et al. The E1E4 protein of HPV 16 associates with a putative RNA helicase through sequences in its C terminus. J Virol 2000;74: 10081-95.

Dyson N, Howley PM, Munger K, et al. The human papillomavirus-16 E7 oncoprotein is able to bind to the retinoblastoma gene product. Science 1989;243: 934-6.

Edmonds C, Vousden K. A point mutational analysis of human papillomavirus type 16 E7 protein. J Virol 1989;63: 2650-6.

Fehrman F, Laimins LA. The E5 protein of HPV 31 acts to augment cell proliferation and activation of differentiation-dependent late viral functions. J Virol 2003;77:2819-31.

Flores E, Allen-Hoffman L, Lee D, et al. The HPV 16 E7 oncogene is required for the productive stage of life cycle. J Virol 2000;74: 6622-33.

Foster S, Demers GW, Etscheid BG, et al. The ability of human papillomavirus E6 proteins to target p53 for degradation in vivo correlates with their ability to abrogate actinomycin D-induced growth arrest. J Virol 1994;68: 5698-5705.

Frattini M, Lim B, Laimins LA. In vitro synthesis of oncogenic human papillomaviruses requires episomal genomes for differentiation-dependent late expression. Proc Natl Acad Sci USA 1996; 93: 3062-7.

Gardiol D, Kuhne B, Glausinger S, et al. Oncogenic human papillomavirus E6 proteins target the discs large tumour suppressor for proteasome-mediated degradation. Oncogene 1999;18: 283-9.

Gewin L, Galloway DA. E box-dependent activation of telomerase by HPV 16 E6 does not require induction of c-myc. J Virol 2001;75:7198-201.

Gius D, Grossman S, Bedell MA, et al. Inducible and constitutive enhancer domains in the noncoding region of human papillomavirus type 18. J Virol 1988;62: 665-72.

Glausinger R, Lee S, Thomas M, et al. Interactions of the PDZ protein MAGI-1 with adenovirus E4-ORF1 and high risk HPV E6 oncoproteins. Oncogene 2000;19: 5270-80.

Gloss B, Bernard H-U, Seedorf K, et al. The upstream regulatory region of HPV 16 contains an E2-independent enhancer which is specific for cervical carcinoma cells. EMBO J 1987;6: 3735-43.

Gu Z, Pim D, Labercque S, et al. DNA damage induced p53 mediated transcription is inhibited by human papillomavirus type 18 E6. Oncogene 1994;9: 629-33.

Hawley-Nelson P, Vousden KH, Hubbert NL, et al. HPV 16 E6 and E7 proteins cooperate to immortalize human foreskin keratinocytes. EMBO J. 1989;8: 3905-10.

Heck D, Yee C, Howley PM, et al. Efficiency of binding the retinoblastoma protein correlates with the transforming capacity of the E7 oncoproteins of the human papillomaviruses. Proc Natl Acad Sci USA 1992;89: 4442-6.

Howley PM. Papillomaviridae: the viruses and their replication. In: Fields BN, Knipe DM, Howley PM, eds. Virology, 3rd ed. Philadelphia, Lippincott-Raven Publishers 1996: 947-78.

Hudson JM, Bedell MA, McCance DJ, et al. Immortalization and altered differentiation of human keratinocytes in vitro by the E6 and E7 open reading frames of human papillomavirus type 18. J Virol 1990;64: 519-26.

Huibregtse JM, Beaudenon SL. Mechanism of HPV E6 proteins in cellular transformation. Sem Canc Biol 1996;7: 317-26.

Huibregtse JM, Scheffner M, Howley PM. A cellular protein mediates association of p53 with the E6 oncoprotein of human papillomavirus types 16 or 18. EMBO J 1991;10: 4129-35.

Hummel M, Hudson JB, Laimins LA. Differentiation-induced and constitutive transcription of human papillomavirus type 31b in cell lines containing viral episomes. J Virol 1992;66: 6070-80.

Hwang E, Naeger L, DiMaio D. Activation of the endogenous p53 growth inhibitory pathway in Hela cervical carcinoma cells by expression of the papillomavirus E2 gene. Oncogene 1996;12: 795-803.

Ishiji T, Lace M, Parkinnen S, et al. Transcriptional enhancer factor (TEF-1) and its cell-specific co-activator activate HPV 16 E6 and E7 oncogene expression in keratinocytes and cervical carcinoma cells. EMBO J 1992;11: 2271-81.

Jones DL, Alani RM, Munger K. The human papillomavirus E7 oncoprotein can uncouple cellular differentiation and proliferation by abrogating $p21^{cip1}$-mediated inhibition of cdk2. Genes Dev 1997;11: 2101-11.

Jones DL, Munger K. Interactions of the human papillomavirus E7 protein with cell cycle regulators. Sem Canc Biol 1996;7: 327-37.

Jones DL, Thompson DA, Munger K. Destabilization of the Rb tumor suppressor protein and stabilization of p53 contribute to HPV type 16 E7-induced apoptosis. Virology 1997; 239: 97-107.

Jones SN, Sands AT, et al. The tumorigenic potential and cell growth characteristics of p53-deficient cells are equivalent in the presence or absence of Mdm2. Proc Natl Acad Sci USA 1996; 93: 14106-11.

Kessis TD, Slebos RJ, Nelson WG, et al. Human papillomavirus 16 E6 expression disrupts the p53-mediated cellular response to DNA damage. Proc Natl Acad Sci USA 1993;90: 3988-92.

Kiyono TS, Foster SA, Koop JI, et al. Both Rb/p16INK4a inactivation and telomerase activity are required to immortalize human epithelial cells. Nature 1998;396(6706): 84-8.

Klingelhutz AJ, Foster SA, McDougall J. Telomerase activation by the E6 gene product of human papillomavirus type 16. Nature 1996;380: 79-82.

Ko L, Prives C. p53: puzzle and paradigm. Genes Dev 1996;10: 1054-72.

Kubbutat MH, Vousden KH. Role of E6 and E7 oncoproteins in HPV induced anogenital malignancies. Sem Virol 1996;7: 295-304.

Kyo S, Klumpp D, Inoue M, et al. Transcriptional activity of HPV 31 enhancer is regulated through synergistic interactions with two novel cellular factors. Virology 1997;211: 184-97.

Laimins LA. Human papillomaviruses target differentiating epithelia for virion production and malignant conversion. Sem Virol 1996;7: 305-13.

Laimins LA. Regulation of transcription and replication by human papillomaviruses. In: McCance DJ, ed. Human Tumor Viruses, Washington, DC, American Society for Microbiology: 1998:201-23.

Lechner MS, Laimins LA. Inhibition of p53 DNA binding by human papillomavirus E6 proteins. J Virol 1994;68: 4262-73.

Lee S, Mantovani L, Banks L, et al. Multi-PDZ domain protein MUPP1 is a cellular target for both adenovirus E4-ORF1 and HPV 16 E6 oncoproteins. J Virol 2000;74: 9680-93.

Li X, Coffino P. High-risk human papillomavirus E6 protein has two distinct binding sites within p53, of which only one determines degradation. J Virol 1996; 70: 4509-16.

Lukas J, Bartkova J, Bartek J. Convergence of mitogenic signalling cascades from diverse classes of receptors at the cyclin D-cyclin-dependent-kinase-pRb-controlled G1 checkpoint. Mol Cell Biol 1996;16: 6917-25.

McIntyre M, Ruesch M, Laimins LA. Human papillomavirus E7 oncoproteins bind a single form of cyclin E in a complex with cdk2 and p107. Virology 1996;215: 73-82.

Meyers G, Lu H, Calef C, et al. Heterogeneity of papillomaviruses. Sem Cancer Biol 1996;7: 349-58.

Mohr I, Clark R, Sun S, et al. Targeting the E1 replication factor to the papillomavirus origin of replication by complex formation with the E2 transactivator. Science 1990; 250: 1694-9.

Munger K, Phelps WC, Bubb V, et al. The E6 and E7 genes of the human papillomavirus type 16 together are necessary and sufficient for transformation of primary human keratinocytes. J Virol 1989; 63: 4417-21.

Munger K, Werness B, Dyson N, et al. Complex formation of human papillomavirus E7 proteins with the retinoblastoma tumor suppressor gene product. EMBO J 1989;8: 4099-4105.

Nees M, Geoghegan T, Hyman S, et al. Papillomavirus type 16 oncogenes downregulate expression of interferon-responsive genes and upregulate proliferation-associated NF-kappaB responsive genes in cervical keratinocytes. J Virol 2001;75: 4283-96.

O'Conner M, Bernard H-U. Oct-1 activates the epithelial-specific enhancer of HPV 16 through synergistic interaction with NF-1 at a conserved regulatory site. Virology 1995;207: 77-88.

Oh S, Kyo S, Laimins LA. Telomerase activation by human papillomavirus 16 E6 protein: induction of telomerase reverse transcriptase expression through Myc and Sp1 sites. J Virol 2001;75: 5559-66.

Pan H, Griep A. Altered cell cycle regulation in the lens of HPV 16 E6 or E7 transgenic mice: implications for tumor suppressor gene function in development. Genes Dev 1994; 8: 1285-99.

Patel D, Huang S, Baglia L, et al. The E6 protein of HPV 16 binds to and inhibits co-activation by CBP and p300. EMBO J 1999;18: 5061-72.

Pattison S, Skalnik D, Roman A. CCAAT displacement protein, a regulator of differentiation-specific gene expression, binds a negative regulatory element at the 5' end of the HPV 6 long control region. J Virol 1997;71: 2013-22.

Perea S, Massimi P, Banks L. HPV 16 E7 impairs the activation of the interferon regulatory factor-1. Int J Mol Med 2000;5: 661-6.

Petti L, DiMaio D. Stable association between BPV E5 transforming protein and the activated platelet-derived growth factor receptor in transformed mouse cells. EMBO J 1992;10:845-55

Phelps W, Munger K, Yee LC, et al. Structure-function analysis of the human papillomavirus type 16 E7 oncoprotein. J Virol 1992;66: 2418-27.

Roberts S, Ashmole G, Johnson J, et al. Cutaneous and mucosal HPV E4 proteins form intermediate filament-like structures in epithelial cells. Virology 1993;197: 176-87.

Ronco LV, Karpova AY, Vidal M, et al. Human papillomavirus 16 E6 oncoprotein binds to interferon regulatory factor-3 and inhibits its transcriptional activity. Genes Dev 1998;12(13): 2061-72.

Scheffner M, Werness B, Huiberegtse JM, et al. The E6 oncoprotein encoded by human papillomavirus types 16 and 18 promotes the degradation of p53. Cell 1990;63: 1129-36.

Schmitt A, Harry JB, Rapp FO, et al. Comparison of the properties of the E6 and E7 genes of low- and high-risk cutaneous papillomaviruses reveals strongly transforming and high Rb-binding activity for the E7 protein of the low-risk human papillomavirus type 1. J Virol 1994; 68: 7051-9.

Spalholz BA, Yang YC, Howley PM. Transactivation of a bovine papilloma virus transcriptional regulatory element by the E2 gene product. Cell 1985;42: 183-91.

Straight S, Herman WB, McCance DJ. The E5 oncoprotein of human papillomavirus type 16 inhibits the acidification of endosomes in human keratinocytes. J Virol 1995;69: 3185-92.

Stubenrauch F, Lim BH, Laimins LA. Differential requirements for conserved E2 binding sites in the life cycle of oncogenic human papillomavirus type 31. J Virol 1998;72: 1071-7.

Thierry F, Carranca S, Yaniv M. Characterization of a transcriptional promoter of HPV 18 and modulation of its expression by SV40 and adenovirus early antigen. J Virol 1987; 64: 5420-9.

Thomas JT, Hubert WG, Ruesch MN, et al. Human papillomavirus type 31 oncoproteins E6 and E7 are required for the maintenance of episomes during the viral life cycle in normal human keratinocytes. Proc Natl Acad Sci USA 1999;96: 8449-54.

Thomas JT, Laimins LA, Ruesch MN. Perturbation of cell cycle control by E6 and E7 oncoproteins of human papillomaviruses. Papillomavirus Report 1998;9: 59-64.

Thompson D, Belinsky G, Chang TH, et al. The human papillomavirus-16 E6 oncoprotein decreases the vigilance of mitotic checkpoints. Oncogene 1997;15: 3025-35.

Ustav M, Stenlund A. Transient replication of BPV-1 requires two viral polypeptides encoded by the E1 and E2 open reading frames. EMBO J 1991;10: 449-57.

Wang H, Liu K, Yaun F, et al. C/EBPbeta is a negative regulator of human papillomavirus type 11 in keratinocytes. J Virol 996;70: 4839-44.

Wang Y, Okan I, Pokrovskaja K, et al. Abrogation of p53-induced G1 arrest by the HPV 16 E7 protein does not inhibit p53-induced apoptosis. Oncogene 1996; 12: 2731-5.

Werness B, Levine AJ, Howley PM. Association of human papillomavirus types 16 and 18 E6 proteins with p53. Science 1990; 248: 76-9.

Woodworth CD, Cheng S, Simpson S, et al. Recombinant retroviruses encoding human papillomavirus type 18 E6 and E7 stimulate proliferation and delay differentiation of human keratinocytes early after infection. Oncogene 1992; 7: 619-26.

Zimmerman H, Degenkolbe H, Bernard H-U, et al. The human papillomavirus type 16 E6 oncoprotein can down-regulate p53 activity by targeting the transcriptional coactivator CBP/p300. J Virol 1999; 73: 6209-19.

zur Hausen H. Papillomaviruses and cancer: from basic studies to clinical application. Nat Rev Cancer 2002;2: 342-50.

Chapter 5

Measurement of Exposure to Human Papillomaviruses

Patti E. Gravitt, M.S., Ph.D.[1] and Raphael P. Viscidi, M.D.[2]
[1]*Department of Epidemiology, Johns Hopkins Bloomberg School of Public Health, and*
[2]*Department of Pediatrics, Johns Hopkins School of Medicine*

INTRODUCTION

A key component of clinical and epidemiologic investigation of exposure-disease associations is accurate and reliable measurement of exposure and outcome. Detection of human papillomavirus (HPV) infection is important both as an outcome of sexually transmitted disease research and natural history studies and as a critical exposure measure in the study of a variety of diseases, including cervical cancer. Measurement of current HPV infection relies on the detection of HPV DNA from tissues at the site of exposure (e.g., anogenital tract). HPV DNA detection assays have evolved over the past 15 years from assays with low sensitivity and specificity (e.g., filter *in situ* hybridization), to assays with increasing specificity but low sensitivity (e.g., Southern blot and dot blot hybridization, including ViraPap and Hybrid Capture Tube assays), to assays with both high sensitivity and specificity (e.g., target and signal amplification systems such as PCR and Hybrid Capture 2). No single gold standard test has emerged for the detection of HPV, although several assays have been well validated for use in the detection of the types commonly found in the genital tract. Evolution of the technology to produce virus like particles (VLPs) has helped advance the

119

development of serologic assays to detect antibodies to the L1 capsid protein of HPV as a cumulative measure of past and some prevalent HPV infections. In addition, a variety of promising new technologies for the detection, genotyping, and quantitation of HPV DNA or RNA, as well as cellular protein disturbances resulting from HPV infection, have been described and are currently being subjected to validation.

The assays discussed in this chapter have been well validated in laboratory, epidemiologic, and clinical diagnostic settings. Each may be uniquely well suited to specific applications (as described below), stemming from the comparative strengths and limitations of each assay system. No test is perfect, and the appropriate HPV exposure measurement tool will depend on the quality and quantity of the source material, the available resources, and the aims of the study or diagnosis. The goal of this chapter is to review the current validated options for genital HPV exposure measurement, indicate the most appropriate application of each technology, and to finally introduce the promising technologies that may comprise the future battery of HPV detection options.

1   DNA DETECTION ASSAYS

Most exposure measurements for HPV are based on detection of the viral DNA from tissues or exfoliated cells collected from the presumptive site of infection. For most types of cell collection, the DNA yield is such that sensitive tests must be used. Positive DNA tests are markers of prevalent infection. The absence of viral DNA is usually interpreted as absence of HPV infection, although undetectable latent infection cannot be ruled out.

More than 40 different HPV genotypes are known to commonly infect the genital tract. A comprehensive measurement of HPV status therefore relies on DNA detection techniques with broad spectrum; that is, assays that can detect multiple genotypes. Except for some unique and very specific research aims, broad spectrum HPV detection is usually necessary for adequate exposure measurement in cervical cancer research. The breadth of the spectrum of types required will be dependent on the specific aims of the research. Sensitive detection of the high-risk HPV types 16, 18, 31, 33, 35, 39, 45, 51, 52, 56, 58, 59, and 68 will allow for the identification of >90% of HPV infections in cervical cancers (Bosch, et al. 1995; Walboomers, et al. 1999). Increasing the spectrum of detectable types beyond this will only incrementally improve risk estimates in epidemiologic studies of invasive cervical cancer. However, natural history investigations of HPV will benefit from study of a wider spectrum of detectable genotypes, as other types may be common in the population under study, and comparison of the natural history of HPV by genotype will help in understanding the determinants of a high risk infection and differences in the role of the host response to infection in predicting malignant outcomes.

Three consensus PCR assays, in addition to HC2, can provide the required sensitivity and spectrum for most applications. Consensus PCR assays are designed as described below, to amplify most genital HPV types in a single PCR reaction. Type-specific discrimination is performed by oligonucleotide probe hybridization following the consensus amplification. However, each assay system has particular strengths and limitations that should be considered when choosing the HPV DNA detection method appropriate for a particular application. Table 1 summarizes the salient characteristics of each assay, and the impact of these on common applications. The following sections will discuss these methods in some detail.

1.1   Signal amplified assays

Hybrid Capture 2 (HC2) is a commercially available, FDA approved HPV DNA detection assay (Digene Diagnostics, Gaithersburg, MD). Full length RNA probes complementary to the target HPV DNA sequences are hybridized in solution after HPV DNA denaturation. The HPV DNA:RNA hybrids are captured in 96-well microtiter plates coated with anti-DNA:RNA capture antibodies. Unbound nucleic acid is washed away, and bound target:probe hybrids are detected with enzyme labeled detection antibodies (also anti-DNA:RNA hybrid). Multiple labeled antibodies can bind a single HPV probe complex, thus generating relative signal amplification per target virus of at least 3000-fold. The current and most commonly used configuration of the HC2 assay utilizes a high-risk probe mix that detects the presence of one, or more, of the 13 most common HPV genotypes found in cancer: HPV 16, 18, 31, 33, 35, 39, 45, 51, 52, 56, 58, 59, or 68. A second probe mix is occasionally used that detects low risk HPV types 6, 11, 40, 42, and 44; however, the remaining discussion of HC2 relates to the high-risk probe pool only. HC2 signal is read on a luminometer in relative light units (RLU). Unknown RLU values are compared relative to a 1.0 pg/ml HPV 16 positive control reaction, and ratios of unknown RLU to control (RLU/CO) greater than 1.0 are considered to be positive. This cut point is equivalent to ~5000 genomes per reaction, and was chosen based on optimal sensitivity and specificity for the detection of prevalent HSIL (Schiffman et al., 2000; Lorincz et al., 2001). HC2 performance using the 1.0 pg/ml control standard has been shown to be comparable to PCR-based assays in multiple comparison studies (Peyton et al., 1998; Terry et al., 2001). Only HPV at very low viral load is likely to be missed by HC2 detection (Gravitt, unpublished data).

Table 1. Characteristics of HPV DNA detection assays

	Multiple infection determination	Archival tissue amplification	Genotype Spectrum*	PCR product length
HC 2	NO	Ok for stored PreservCyt; Unknown for paraffin tissue	16, 18, 31, 33, 35, 39, 45, 51, 52, 56, 58, 59, 68	N/A
MY09/11	Limited relative to PGMY09/11 and SPF(10)	Modest	2, 6, 11, 13, 16, 18, **26**, 31, 32, 33, <u>**35**</u>, 39, 40, 42, 43, 44, **45**, 51, **52**, 53, 54, **55**, 56, 57, 58, **59**, 61, 62, 66, 67, **68**, 69, 70, 71, 72, **73**, 81, 82, **83**, 84, 86	~ 450 bp
PGMY09/11	YES	Modest	6, 11, 16, 18, 26, 31, 33, 35, 39, 40, 42, 45, 51, 52, 53, 54, 55, 56, 58, 59, 61, 62, 64, 66, 67, 68, 69, 70, 71, 72, 73, 82, 83, 84, 86	~ 450 bp
GP5+/6+	Limited	Good	6, 11, 16, 18, 26, 31, 33, 34, 35, 39, 40, 42, 43, 44, 45, 51, 52, <u>53</u>, 54, 55, 56, 57, 58, 59, <u>61</u>, 66, 68, 70, 71, 72, 73, 81, 82, 83, 84, 86	~ 150 bp
SPF (10)	YES	Excellent	6, 11, 16, 18, 31, 33, 35, 39, 40, 42, 43, 44, 45, 51, 52, 53, 54, 56, 58, 59, 66, 68, 70, 73, 74	~ 62 bp

*The spectrum of PCR genotypes is derived from the following sources: MY09/11 (Castle et al., 2002); PGMY09/11 (Peyton et al., 2001); GP5+/6+ (van den Brule et al., 2002); SPF (10) (van Doorn et al., 2002).

    BOLD types represent HPV genotypes shown to amplify with less efficiency in a comparison between MY09/11 and PGMY09/11 (Gravitt et al., 2000).

    <u>UNDERLINED</u> types represent types shown to amplify with less efficiency in a comparison between MY09/11 and GP5+/6+ (Qu et al., 1997).

    HIGHLIGHTED types represent types shown to amplify with less efficiency in a comparison between PGMY09/11 and SPF (10) (van Doorn et al., 2002).

For clinical applications with a goal of detecting prevalent HSIL and cancer, HC2 has demonstrated a sensitivity of 88-89% with specificity of 64-89% (Schiffman et al., 2000; Manos et al., 1999). The optimum cutpoint for the HC2 assay was determined in a population-based screening study, with clear performance advantage at the 1.0 pg/ml level. Increasing the number of genotypes included in the high-risk probe cocktail would not substantially increase the sensitivity of the test for detection of HSIL/cancer. The specificity of the assay is affected by the known cross-reactivity of the high risk probe pool to some common, low risk HPV genotypes, including HPV 30, 53, 66, and 69 (Peyton et al., 1998; Terry et al., 2001). Digene is currently developing a third generation assay, HC3, which attempts to decrease the cross-reactivity by employing oligonucleotide capture probes (Lorincz et al., 2001). Preliminary comparison studies have shown that the increased specificity afforded by the new format facilitates a lower cutpoint for positivity. Performance data comparing HC3 using the lower threshold and HC 2 at the 1.0 pg/ml threshold shows a increase in clinical sensitivity with HC3 with no substantial decrease in clinical specificity (Castle, unpublished data).

The utility of HC2 HPV DNA exposure measurement in research studies may be more variable. When conducting a case-control study of cervical cancer, adequate control for the presence of cancer-associated HPV can be achieved using HC2 assays. However, HC2 will not detect high risk HPVs present at very low copy (which will be disproportionately higher among control women). Therefore, risk estimates (by odds ratio) for HPV cancer associations are likely to be higher when using HC2 relative to more sensitive PCR methods. Residual confounding resulting from undetected HPV should, however, be negligible when employing case-control study designs. Given the spectrum of HPV types that infect the cervix, often as multiple infections, type-specific association studies are often desirable, and the pooled probe configuration of HC2 does not facilitate this application. Similarly, HPV persistence (vs. sequential new infections), immune response, and attributable risk of SIL/cancer by type will not be possible to estimate using an HC2 measure.

Finally, HC2 assays are semi-quantitative, allowing for some assessment of viral load and SIL/cancer risk. In the context of single infections, the HC2 value is a good marker of viral load (Gravitt et al., 2003). However, in the case of multiple HPV infections, HC2 values will mark the cumulative load measure, and since multiple infections are less common in prevalent HSIL/cancer than low grade lesions (at least in some studies) (Fife et al., 2001; Gravitt et al., 2003), HC2 load measurements are likely to cause differential misclassification bias in the analysis of viral load association with cervical cancer in a case control design, where low grade lesions are included in the control definition. The extent of HC2 viral load applicability in a given study can only be assessed if concomitant type-specific information is available.

1.2   Target amplified consensus PCR assays

Since the PCR revolution, countless primer systems have been developed and used to detect HPV DNA. Type-specific PCR assays are too numerous to discuss individually, but the performance of many of them has been shown to be quite good. The only limitation of type-specific PCR is the limited type spectrum available, unless upwards of 13 different PCR assays are employed for HPV DNA exposure assessment. As this is not currently feasible in clinical or large epidemiologic studies, the most broadly applicable PCR assays involve the use of consensus primer systems. Consensus primers are essentially designed to amplify HPV DNA under relatively low stringency annealing conditions to allow amplification of all genital HPV types. The four most well validated systems all target a region of the L1 open reading frame (ORF) encoding the major capsid protein, which is highly conserved across the genital HPV types (Figure 1). Amplification results in positive PCR product formation from practically all HPV genotypes infecting the genital tract, and subsequent hybridization analysis to type-specific oligonucleotide probes allows for genotype discrimination. The four consensus PCR systems described below perform similarly, but vary in the primer design/amplification strategy, the ability to detect multiple infections, the amplification product length, and the method of genotyping. These differences make each method uniquely suited to specific applications, as outlined in Table 1.

1.2.1   MY09/11

The MY09/11 primer system uses degenerate primers to maximize the spectrum of HPV types detected among related, but substantially different HPV genotypes (Manos et al., 1989; Bauer et al., 1992). Even in the most conserved region of the HPV genome, no more than 9-10 contiguous base pairs of perfect homology exist, even among the most related HPV genotypes (i.e., same phylogenetic clade) (Gravitt et al., 2000). Efficient priming in PCR requires a minimal primer length of approximately 17-18 bases, so that primers designed to target the most conserved sequence must still accommodate hetereogeneity between the types for consensus amplification across the genotype spectrum. Degenerate primer designs allow a random insertion of nucleotides at positions of heterogeneity during oligonucleotide synthesis. What results from a degenerate primer synthesis is essentially a primer mix of all possible combinations of sequences given the

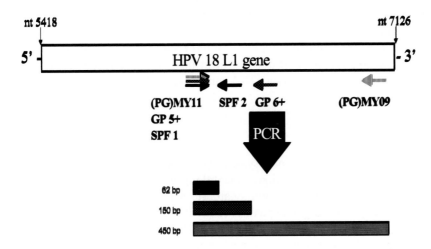

Figure 1. Schematic of L1 consensus primer alignments.

degenerate base sites. For the MY09/11 system, this results in a mixture of 24 different primer sequences. Because of the degenerate sites, most HPV types are reasonably well matched to at least one of the degenerate sequence combinations; a remarkable feat considering that the primers were designed knowing the L1 sequence of only 5 HPV genotypes.

The MY09/11 primers amplify a broad spectrum of genital HPV types, resulting in a product length of approximately 450 bp. The sensitivity of the MY09/11 system is quite high in general, but varies by type (Qu et al., 1997; Gravitt et al., 2000). Some types (like HPV 16 and 18) are amplified with sensitivity around 10 genomes/PCR, while others are inefficiently amplified, with sensitivity limits around 10,000 genomes/PCR (e.g., HPV 35 and 59). The specificity of amplification is poor, as many non-HPV specific products are formed. This is why analysis by electrophoretic gel detection alone is insufficient. Specificity is achieved by probing amplification products with an HPV specific probe. The detection of PCR products will be discussed in more detail in subsequent sections.

For clinical diagnostic purposes, the MY09/11 amplification is usually comparable in performance to the HC2 assay (Peyton et al., 1998). However, in populations where HPV types that are inefficiently amplified comprise a larger fraction of SIL/cancer, this system may be limited in sensitivity (Gravitt et al., 2002). For research purposes, the MY09/11 primer system has been instrumental in defining new HPV genotypes, as well as the natural history of HPV (Manos et al., 1994; Bernard et al., 1994). However, this system is not desirable when estimating type-specific population prevalence or attributable fractions of disease by genotype, since some types will be substantially underdetected (Qu et al., 1997; Gravitt et al., 2000). Because the length of the product generated from MY09/11 amplification is relatively long (450 bp), this method may result in false negative results if applied to archival specimens with poor DNA quality (e.g., fixed tissue) (Greer et al., 1994).

1.2.2   PGMY09/11

The PGMY09/11 primer system is a modification of the MY09/11 primers with 18 pooled oligonucleotide primer sequences replacing the degenerate base sites to accommodate the heterogeneity between the HPV types in the primer target sequences (Gravitt et al., 2000). PGMY09/11 sit in the same relative sites of the L1 ORF as MY09/11, but are more closely matched to all sequenced genotypes, so that the sensitivity of amplification is similar across the genotype spectrum. Multiple studies have validated the improved performance of PGMY09/11 to MY09/11, particularly in the detection of HPV types 26, 35, 42, 52, 54, 55, 59, 66, 68, 73, and 83 (Gravitt et al., 2000; Coutlee et al., 2002). The overall prevalence of HPV detection using these primers is only incrementally increased, but type-specific prevalences can be dramatically increased, and proportion of multiple infections are much higher compared to MY09/11 (40 vs. 33%), due to less competition between types in amplification. The PGMY09/11 system can be used in the same applications favoring MY09/11. It is the preferred method of detection for type-specific prevalence and cohort studies, because of the increased detection of HPV types in multiple infections. The 450 bp product length from PGMY09/11 amplification may preclude the utility of these primers in HPV detection from archival DNA.

1.2.3   GP5+/6+

The GP5+/6+ primers target the same L1 ORF consensus region, with the GP5+ primer essentially mapping to the same location as MY- and PGMY11 (de Roda Husman et al., 1995). The downstream primer targets another conserved region ~150 bp downstream. This primer pair consists of just two oligonucleotides, rather than the mixture of degenerate sequences of MY09/11 or the primer pool of PGMY09/11. Broad-spectrum amplification from genital types heterogeneous in the primer binding-region is effected by low stringency annealing during PCR (temperature of annealing = 45°C). The sensitivity and spectrum of amplification using this primer system is similar to MY09/11, with the propensity for non-specific product formation similarly affecting the amplification specificity of GP5+/6+ such that subsequent HPV specific probe hybridization is also required. The low stringency annealing of just two primers creates a greater likelihood of competitive inhibition of amplification of HPV types with more mismatches to the primer sequence in the presence of HPV types better matched in the primer binding regions. This results in lower frequency of multiple infections (MY09/11 was shown to be 5.3 times more likely to detect infection with multiple genotypes than GP5+/6+ (Qu et al., 1997)), and underestimation of type-specific prevalence for types with greater number of primer mismatches. Such competitive inhibition is unlikely to obscure the ability to detect significant HPV associations with cervical cancer, but can be detrimental when examining type-specific infections over time, and estimating total population prevalence of HPV by type. However, the shorter product length makes GP5+/6+ a preferable primer system, compared to MY- or PGMY09/11, when using archival DNA.

1.2.4 SPF (10)

The SPF, or short PCR fragment, primer system also targets the L1 ORF, where the upstream primer maps to the same site as MY- and PGMY11 (Kleter et al., 1998; Kleter et al., 1999). However, in this system the lower primer sits only 22 bp downstream, generating a short PCR fragment length of only ~62 bp. The SPF system is a mixture of ten primers, with inosine base substitution at some of the common sites of base heterogeneity. Inosine allows for promiscuous base pairing, which facilitates broad-spectrum amplification at relatively high stringency annealing of 52°C. The performance of the SPF primers have been compared to GP5+/6+ (Kleter et al., 1998; Kleter et al., 1999) and PGMY09/11 (van Doorn et al., 2002), showing increased and comparable sensitivity to each system respectively. The short product length makes this the preferred system for archival DNA amplification, but also results in the inability to discriminate between a few genotypes. The ability to detect multiple infections is slightly, but non-significantly compromised relative to PGMY09/11.

1.2.5 Detection and genotyping of broad spectrum HPV amplification products

All of the amplification assays described have used a variety of methods to detect the presence of HPV specific amplified product. Separation of PCR products by gel electrophoresis can help in identification of the targeted fragment length, but is relatively insensitive, and some assays (e.g., MY09/11) will generate non-specific fragments indistinguishable by gel separation from the target HPV product. Therefore, specificity of these assays is obtained only through post-PCR sequence analysis or type-specific probe hybridization.

Generic probe detection by Southern blot (Herrero et al., 2000), dot-blot (Bauer et al., 1992; Hildesheim et al., 1994), or microwell plate (Jacobs et al., 1997; Kornegay et al., 2001; Quint et al., 2001) hybridization has been described for consensus PCR systems. This method identifies any HPV amplification by positive hybridization to pools of HPV specific probes. Consensus PCR amplification followed by generic probe hybridization has historically led to the discovery of many new HPV genotypes. Many investigators have subsequently isolated, sequenced, and designed probes for the types previously determined only as HPV 'X'. After such an exhaustive effort, it is unlikely that a significant proportion of HPV types infecting the genital tract are still unidentified, at least in immunocompetent individuals (Broker et al., 2001). With current HPV typing systems including probes for most known genital HPV types, few additional positive results are expected by inclusion of generic probe detection methods. However, it may be cost-effective to screen low prevalence populations using generic probe-based, high-throughput microwell formats to avoid expensive genotyping of HPV negative samples.

PCR products can be genotyped by restriction fragment length polymorphism (RFLP), direct sequencing, or dot blot/line blot hybridization with type-specific oligonucleotide probes. All of these methods can discriminate between most genital HPVs when present as single infections. RFLP lacks sensitivity at low target concentration where the PCR product is below the limit of gel visualization (Bernard et al., 1994). Resolution of the restriction patterns in the presence of multiple genotype infections or significant non-specific product formation is difficult. Direct sequencing, by standard or novel "pyrosequencing" techniques, has been shown to perform well in comparison with other detection methods, and affords the ability to examine subtle variations of sequence within types. However, sequences of PCR products generated from multiple HPV infections are not easily resolved (Vernon et al., 2000; Gharizadeh et al., 2001). Dot blot hybridization of PCR products with labeled oligonucleotide probes has been widely used (Bauer et al., 1992; Thomas et al., 2000), but is labor intensive, requiring separate hybridizations for each genotype (>40 different hybridizations per sample for comprehensive genotyping). Reverse hybridization to HPV type-specific probes arrayed on strips has been described for all the consensus PCR systems, and allows comprehensive genotyping of PCR products in a single hybridization reaction (Gravitt et al., 1998; Kleter et al., 1999; van den Brule et al., 2002). This method offers the most utility to broad spectrum typing either clinically, or in epidemiologic applications. Dot blot and reverse line blot assays can easily determine the presence of multiple HPV genotypes. Recently, a chip-based reverse hybridization assay has been described (Kim et al., 2003) which, if adequately validated, could allow high-throughput genotyping using standard microarray technologies.

2   SEROLOGIC ASSAYS

Serologic assays for HPV detection have advanced in the past decade, as described below, and offer a cumulative estimate of HPV exposure. The current assay measures type-specific antibody response to an HPV genotype. Women who seroconvert have been shown to have detectable antibody responses for a long time period, even after HPV DNA becomes undetectable. However, limited data suggests a significant fraction of women (30–50%) with positive HPV DNA tests do not appear to seroconvert. Therefore, serology is a relatively insensitive marker of HPV infection, and would not be useful for clinical diagnosis of HPV infection. The utility of HPV serology as an HPV exposure measure in epidemiologic investigations depends on the study design and aim, where the extent of residual confounding from the unmeasured HPV (i.e., the non-seroconverters) is difficult to estimate. However, seromeasures will provide a good estimate of the relative HPV type specific disease burden in targeted populations which is useful for planning in vaccine studies and eventual program implementation. Additionally, cohort studies linking sero-conversion to HPV incidence are helpful in understanding the nature of the host response to HPV following natural infection.

2.1   Serologic Reagents

The development of HPV serological assays has lagged behind that of assays for HPV DNA. The principal reason for this is that HPVs cannot be propagated in tissue culture and thus there is no reliable source for authentic viral proteins. A significant advance in reagent production for serological assays was achieved with the demonstration that the major papillomavirus capsid protein, L1, has the intrinsic capacity to self assemble into virus-like-particles (VLPs) when expressed via recombinant baculoviruses or other eukaryotic expression systems (Kirnbauer et al., 1992). These VLPs are morphologically indistinguishable from authentic virions except that they lack the viral genome. VLPs retain conformational neutralizing epitopes as defined by monoclonal antibodies and they induce the formation of neutralizing antibodies, suggesting that VLPs can substitute for native virions in the development of serodiagnostic assays (Rose et al., 1994; Christensen et al., 1994).

HPV VLPs have been generated for many HPV types, including types 1, 6, 8, 11, 16, 18, 31, 33, 35, 39, 45, 51, 52, 53, 58, and 73. Because of its versatility and suitability for large scale testing, enzyme immunoassay technology is the preferred method to measure anti-viral antibodies. VLPs-based enzyme immunoassays have been established in many laboratories and applied extensively to studies of the humoral immune response to HPV. Because of the clinical importance of HPV type 16, most serodiagnostic studies have been done using HPV 16 VLPs.

2.2   Sensitivity of VLP-Based Enzyme Immunoassays

The sensitivity of VLP-based enzyme immunoassays has been measured using serum samples obtained from individuals with documented HPV infections determined by viral DNA detection methods. In general, the sensitivity of HPV 16 VLP-based enzyme immunoassays for identification of prevalent HPV infection, determined by PCR, is approximately 50% or greater (Table 2). The titers of antibody to HPV 16 VLPs are low, with the majority of seropositive samples having OD values close to the cut point for seropositivity.

Sensitivity appears to be strongly influenced by viral load and persistence. Women with prevalent low viral loads have ~35% sero-prevalence for HPV 16, compared to ~65% seroprevalence among women with high viral load (Kirnbauer et al., 1994; Viscidi et al., 1997). Similarly, only ~25% of women with a transient HPV 16 infection are seropositive, relative to >70% seropositives among women shown to have persistently detectable HPV DNA (Wideroff et al., 1994; de Gruijl et al., 1997). The lower seroprevalence in women with weakly detectable or transiently detectable HPV DNA may result from insufficient production of viral antigen to effectively stimulate an immune response. In addition, the presence of viral DNA may not be associated with production of capsid proteins either because HPV virions are cleared before an infection is established, or infection is confined to the basal layer of the epithelium where only early genes are expressed. Another explanation is the long delay between the detection of HPV DNA by PCR and seroconversion. In a prospective study by Carter and colleagues (Carter et al., 2000), among women with incident HPV infections, the median time to seroconversion was approximately 12 months for the three HPV types; 59%, 54% and 69% seroconverted for HPV types 16, 18 and 6, respectively, within 18 months of detecting the corresponding HPV DNA. Transient HPV DNA was associated with a failure to seroconvert following incident infection; however, some women with persistent HPV DNA also did not seroconvert. None of the factors other than DNA persistence examined in this study, which included site of infection, presence of other HPV DNAs, detection and treatment of squamous intraepithelial lesions, and HPV variants, were shown to contribute to failure to seroconvert. Consideration of these alternative explanations for seronegative results in the context of the natural history of HPV infection is important when making etiologic inference based on HPV serostatus.

Table 2. Prevalence of HPV 16 VLP antibodies in relation to cervical HPV DNA by PCR

Study Population	Age (yrs)	HPV DNA	No. Women	% Positive	Reference
Population- based cases/controls	25-59	Negative Other types Type 16	376 112 52	26 30 65	Kjellberg et al., 1999
GYN and student health clinic	18-42	Negative Other types Type 16	31 37 54	6 27 59	Kirnbauer et al., 1994
University students	18-40	Negative Other types Type 16	247 101 28	19 30 46	Viscidi et al., 1997
University students	18-20	Negative Other types Type 16	216 58 19	7 5 53	Carter et al., 1996
GYN clinic	19-83	Negative Other types Type 16	97 24 67	12 17 46	Tachezy et al., 1999

2.3   Specificity of VLP-Based Enzyme Immunoassays

The specificity of VLP-based enzyme immunoassays has been examined in studies with animal sera of known specificity and by comparing the reactivity of serum from women with the same HPV type, women infected with other HPV types, and women presumably not exposed to HPV. A number of observations from human studies support the type specificity of HPV VLP seroreactivity. The reactivity of human sera to bovine papillomavirus VLPs is negligible, suggesting that there are no genus specific epitopes displayed on intact VLPs (Heim et al., 1995). The low HPV 16 seroprevalence in children (3-5% (af Geijersstam et al., 1999;

Manns et al., 1999; Marais et al., 1997)) argues against significant cross-reactivity between HPV 16 and cutaneous HPV types associated with skin warts, which occur commonly in children. The strong positive association of HPV 16 VLP seroreactivity with sexual behavior is also evidence for the lack of cross-reactivity with cutaneous HPV types (Andersson-Ellstrom et al., 1996; Viscidi et al., 1997). It also confirms the sexual mode of transmission of HPV 16 and suggests that women have no important extracervical sites that harbor nonsexually transmitted HPV 16 infections.

Cross-sectional studies measuring reactivity to multiple HPV VLP types have found that seroreactivity to one type is strongly associated with seroreactivity to other types. However, the type specificity of VLP reactivity for individual genital HPV types is supported by the observation of a stronger association of HPV 16 seroreactivity with HPV 16 DNA than with DNA of other types (Table 2). In most of the studies cited in Table 1, women positive for DNA of other types had an HPV 16 seroprevalence similar to that of HPV DNA negative women. In addition, if there were serological cross-reactivity among HPV types, one might expect greater cross-reactivity between genetically similar HPV types, such as between HPV 16 and 31 or between HPV 18 and 45. However, in a study reported by Wideroff, et al. (1999), stronger associations were not observed for genetically similar pairs. The most likely explanation for this reactivity is cumulative exposure to multiple HPV types, rather than serologic cross-reactivity between types.

One of the most convincing demonstrations of the type specificity of VLP seroreactivity comes from serologic studies of women with incident HPV infection. In the study of Carter et al. (1996), 67% of women with an incident HPV 16 DNA positive infection seroconverted within 15 months, while only 5% of women with incident infections positive for HPV DNA of other types and 4% of women in whom no DNA was detected developed HPV 16 antibodies over the same time period.

Finally, two experimental observations support the type specificity of HPV 16 VLP seroreactivity of human sera. The HPV 16 type specific monoclonal antibody designated V5 is capable of inhibiting the reactivity of more than 75% of reactive human sera (Wang et al., 1997). Studies with a small number of human sera have shown that absorption with heterotypic VLPs has only a minor effect on the homotypic HPV 16 VLP reactivity (Combita et al., 2002).

Given the strong type-specificity of the serologic assays, the total number of serotypes tested will affect the sensitivity of serostatus as a marker of HPV exposure. For example, when measuring HPV 16 serostatus, women exposed to other HPV types but not to HPV 16, in addition to the HPV 16 exposed women who did not seroconvert, will be misclassified as 'unexposed' to HPV. The effect of these false negative results in epidemiologic inference will depend on the relative genotype distribution in the study population and the nature of the association under investigation.

2.4   Biological and Assay Variability of VLP-Based Enzyme Immunoassays

Studies of the reactivity of human sera to HPV VLPs of types other than 16 are limited, but in general have shown that the performance characteristics of VLP-based enzyme immunoassays using these types are similar to those of HPV 16 VLP assays (Dillner et al., 1996; Heim et al., 1995; Kjellberg et al., 1999). One exception to this generalization is the lower sensitivity of HPV 18 VLP-based assays; the sensitivity of HPV 18 VLP assays for HPV 18 DNA positive women is lower (20-35%), relative to the sensitivity of HPV 16 VLP assays in the same studies (50-70%) (Tachezy et al., 1999; Wideroff et al., 1999; Carter et al., 2000). It is unknown whether the lower sensitivity is due to a biological difference in the immune response to HPV 18 compared to HPV 16 or differences in the quantity or quality of the VLP protein used in the assays. The sensitivity of VLP-based assays is highly dependent on having intact VLPs, as partial disruption of VLPs results in loss of reactivity of human sera (Kirnbauer et al., 1994; Wang et al., 1997; Christensen et al., 1996).

2.5   Serological Assays for HPV E6 and E7 Proteins

The early HPV proteins, E6 and E7, are consistently expressed in cancer cells. Serological studies using bacterially expressed proteins or synthetic peptides first established an association between antibodies to these proteins and cervical cancer (Jochmus-Kudielka et al., 1989; Muller et al., 1992). However, the sensitivity and specificity of assays using the above reagents was low. Improvements in sensitivity and specificity were realized by using full-length E6 and E7 proteins produced by in vitro transcription and translation or by using full-length proteins produced in yeast (Viscidi et al., 1993; Sun et al., 1994b; Meschede et al., 1998). Approximately 60-70% of women with HPV 16 DNA positive invasive cervical cancer have antibodies to HPV 16 E6 or E7 protein. The specificity of assays for antibodies to E6 and E7 is high; seroreactivity among women without cervical cancer ranges from 1-5%. Seroreactivity to the E6 and E7 proteins is a diagnostic marker for invasive disease; the reactivity of sera from women with high-grade cervical intraepithelial neoplasia does not differ from that of women with no cytological abnormalities. The antibody responses to the E6 and E7 proteins appear to be independent since not all women who react to one protein react with the other protein. The specificity of the assays with respect to HPV type is supported by the observation that antibodies to HPV 16 E6 and E7 are not seen in women with HPV 18 associated cancers. In some studies the antibody response to E6 and E7 is increased in women with advanced stages of disease (Sun et al., 1994a; Meschede et al., 1998). However, in a multivariate analysis that included stage, age and histology, antibodies to E6 and E7 did not appear to be useful indicators of cervical cancer prognosis (Silins et al., 2002).

3   REPRODUCIBILITY OF HPV EXPOSURE MEASURES

The ability to compare results across multiple studies is important for interpretation of cumulative epidemiologic evidence. The HC 2 assay reagents are commercially available with validated internal controls, maximizing the comparability of these results across studies (Clavel et al., 2000; Terry et al., 2001; Castle et al., 2002). The PCR-based assays, however, are not standardized, and while using the same primer and probe sequences, the core protocol has varied from study to study in key parameters that will influence the performance of the system significantly. For example, the sensitivity of amplification using MY09/11 primers is compromised at $MgCl_2$ concentrations below 4.0 mM, explaining the poor comparative performance of the MY09/11 in studies using $MgCl_2$ from 1.5– 2.5 mM (Perrons et al., 2002; Husnjak et al., 2000; Karlsen et al., 1996). Careful examination of the experimental conditions is warranted for each published report. Standards are needed to allow for relative performance assessment of these methods across laboratories and applications.

A comparison of VLP-based enzyme immunoassays for HPV 16 performed in three laboratories showed Pearson's correlation values ranging between 0.6 and 0.8, indicating that OD levels in the three laboratories were linearly related (Strickler et al., 1997). When agreement was measured according to the categorical interpretations of assay values in each laboratory, there was little discordance between laboratories when OD values near seropositive cutpoints were treated as indeterminate. The results show that even when assay protocols were not standardized, HPV 16 VLP based enzyme immunoassays perform similarly in different laboratories and suggest that comparisons across studies using VLP-based enzyme immunoassays are likely to be valid. Antibody levels to HPV 16 VLPs have been demonstrated to be stable after more than 2 years of follow-up (af Geijersstam et al., 1998).

4   SAMPLE COLLECTION, PROCESSING, AND STORAGE

As mentioned in the preceding sections, the quality of the material collected will dictate the choice of DNA testing method, and may influence the sensitivity and specificity of the test. Multiple collection buffers are available for exfoliated cervical cell samples. Generic buffers such as PBS and TE are valid if samples are stored at -70°C and processed by proteinase K digestion (Bauer et al., 1992) or boiling (van den Brule et al., 2002). Samples collected in Digene STM are stable for HC 2 and PCR testing if stored untreated for up to 3 weeks at room temperature, and over several years at -70°C. However, once the STM has been treated with NaOH for HC 2 testing, the DNA becomes unstable (AT Lorincz, personal communication). Aliquots should be taken prior to preparation for HC 2 testing if subsequent DNA analysis is desired. Extraction of the sample after proteinase K digestion via ethanol precipitation is required due to the presence of PCR inhibitors in the STM formulation. Samples stored in liquid cytology buffers (e.g., PreservCyt and AutoRich) are also valid for near term HPV DNA testing. The longer term stability of these samples stored at room temperature for either HC2 or PCR testing is questionable and stability of frozen samples has not been widely reported.

For HPV serology, both plasma and serum samples may be used. In general, the stability of these samples for future antibody testing is less susceptible to storage conditions, though freezing is the preferred option.

5   NEW METHODS OF HPV EXPOSURE MEASUREMENT

Most of the new HPV detection methods are directed to variant determination, viral load measurement, or HPV gene expression measurement. These are generally type-specific assays, relying on a PCR amplification of the target region. Variant determination is generally accomplished by sequencing the LCR, E6, and/or L1 open reading frames (ORF) (Villa et al., 2000), although probe-based assays (Emeny et al., 1999) and single strand conformational polymorphism (SSCP) analysis (Xi et al., 1993) have been employed. Viral load can be estimated by HC 2 RLU/CO as discussed previously, although type-specific viral load using TaqMan real-time PCR assays may be more relevant for use in epidemiologic investigations, since viral load associations with disease may differ by HPV genotype (Swan et al., 1999). Real-time PCR viral load systems have been described that use TaqMan probes (Swan et al., 1999; Tucker et al., 2001;

Josefsson et al., 1999), Molecular Beacon probes (Szuhai et al., 2001), and Scorpions (Hart et al., 2001), targeting a variety of ORFs. Some of the quantitative PCR methods use multiplexed primer amplification, where up to four different type-specific probes, each with a unique dye, can discriminate genotypes in a single reaction by measuring multiple wavelengths. It would be prudent to consider the effect of amplification competition, since the accuracy of quantitation will depend on the relative efficiency of amplification. Similar quantitative assays incorporating a reverse-transcription step are being increasingly employed to measure viral gene expression. Few of these tests, however, have been formally validated, and the unavailability of standards make inter-assay comparisons difficult.

CONCLUSION

In conclusion, a variety of options are available for the detection and genotyping of both prevalent HPV infections (using DNA assays), and cumulative HPV exposure (using serologic assays). Newer methods are under development to quantitate HPV DNA and mRNA, and to determine genotype-specific variants. Validation of the assays will be important in their broad application in continued research into the HPV associated patho-genesis of cervical cancer. Development of an international reference standard for HPV DNA and serologic assays would be valuable to allow a more confident interpretation of observations from multiple studies. Utilization of HPV DNA and serologic detection of HPV antibodies in prospective studies involving repeated measurement of exposure will allow for a much better understanding of HPV natural history and host response. In addition, population-based, longitudinal correlation of DNA and serologic measures will help to determine the most appropriate HPV exposure marker for future epidemiologic investigations.

REFERENCES

af Geijersstam V, Kibur M, Wang Z, et al. Stability over time of serum antibody levels to human papillomavirus type 16. J Infect Dis 1998; 177: 1710-14.

af Geijersstam V, Eklund C, Wang Z, et al. A survey of seroprevalence of human papillomavirus types 16, 18 and 33 among children. Int J Cancer 1999; 80:489-93.

Andersson-Ellstrom A, Dillner J, Hagmar B, et al. Comparison of development of serum antibodies to HPV16 and HPV33 and acquisition of cervical HPV DNA among sexually experienced and virginal young girls. A longitudinal cohort study. Sex Transm Dis 1996; 23:234-8.

Bauer HM, Greer CE, Manos MM. Determination of genital human papillomavirus infection using consensus PCR. In: Herrington CS, McGee JOD, eds, Diagnostic molecular pathology: a practical approach. Oxford:Oxford University Press, 1992, pp. 132-152.

Bernard HU, Chan SY, Manos MM, et al. Identification and assessment of known and novel human papillomaviruses by polymerase chain reaction amplification, restriction fragment length polymorphisms, nucleotide sequence, and phylogenetic algorithms. J Infect Dis 1994; 170:1077-85.

Bosch FX, Manos MM, Munoz N, et al. Prevalence of human papillomavirus in cervical cancer: a worldwide perspective. J Natl Cancer Inst 1995; 87:796-802.

Broker TR, Jin G, Croom-Rivers A, et al. Viral latency--the papillomavirus model. Dev Biol (Basel) 2001;106:443-5; discussion 452-3, 465-75.

Carter JJ, Koutsky LA, Wipf GC, et al. The natural history of human papillomavirus type 16 capsid antibodies among a cohort of university women. J Infect Dis 1996; 174:927-36.

Carter JJ, Koutsky LA, Hughes JP, et al. Comparison of human papillomavirus types 16, 18, and 6 capsid antibody responses following incident infection. J Infect Dis 2000; 181:1911-19.

Castle PE, Schiffman M, Gravitt PE, et al. Comparisons of HPV DNA detection by MY09/11 PCR methods. J Med Virol 2002; 68:417-23.

Castle PE, Lorincz AT, Mielzynska-Lohnas I, et al. Results of human papillomavirus DNA testing with the hybrid capture 2 assay are reproducible. J Clin Microbiol 2002; 40:1088-90.

Christensen ND, Dillner J, Eklund C, et al. Surface conformational and linear epitopes on HPV 16 and HPV 18 L1 virus-like particles as defined by monoclonal antibodies. Virology 1996; 223:174-84.

Christensen ND, Hopfl R, DiAngelo SL, et al. Assembled baculovirus-expressed human papillomavirus type 11 L1 capsid protein virus-like particles are recognized by neutralizing monoclonal antibodies and induce high titres of neutralizing antibodies. J Gen Virol 1994; 75:2271-76.

Clavel C, Masure M, Levert M, et al. Human papillomavirus detection by the hybrid capture II assay: a reliable test to select women with normal cervical smears at risk for developing cervical lesions. Diagn Mol Pathol 2000; 9:145-50.

Combita AL, Bravo MM, Touze A, et al. Serologic response to human oncogenic papillomavirus types 16, 18, 31, 33, 39, 58 and 59 virus-like particles in Colombian women with invasive cervical cancer. Int J Cancer 2002; 97:796-803.

Coutlee F, Gravitt P, Kornegay J, et al. Use of PGMY primers in L1 consensus PCR improves detection of human papillomavirus DNA in genital samples. J Clin Microbiol 2002;40:902-7.

de Gruijl TD, Bontkes HJ, Walboomers JM, et al. Immunoglobulin G responses against human papillomavirus type 16 virus-like particles in a prospective nonintervention cohort study of women with cervical intraepithelial neoplasia. J Natl Cancer Inst 1997; 89:630-38.

de Roda Husman AM, Walboomers JMM, van den Brule AJC, et al. The use of general primers GP5 and GP6 elongated at their 3' ends with adjacent highly conserved sequences improves human papillomavirus detection by polymerase chain reaction. J Gen Virol 1995; 76:1057-62.

Dillner J, Kallings I, Brihmer C, et al. Seropositivities to human papillomavirus types 16, 18, or 33 capsids and to Chlamydia trachomatis are markers of sexual behavior. J Infect Dis 1996; 173:1394-98.

Emeny RT, Herron JR, Xi LF, et al. Comparison of variant-specific hybridization and single-strand conformational polymorphism methods for detection of mixed human papillomavirus type 16 variant infections. J Clin Microbiol 1999; 37:3627-33.

Fife KH, Cramer HM, Schroeder JM, et al. Detection of multiple human papillomavirus types in the lower genital tract correlates with cervical dysplasia. J Med Virol 2001; 64:550-59.

Franco EL, Villa LL, Sobrinho JP, et al. Epidemiology of acquisition and clearance of cervical human papillomavirus infection in women from a high-risk area for cervical cancer. J Infect Dis 1999;180:1415-23.

Gharizadeh B, Kalantari M, Garcia CA, et al. Typing of human papillomavirus by pyro-sequencing. Lab Invest 2001; 81(5):673-9.

Gravitt PE, Peyton CL, Apple RJ, et al. Genotyping of 27 human papillomavirus types by using L1 consensus PCR products by a single-hybridization, reverse line blot detection method. J Clin Microbiol 1998; 36:3020-7.

Gravitt PE, Peyton CL, Alessi TQ, et al. Improved amplification of genital human papillomaviruses. J Clin Microbiol 2000; 38(1):357-61.

Gravitt PE, Kamath A, Gaffikin L, et al. HPV genotype prevalence in HSIL and colposcopically normal women from Zimbabwe. Int J Cancer 2002; 100:729-32.

Greer CE, Wheeler CM, Manos MM. Sample preparation and PCR amplification from paraffin-embedded tissues. PCR Methods Appl 1994; 3(6):S113-22.

Hart KW, Williams OM, Thelwell N, et al. Novel method for detection, typing, and quantification of human papillomaviruses in clinical samples. J Clin Microbiol 2001; 39:3204-12.

Heim K, Christensen ND, Hoepfl R, et al. Serum IgG, IgM, and IgA reactivity to human papillomavirus types 11 and 6 virus-like particles in different gynecologic patient groups. J Infect Dis 1995; 172:395-402.

Herrero R, Hildesheim A, Bratti C, et al. Population-based study of human papillomavirus infection and cervical neoplasia in rural Costa Rica. J Natl Cancer Inst 2000;92(6):464-74.

Hildesheim A, Schiffman MH, Gravitt PE, et al. Persistence of type-specific human papillomavirus infection among cytologically normal women. J Infect Dis 1994; 169:235-40.

Husnjak K, Grce M, Magdic L, et al. Comparison of five different polymerase chain reaction methods for detection of human papillomavirus in cervical cell specimens. J Virol Methods 2000;88:125-34.

Jacobs MV, Walboomers JMM, van Beek J, et al. A quantitative polymerase chain reaction-enzyme immunoassay for accurate measurements of human papillomavirus type 16 DNA levels in cervical scrapings. Br J Cancer 1999; 81:114-21.

Jochmus-Kudielka I, Schneider A, Braun R, et al. Antibodies against the human papillomavirus type 16 early proteins in human sera: correlation of anti-E7 reactivity with cervical cancer. J Natl Cancer Inst 1989; 81:1698-704.

Josefsson A, Livak K, Gyllensten U. Detection and quantitation of human papillomavirus by using the fluorescent 5' exonuclease assay. J Clin Microbiol 1999; 37:490-6.

Karlsen F, Kalantari M, Jenkins A, et al. Use of multiple PCR primer sets for optimal detection of human papillomavirus. J Clin Microbiol 1996; 34:2095-100.

Kim CJ, Kim JJ, Park M, et al. HPV oligonucleotide microarray-based detection of HPV genotypes in cervical neoplastic lesions. Gynecol Oncol 2003; 89:360-8.

Kirnbauer R, Booy F, Cheng N, et al. Papillomavirus L1 major capsid protein self-assembles into virus-like particles that are highly immunogenic. Proc Natl Acad Sci USA 1992; 89:12180-4.

Kirnbauer R, Hubbert NL, Wheeler CM, et al. A virus-like particle enzyme-linked immunosorbent assay detects serum antibodies in a majority of women infected with human papillomavirus type 16. J Natl Cancer Inst 1994; 86:494-9

Kjellberg L, Wang Z, Wiklund F, et al. Sexual behaviour and papillomavirus exposure in cervical intraepithelial neoplasia: a population-based case-control study. J Gen Virol 1999; 80:391-8.

Kleter B, van Doorn L-J, ter Schegget J, et al. Novel short-fragment PCR assay for highly sensitive broad-spectrum detection of anogenital human papillomaviruses. Am J Pathol 1998; 153:1731-9.

Kleter B, van Doorn L-J, Schrauwen L, et al. Development and clinical evaluation of a highly sensitive PCR-reverse hybridization line probe assay for detection and identification of anogenital human papillomavirus. J Clin Microbiol 1999; 37:2508-17.

Kornegay JR, Shepard AP, Hankins C, et al. Nonisotopic detection of human papillomavirus DNA in clinical specimens using a consensus PCR and a generic probe mix in an enzyme-linked immunosorbent assay format. J Clin Microbiol 2001; 39:3530-6.

Lorincz AT, Anthony J. Advances in HPV detection by Hybrid Capture. Papillomavirus Report 2001; 12:145-54.

Manns A, Strickler HD, Wikktor SZ, et al. Low incidence of human papillomavirus type 16 antibody seroconversion in young children. Pediatr Infect Dis J 1999; 18:833-835.

Manos MM, Ting Y, Wright DK, et al. Use of polymerase chain reaction amplification for the detection of genital human papillomaviruses. Cancer Cells 1989; 7:209-14.

Manos MM, Waldman J, Zhang TY, et al. Epidemiology and partial nucleotide sequence of four novel genital human papillomaviruses. J Infect Dis 1994; 170:1096-9.

Manos MM, Kinney WK, Hurley LB, et al. Identifying women with cervical neoplasia using human papillomavirus DNA testing for equivocal Papanicolaou results. JAMA 1999; 281: 1605-10.

Marais D, Rose RC, Williamson AL. Age distribution of antibodies to human papillomavirus in children, women with cervical intraepithelial neoplasia and blood donors from South Africa. J Med Virol 1997; 51:126-31.

Meschede W, Zumbach K, Braspenning J, et al. Antibodies against early proteins of human papillomaviruses as diagnostic markers for invasive cervical cancer. J Clin Microbiol 1998; 36:475-80.

Muller M, Viscidi RP, Sun Y, et al. Antibodies to HPV 16 E6 and E7 proteins as markers for HPV 16- associated invasive cervical cancer. Virology 1992; 187:508-14.

Perrons C, Kleter B, Jelley R, et al. Detection and genotyping of human papillomavirus DNA by SPF10 and MY09/11 primers in cervical cells taken from women attending a colposcopy clinic. J Med Virol 2002; 67:246-52.

Peyton CL, Schiffman MH, Lorincz AT, et al. Comparison of PCR- and Hybrid Capture-based human papillomavirus detection systems using multiple cervical specimen collection strategies. J Clin Microbiol 1998; 36:3248-54.

Peyton CL, Gravitt PE, Hunt WC, et al. Determinants of genital human papillomavirus detection in a US population. J Infect Dis 2001;183:1554-64.

Qu W, Jiang G, Cruz Y, et al. PCR detection of human papillomavirus: comparison between MY09/MY11 and GP5+/GP6+ primer systems. J Clin Microbiol 1997;35:1304-10.

Quint WGV, Scholte G, van Doorn LJ, et al. Comparative analysis of human papillomavirus infections in cervical scrapes and biopsy specimens by general SPF10 PCR and HPV genotyping. J Pathol 2001; 194:51-8.

Rose RC, Reichman RC, Bonnez W. Human papillomavirus (HPV) type 11 recombinant virus-like particles induce the formation of neutralizing antibodies and detect HPV specific antibodies in human sera. J Gen Virol 1994; 75:2075-9.

Schiffman M, Herrero R, Hildesheim A, et al. HPV DNA testing in cervical cancer screening: results from women in a high-risk province of Costa Rica. JAMA 2000;283:87-93.

Silins I., Avall-Lundqvist E., Tadesse A., et al. Evaluation of antibodies to human papillomavirus as prognostic markers in cervical cancer patients. Gynecol Oncol 2002; 85:333-8.

Strickler HD, Hildesheim A, Viscidi RP, et al. Interlaboratory agreement among results of human papillomavirus type 16 enzyme-linked immunosorbent assays. J Clin Microbiol 1997; 35:1751-6.

Sun Y, Eluf-Neto J, Bosch FX, et al. Human papillomavirus-related serological markers of invasive cervical carcinoma in Brazil. Cancer Epidemiol Biomarkers Prev 1994a; 3:341-7.

Sun Y, Shah KV, Muller M, et al. Comparison of peptide enzyme-linked immunosorbent assay and radioimmunoprecipitation assay with in vitro-translated proteins for detection of serum antibodies to human papillomavirus type 16 E6 and E7 proteins. J Clin Microbiol 1994b; 32:2216-20.

Swan DC, Tucker RA, Tortolero-Luna G, et al. Human papillomavirus (HPV) DNA copy number is dependent on grade of cervical disease and HPV type. J Clin Microbiol 1999; 37:1030-4.

Szuhai K, Sandhaus E, Kolkman-Uljee SM, et al. A novel strategy for human papillomavirus detection and genotyping with SybrGreen and molecular beacon polymerase chain reaction. Am J Pathol 2001; 159:1651-60.

Tachezy R, Hamsikova E, Hajek T, et al. Human papillomavirus genotype spectrum in Czech women: correlation of HPV DNA presence with antibodies against HPV 16, 18, and 33 virus-like particles. J Med Virol 1999; 58:378-86.

Terry G, Ho L, Londesborough P, et al. Detection of high-risk HPV types by the Hybrid Capture 2 test. J Med Virol 2001; 65:155-62.

Thomas KK, Hughes JP, Kuypers JM, et al. Concurrent and sequential acquisition of different genital human papillomavirus types. J Infect Dis 2000;182(4):1097-102.

Tucker RA, Unger ER, Holloway BP, et al. Real-time PCR-based fluorescent assay for quantitation of human papillomavirus types 6, 11, 16, and 18. Mol Diagn 2001; 6:39-47.

van den Brule AJC, Pol R, Fransen-Daalmeijer N, et al. GP5+/6+ PCR followed by reverse line blot analysis enables rapid and high-throughput identification of human papillomavirus genotypes. J Clin Microbiol 2002;40(3):779-87.

van Doorn L-J, Quint W, Kleter B, et al. Genotyping of human papillomavirus in liquid cytology cervical specimens by the PGMY line blot assay and the SPF_{10} line probe assay. J Clin Microbiol 2002; 40(3):979-83.

Vernon SD, Unger ER, Williams D. Comparison of human papillomavirus detection and typing by cycle sequencing, line blotting, and Hybrid Capture. J Clin Microbiol 2000; 38:651-5.

Villa LL, Sichero L, Rahal P, et al. Molecular variants of human papillomavirus types 16 and 18 preferentially associated with cervical neoplasia. J Gen Virol 2000;81:2959-68.

Viscidi RP, Sun Y, Tsuzaki B, et al. Serologic response in human papillomavirus-associated invasive cervical cancer. Int J Cancer 1993; 55:780-4.

Viscidi RP, Kotloff KL, Clayman B, et al. Prevalence of antibodies to human papillomavirus (HPV) type 16 virus-like particles in relation to cervical HPV infection among college women. Clin Diagn Lab Immunol 1997; 4:122-6.

Walboomers JMM, Jacobs MV, Manos MM, et al. Human papillomavirus is a necessary cause of invasive cervical cancer worldwide. J Pathol 1999;189:12-9.

Wang Z, Christensen N, Schiller JT, et al. A monoclonal antibody against intact human papillomavirus type 16 capsids blocks the serological reactivity of most human sera. J Gen Virol 1997; 78: 2209-15.

Wideroff L, Schiffman MH, Nonnenmacher B, et al. Evaluation of seroreactivity to human papillomavirus type 16 virus-like particles in an incident case-control study of cervical neoplasia. J Infect Dis 1995; 172:1425-30.

Wideroff L, Schiffman M, Haderer P, et al. Seroreactivity to human papillomavirus types 16, 18, 31, and 45 virus- like particles in a case-control study of cervical squamous intraepithelial lesions. J Infect Dis 1999; 180:1424-8.

Xi LF, Demers GW, Kiviat NB, et al. Sequence variation in the noncoding region of human papillomavirus type 16 detected by single-strand conformation polymorphism analysis. J Infect Dis 1993; 168:610-7.

Chapter 6

The Epidemiology of Human Papillomavirus Infections

Rachel L. Winer, M.P.H. and Laura A Koutsky, Ph.D.

Department of Epidemiology, University of Washington

INTRODUCTION

Genital human papillomavirus (HPV) is one of the most common sexually transmitted infections in the United States, and current estimates suggest that at least 50% of sexually active women have been infected with one or more types (Koutsky and Kiviat, 1999). More than 84 types of HPV have been identified, and at least 38 are known to primarily infect genital epithelium (Wheeler, 2002). Individual HPV types are associated with varied clinical manifestations (de Villiers, 1989) and genital types have been classified as high-risk or low-risk based on their oncogenic potential (zur Hausen, 1985). For example, genital warts are most often positive for HPV 6 (Greer et al., 1995, Langenberg et al., 1993, Sugase et al., 1991), while 16, 18, 31, and 45 are the types most frequently associated with the development of invasive anogenital cancers (Bosch et al., 1995). Recent international evidence has shown that HPV DNA is present in 99.7% of cervical cancer specimens, supporting a causal link between HPV infection and the development of cervical neoplasia (Bosch et al., 1995, Walboomers et al., 1999, Walboomers and Meijer, 1997). While progress has been made in defining the epidemiology and natural history of HPV infection, data are limited by a combination of factors (Tortolero-Luna, 1999), including the subclinical and transient nature of most HPV infections (Ho et al., 1995, Ho et al., 1998c, Villa, 1997), limited surveillance (Tortolero-Luna, 1999), and a limited number of prospective studies.

1   DEFINITIONS

Genital HPV infections are commonly defined using clinical, molecular, and serologic detection methods (Table 1). Clinical manifestations are characterized by the presence of grossly visible genital warts or by the presence of squamous intraepithelial lesions (SIL) detected either by microscopically visible cytologic and histologic features or by colposcopic visualization of aceto-white areas of genital epithelium after application of a 3 to 5 percent vinegar solution (Koutsky and Kiviat, 1999). Molecular detection of HPV DNA in genital tract specimens is achieved using either PCR-based amplification methods (Saiki et al., 1988) or by direct DNA hybridization with or without amplification of the hybrid (see Chapter 5). Serologic methods are used to detect serum antibodies to certain viral proteins produced by specific HPV types.

Table 1. Definitions of human papillomavirus infections

Detection Method	Definition
Clinical	Grossly visible
	(i) Genital warts
	Microscopically visible
	(i) Squamous intraepithelial lesions
Molecular	HPV DNA or RNA detected in the genital tract
Serologic	Serum antibodies to specific HPV types

2   PREVALENCE

HPV prevalence is defined as the proportion of individuals with detectable infection at a given point or period in time. Estimates vary based on the method of HPV detection. Studies relying on grossly visible genital warts as the marker of infection typically yield the lowest prevalence estimates, whereas the highest estimates have been reported in studies using PCR-based methods for detecting HPV DNA in the genital tract (Koutsky, 1997). Even among studies using highly sensitive PCR-based methods for HPV DNA detection, differences in specimen collection methods (Goldberg et al., 1989), populations sampled, and protocols, primers, and probes used make it difficult to compare estimates from different studies (Xi and Koutsky, 1997).

2.1 Genital warts

Virtually all genital warts are caused by HPV 6 or 11, with 70 to 100 percent of genital wart tissues containing one or both of these types (Brown et al., 1999, Coleman et al., 1994, Cui et al., 1994, Greer et al., 1995, Li et al., 1995, Tsao et al., 1994). Roughly 1 percent of sexually active adults (15 to 49 years of age) in the United States have clinically visible external genital warts (condylomata acuminata) (Koutsky et al., 1988). Genital warts tend to be more common in men than in women, and the highest prevalence estimates have been reported in persons attending sexually transmitted disease (STD) clinics. Prevalence estimates among patients attending STD clinics in the United States, United Kingdom, and Australia have ranged between 4 and 13 percent (Koutsky et al., 1988). In a study conducted at a Seattle-King County STD clinic, 13 percent of men and 9 percent of women had evidence of genital warts on examination (Koutsky et al., 1988). Among 545 women visiting a university health center for an annual exam, 2 percent had macroscopically visible genital warts (Kiviat et al., 1989). Available data suggest a lower prevalence in women over 30 years of age. Among women attending an STD clinic, the prevalence of genital warts in women 16 to 29 years of age was more than double that in women aged 30 to 50 (Kiviat et al., 1989). Additionally, among women examined at a health maintenance organization, the prevalence of genital warts was 0.8 percent for women between the ages of 21 and 29 and 0.6 percent for women 30 to 39 years of age (Koutsky et al., 1988).

Condylomata acuminata tends to be more prevalent in immunosuppressed populations. In one large cohort study, 9.8 percent of women seropositive for the human immunodeficiency virus (HIV) had genital warts detected at baseline, compared to 3.1 percent of HIV-seronegative women (Silverberg et al., 2002). Studies estimating the prevalence of genital warts in HIV-infected women have reported values ranging from 5.6 to 37 percent (Byrne et al., 1989, Chiasson et al., 1997, Chirgwin et al., 1995, Conley et al., 2002, Silverberg et al., 2002).

2.2   Squamous intraepithelial lesions (SIL)

All genital HPV types have been linked with the development of cervical SIL, the precursor lesions to invasive cervical cancer (Wright et al., 1994b). Pap smear screening is the most common method for detecting cervical SIL. Variations in interpretation and reporting of cytologic findings make it difficult to compare prevalence estimates across countries, laboratories, and time periods (Schiffman et al., 1995). Prevalence estimates have ranged from 0.43 to 24 percent (Bjorge et al., 1994, Edelman et al., 1999, Engels et al., 1992, Fonn et al., 2002, Healey et al., 2001, Heystek et al., 1995, Hurley et al., 1997, Kamb, 1995, Kiviat et al., 1989, Martinez et al., 1988, McKinnon et al., 1991, Mount and Papillo, 1999, Paavonen et al., 1990, Robertson et al., 1991, Sadeghi et al., 1989, Temmerman et al., 1998, Utagawa et al., 1998). Estimates vary according to the population studied, with most STD clinics reporting prevalences between 5 and 13 percent (Edelman et al., 1999, Brish Cooperative Clinical Group, 1987, Kamb, 1995, McKinnon et al., 1991, Paavonen et al., 1990, Robertson et al., 1991) and the majority of gynecologic clinics reporting prevalences of around 2 percent (Kiviat et al., 1999).

Whereas invasive cervical cancer is more common in older women, SIL is detected more frequently in younger women, with peak prevalence estimates occurring in the mid 20s. One study reported that the prevalence of mild-to-moderate dysplasia was highest in women between the ages of 25 and 29, whereas severe dysplasia and carcinoma in situ were most common in women aged 35 to 39 (Sadeghi et al., 1989). (Most laboratories now use the term SIL in place of the term dysplasia. See Chapter 1 for a detailed discussion of the terminology for cervical intraepithelial lesions.) A similar trend was observed in a multi-center prevalence study in South Africa (Fonn et al., 2002). Studies of sexually active adolescent populations have reported prevalence estimates that are comparable to or higher than those observed in populations of adult women (Edelman et al., 1999, Mount and Papillo, 1999, Simsir et al., 2002). Simsir et al. (2002) reported that while the prevalence of lesions was similar among populations of sexually active adolescents (aged 13 to 17 years) and adult women, the ratio of high-grade to low-grade lesions was much higher among the adult women.

Cervical SIL is prevalent among immunosuppressed populations. Schafer et al. (1991) reported dysplasia in 41 percent of HIV-positive women, compared to only 4 percent in a general outpatient population. In another study, evidence of squamous abnormalities was present in 31 percent of HIV-positive and 4 percent of HIV-negative women (Schrager et al., 1989).

2.3 Prevalence of HPV DNA

Using data from PCR-based studies conducted between 1990 and 1996, Xi and Koutsky (1997) determined that the weighted average of HPV prevalence among 12,595 cytologically normal women was 16.2 percent. The prevalence of genital HPV infection detected by PCR-based methods has ranged from 1.5 to 44.3 percent in cytologically normal women, depending on the population sampled (Bauer et al., 1993, Bauer et al., 1991, Becker et al., 1994a, Bosch et al., 1993, Brisson et al., 1996, Burk et al., 1996a, Chang et al., 1997, Coker et al., 1993, Critchlow and Koutsky, 1995, Czegledy et al., 1992, Engels et al., 1992, Hildesheim et al., 1993, Hildesheim et al., 1994, Hinchliffe et al., 1995, Jacobs et al., 2000, Kjaer et al., 1990, Lambropoulos et al., 1994, Maehama et al., 2000, Melkert et al., 1993, Munoz et al., 1992, Munoz et al., 1996b, Nishikawa et al., 1991, Pao et al., 1990, Pasetto et al., 1992, Peyton et al., 2001, Rylander et al., 1994, Schiffman et al., 1993, Seck et al., 1994, Tachezy et al., 1999, van Doornum et al., 1992, Vandenvelde et al., 1992, Wheeler et al., 1993). The highest estimate was reported among a population of sexually active young women (Wheeler et al., 1993), and the lowest estimate was reported among women who had reported that they had not yet engaged in sexual intercourse (Rylander et al., 1994).

Using PCR-based methods, a handful of international studies have estimated the prevalence of HPV infection in otherwise healthy males. Among 105 male Swedish Army recruits between the ages of 18 and 23, urethral samples from 12 percent of men with normal penile epithelium and 26 percent of men with visible lesions tested positive for HPV DNA (Kataoka et al., 1991). Among voluntary Finnish Army conscripts, 16.5 percent of 285 penile shaft or urethral samples were positive for HPV DNA, including 7.1 percent of 168 samples from men with no peniscopic abnormalities (Hippelainen et al., 1993). In Mexico, urethral and coronal sulcus samples were collected from 120 men, and HPV DNA was detected only in men reporting previous sexual activity (42.7 percent of 96 subjects). 46.3 percent of infections were positive for high-risk types (Lazcano-Ponce et al., 2001b). Higher prevalence estimates have been observed in males attending STD clinics, with estimates ranging from 28 to 84 percent (Baken et al., 1995, van Doornum et al., 1992, Weaver et al., 2002, Wikstrom et al., 1991). In cervical cancer case-control studies, urethral, glans, and coronal sulcus samples obtained from husbands of women with cervical cancer have consistently demonstrated higher HPV prevalence than samples obtained from husbands of control women (Bosch et al., 1996, Franceschi et al., 2002, Munoz et al., 1996a).

2.3.1   Type-specific prevalence of HPV DNA

HPV 16 is the most common type detected among cytologically normal women (Schiffman, 1992). Studies using type-specific probes have reported that 0.5 to 44.4 percent of infections in sexually active, cytologically normal women are positive for HPV 16 or 18 (Becker et al., 1994a, Bosch et al., 1993, Chang et al., 1997, Critchlow and Koutsky, 1995, Czegledy et al., 1992, Hildesheim et al., 1994, Jacobs et al., 2000, Kjaer et al., 1990, Lambropoulos et al., 1994, Melkert et al., 1993, Munoz et al., 1992, Nishikawa et al., 1991, Pao et al., 1990, Tachezy et al., 1999, van Doornum et al., 1992, Wheeler et al., 1993). In general, high-risk types tend to be detected more frequently than low-risk types. Among women attending a clinic in New Mexico for routine gynecologic care, 23.8 and 13.2 percent were positive for high- and low-risk HPV types, respectively (Peyton et al., 2001). A similar trend was observed in a population-based study in the Netherlands (Jacobs et al., 2000), even though the reported overall prevalence of HPV DNA was much lower (4.6 percent compared to 36.1 percent among clinic patients in New Mexico). Detection of multiple HPV types is common, with several studies reporting that around 16 to 38 percent of HPV infections are positive for more than one type (Chang et al., 1997, Jacobs et al., 2000, Tachezy et al., 1999).

2.3.2   Age-specific prevalence of HPV DNA

Genital HPV DNA tends to be detected most frequently in younger women, with the highest prevalence estimates reported among sexually active women <30 years of age (Bauer et al., 1993, Burk et al., 1996b, Hildesheim et al., 1993, Jacobs et al., 2000, Ley et al., 1991, Melkert et al., 1993, Peyton et al., 2001). Prevalence appears to decline with age. Melkert et al. (1993) found that the overall prevalence of HPV DNA decreased from 25 percent in women aged 20 to 25 years to 4.6 percent in women ≥35 years of age. Jacobs et al. (2000) reported that the prevalence of HPV DNA was highest among women 25 to 29 years of age (19.6 percent) and decreased to 4.3 percent in women ≥30 years of age. When high-risk and low-risk HPV types are considered separately, the trend of decreasing prevalence with age is more pronounced for high-risk HPV types (Jacobs et al., 2000, Peyton et al., 2001). It should be noted, however, that these trends were observed among populations of cytologically-normal women. Since persistent infections with high-risk types are more likely to cause lesions that are subsequently treated, we might expect to find fewer high-risk than low-risk infections among older women (Jacobs et al., 2000). A couple of studies have reported an additional, albeit smaller peak in the overall prevalence of HPV infection among women ≥60 years of age (Herrero et al., 1997, Sellors et al., 2002). HPV infections in this age group of women are likely to represent persistent infections acquired at a younger age. Such persistent infections are often associated with previously undetected, persistent lesions.

2.3.3   International differences in HPV DNA prevalence

Geographic trends in HPV DNA prevalence across studies are not readily apparent. One study that compared populations of women from Spain, Colombia, and Brazil, however, reported higher prevalence estimates in Brazil (17 percent) and Colombia (13 percent) than in Spain (4.9 percent), reflecting the differing rates of cervical cancer in these countries (Munoz et al., 1996b). Differing prevalence estimates for Colombia and Spain were also observed among husbands of women with cervical cancer and among husbands of control women (Bosch et al., 1996, Munoz et al., 1996a).

2.3.4   Prevalence of HPV 16 variants

HPV 16 variants have been categorized into 5 major lineages according to homology and region of the world where they were originally isolated. Since the prototype variant of HPV 16 was first detected in a cervical cancer specimen from a woman in Europe, this variant established the European lineage. Non-prototype HPV 16 variants are classified into one of four lineages, including Asian, Asian-American, African-1, and African-2 (Chan et al., 1992, Yamada et al., 1995). Non-prototype-like HPV 16 variants generally contain multiple nucleotide alterations (Koutsky and Kiviat, 1999). Among women with cervical cancer, European variants predominate in Europe, North America, and Australia, and African-1 and -2 variants are more common in Africa (Berumen et al., 2001, Watts et al., 2002, Yamada et al., 1997). In a study conducted among female university students in Washington State, there was an association between non-white ethnicity and an increased cumulative incidence of non-prototypic HPV 16 variants (Xi et al., 2002). Recent evidence suggests that non-prototypic HPV 16 variants are associated with an increased risk of high-grade cervical or anal dysplasia and cervical cancer (Xi et al., 2002, Xi et al., 1998, Xi et al., 1997, Yamada et al., 1997).

2.3.5   Prevalence in immunosuppressed individuals

HIV-positive individuals tend to have a higher prevalence of genital HPV DNA than do HIV-negative individuals. Studies comparing groups of women by HIV status using PCR-based methods have reported an HPV prevalence range of 40 to 77.4 percent for HIV-positive women and 14 to 62 percent for HIV-negative women (Ahdieh et al., 2001, Critchlow and

Koutsky, 1995, Ellerbrock et al., 2000, Hankins et al., 1999, Langley et al., 1996, Maiman et al., 1998, Massad et al., 1999, Minkoff et al., 1998, Moscicki et al., 2000, Palefsky et al., 1999, Rezza et al., 1997, Shah et al., 1997, Silverberg et al., 2002, Sun et al., 1995, Sun et al., 1997, Temmerman et al., 1999, Wright et al., 1994a). A similar increase in prevalence has been observed in populations of HIV-positive men (Breese et al., 1995, Critchlow et al., 1992, Kiviat et al., 1993, Law et al., 1991, Palefsky et al., 1994). Renal allograft recipients also appear to be at an increased risk of HPV infection, with recipients demonstrating consistently higher prevalence of HPV 16 or 18 DNA than controls (Alloub et al., 1989, Fairley et al., 1994a, Ogunbiyi et al., 1994).

2.3.6   Prevalence in adolescents, children, and infants

Prevalence data specific to adolescents and young children are limited. Adolescent data come mostly from sexually active clinic populations, and suggest that HPV is highly prevalent among high-risk adolescents (Moscicki, 1996, Moscicki et al., 1990, Rosenfeld et al., 1989). Prevalence data in children are variable. Several studies have reported up to 56 percent prevalence of HPV 16 (Jenison et al., 1990, Mund et al., 1997, Rice et al., 2000), whereas other studies have reported little to no HPV DNA in oral or genital samples taken from children (Koch et al., 1997, Watts et al., 1998). These variations may reflect differences in populations or the accuracy of the testing methods.

Several studies have tested infants for HPV DNA using oral or genital samples, with estimates from the first couple of days of life ranging from 4 to 72 percent among infants born to mothers testing positive for HPV DNA during pregnancy, and 0.6 to 20 percent among those born to mothers with no detectable HPV infection during pregnancy (Cason et al., 1995, Pakarian et al., 1994, Sedlacek et al., 1989, Smith et al., 1995, Watts et al., 1998). While there has been an association between maternal HPV infection during pregnancy and HPV status in the infant at birth, these associations have not always been present 6 weeks post delivery (Carter et al., 1995, Fredericks et al., 1993, Pakarian et al., 1994). Furthermore, no clear evidence of HPV infection was found among 143 infants followed longitudinally for up to 3 years post delivery, even though 74 percent of their mothers had confirmed evidence of infection when followed prospectively during pregnancy (Watts et al., 1998).

2.4   Seroprevalence

Serologic assays for specific HPV types have been used to detect antibodies to virus-like particles (VLPs), with the majority of studies testing for antibodies to HPV 16. HPV seropositivity tends to be more prevalent in females than in males (Slavinsky et al., 2001, Stone et al., 2002, Strickler et al., 1999, Svare et al., 1997, van Doornum et al., 1998). Strickler et al. (1999) reported that the seroprevalence of HPV 16 was consistently higher in women than in men in both STD clinic and blood donor populations. Women attending STD clinics in Denmark and Greenland were also more likely than men to be seropositive for HPV 16, despite the fact that men reported significantly higher lifetime numbers of sex partners than women (Svare et al., 1997).

2.4.1   Seroprevalence of HPV types in women and men

Among women with no clinical evidence of HPV-related disease, the seroprevalence of HPV 16 has ranged from 2 to 66 percent (af Geijersstam et al., 1998, Carter et al., 1996, Combita et al., 2002, Dillner et al., 1997, Hagensee et al., 1999, Lehtinen et al., 1996, Marais et al., 2000, Matsumoto et al., 1997, Nonnenmacher et al., 1995, Nonnenmacher et al., 1996, Park et al., 1998, Shah et al., 1997, Strickler et al., 1999, Svare et al., 1997, Tachezy et al., 1999, Viscidi et al., 1997, Wideroff et al., 1995). The highest estimates have been reported among STD clinic populations, with 42 to 66 percent of female clinic attendees demonstrating seropositivity to HPV 16 antibodies (Nonnenmacher et al., 1996, Slavinsky et al., 2001, Svare et al., 1997). In male STD clinic attendees, the seroprevalence of HPV 16 has ranged from 18 to 36 percent (Slavinsky et al., 2001, Strickler et al., 1999, Svare et al., 1997, van Doornum et al., 1998). Cervical cancer case-control studies have provided another source of seroprevalence estimates; in these studies, HPV 16 antibodies have been present in 2 to 43 percent of cancer-free control women (Combita et al., 2002, Dillner et al., 1997, Lehtinen et al., 1996, Matsumoto et al., 1997, Nonnenmacher et al., 1995, Park et al., 1998, Shah et al., 1997, Wideroff et al., 1995). Recent data from the National Health and Nutrition Examination Survey suggest that roughly 18 percent of women and 8 percent of men in the general United States population are seropositive for HPV 16 (Stone et al., 2002). There has been some evidence of an increase in HPV seroprevalence over time. In Sweden, the seroprevalence of HPV 16 among pregnant women rose from 16 percent in 1969 to 22 percent in 1983, and remained constant at 21 percent in 1989 (Strickler et al., 1999).

A handful of studies have assessed the seroprevalence of other HPV types in women. Nine to 25 percent of women have demonstrated antibodies to HPV 6 or 11 (Carter et al., 1995, Heim et al., 1995, Shah et al., 1997), and seroprevalence estimates for individual HPV 18, 31, 33, 39, 45, 58, 59, and 73 have ranged from 8 to 23 percent (Combita et al., 2002, Dillner et al., 1997, Marais et al., 2000, Matsumoto et al., 1997, Wallin et al., 2000, Wang et al., 1997).

2.4.2   Age-specific seroprevalence

Whereas HPV DNA tends to be detected more frequently in women <25 years of age, seroprevalence tends to be highest among women ≥25 years of age (Nonnenmacher et al., 1996, Slavinsky et al., 2001, Strickler et al., 1999). In men, HPV seroprevalence tends to peak after age 30 (Slavinsky et al., 2001, Stone et al., 2002). Recent population-based data were used to estimate the age-specific seroprevalence of HPV 16 among women and men in the United States (Figure 1). These data suggest that detection of HPV 16 antibodies plateaus in adult women by age 20 and does not decline until after age 50. In men, HPV 16 seroprevalence seems to remain steady after age 30. While HPV 16 seroprevalence is consistently higher in women than in men at every age interval from 12 to 49 years, antibodies seem to be detected in roughly equal proportions by age 50.

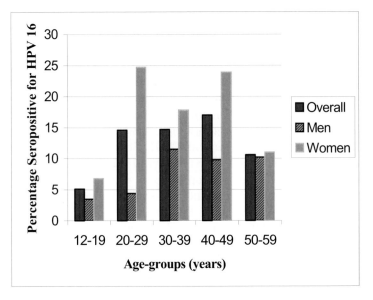

Figure 1. Seroprevalence of HPV 16 in the general United States population, 1991-1994 (Data adapted from Stone et al., 2002).

HPV 16 antibodies have also been detected in younger children. Several studies have reported on the prevalence of antibodies to VLP-16 in children less than 13 years of age, with most estimates ranging from 3 to 8 percent (af Geijersstam et al., 1999, Cubie et al., 1998, Manns et al., 1999, Marais et al., 1997). Studies measuring antibodies to HPV 16 E4, E7, L1, or L2 proteins have reported even higher estimates (Marais et al., 1997, Muller et al., 1995).

2.4.3   International variations in HPV seroprevalence

There is some evidence to suggest that antibodies to HPV 16 are more prevalent in countries with higher rates of cervical cancer. Strickler et al. (1999) reported that the prevalence of HPV 16 antibodies was higher in populations of both male and female Jamaican blood donors than in U.S. blood donors. In addition, Nonnenmacher et al. (1995) found that women enrolled as controls in a case-control study in Colombia demonstrated higher seroprevalence than similar women in Spain, and Svare et al. (1997) reported that the seroprevalence among male and female STD clinic patients in Greenland was higher than that in Denmark.

2.4.4   HPV seroprevalence in HIV-positive individuals

There are limited data on the relationship between HPV seropositivity and HIV infection. Hagensee et al. (1997) reported no associations between HIV infection and seropositivity to either HPV 16 or HPV 6 in homosexual men in Washington State. In contrast, Petter et al. (2000) found strong associations between HPV seropositivity and HIV status among women in Austria. Fifty-eight percent of HIV infected women were seropositive for a high-risk HPV type (16, 18, or 31) as compared to only 19 percent of healthy HIV-negative women. Even when compared to HIV-negative women with cervical intraepithelial neoplasia (CIN)/cancer, HIV-positive women with no clinically evident HPV-related lesions had significantly higher sero-prevalence estimates.

3   INCIDENCE

Incidence refers to the number of new HPV infections occurring in an at-risk population during a specified time interval. Cumulative incidences and incidence rates quantify the risk and rate of new infection, respectively. While incidence measures provide more accurate estimates of acquisition and risk factors for HPV infection, a limited number of studies have been designed to quantify new HPV infections.

3.1   Genital warts

A handful of studies have estimated the incidence of clinically visible genital warts. In a population-based study conducted in Rochester, Minnesota, the annual age- and gender-adjusted incidence of genital warts rose from 13 per 100,000 in the early 1950s to 106 per 100,000 in the late

1970s (Chuang et al., 1984). Other data from private physician offices and STD clinics in the United States and Europe have demonstrated 2.5- to 4.5-fold increases in the incidence of genital warts for males and females between the late 1960s/early 1970s and the late 1970s/early 1980s (Aral and Holmes, 1999, Becker et al., 1987, Koutsky et al., 1988).

Researchers in Norway recently reported that the incidence rate of genital warts among sexually active young women screened at 6-month intervals was 3.6 per 1000 per year (Turpin et al., 2002). Data from a Swedish study reported that the overall incidence of genital warts in men and women was 2.4 per 1000, with the highest incidence reported among individuals aged 15 to 29 years (Persson et al., 1996). Another recent study reported an age-standardized incidence of 1.6 per 1000 among privately insured individuals in the United States in 1999, with the highest incidence observed among individuals aged 15 to 34 years (Insinga and Dasbach, 2002). In both of these studies, the peak age of incidence was lower in women than in men.

3.2   Squamous intraepithelial lesions

Two recent studies have estimated the incidence of SIL among young women acquiring incident HPV infections. Moscicki et al. (2001) reported that 15 percent of women developed low-grade SIL within 3 years of initial HPV infection. Woodman et al. (2001) reported that the cumulative risk of any cytologic abnormality was 33 percent at 3 years after detection of an incident HPV infection. These results suggest a high rate of HPV-related lesions in young women with incident HPV infection.

3.3   Subclinical HPV infection

Between 1985 and 1986, 22-year-old Finnish women were mass screened and the crude annual incidence of HPV infection based on cytology was roughly 7 percent (Syrjanen et al., 1990). More recent studies have been designed to follow-up women who test negative for HPV DNA at an enrollment visit. Ho et al. (1998c) followed 399 female university students in New Jersey every 6 months, and reported that the cumulative incidence of HPV infection was 43 percent at 36 months. Comparable rates were reported in similarly designed studies, one conducted among women aged 15 to 19 years in the United Kingdom (44 percent at 36 months) (Woodman et al., 2001), and another conducted among a population of female university students in Seattle, Washington (43 percent at 36 months) (Winer et al., 2003). Figure 2 illustrates the cumulative incidence of HPV infection among enrolled sexually active women in the Seattle cohort. A slightly higher cumulative incidence of 55 percent at 36 months was reported in a population of 13 to 21 year old women attending family planning clinics in

San Francisco, California (Moscicki et al., 1998). A study enrolling a wider age range of women (18 to 60 years) in Brazil found that the incidence of infection was higher in women <35 years of age than in women ≥35 years (Franco et al., 1999). Incidence rates are greater for high-risk types than for low-risk types (Ho et al., 1998c, Moscicki et al., 1998, Winer et al., 2003, Woodman et al., 2001), with the highest rates typically reported for HPV 16

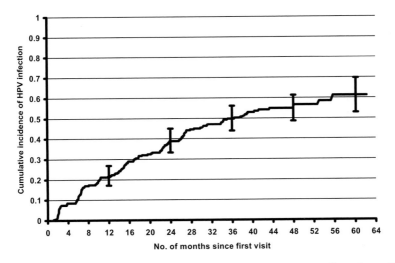

Figure 2. Cumulative incidence of HPV infection among women sexually active and HPV DNA negative at enrollment, Washington State, 1990-2000 (Data adapted from Winer et al., 2003).

(Giuliano et al., 2002, Winer et al., 2003, Woodman et al., 2001). Infection with multiple types seems to be common (Franco et al., 1999, Ho et al., 1998c, Rousseau et al., 2001, Thomas et al., 2000), as does sequential infection with new HPV types (Ho et al., 2002, Rousseau et al., 2001, Thomas et al., 2000).

The incidence of HPV infection in men has not been evaluated. Data from one small study of STD clinic attendees with multiple sex partners suggest that incidence rates may be similar for men and women (Franco et al., 1999), but further investigation of male populations is necessary to estimate the incidence of HPV infection in susceptible men.

4 RISK FACTORS FOR TRANSMISSION

The sexual transmission of genital HPV infection has been confirmed through clinical, molecular, and epidemiologic evidence. Possible routes of non-sexual transmission have also been explored, with conflicting results. Recent data from longitudinal studies have helped to elucidate potential demographic, behavioral, and host-susceptibility risk factors that have been identified in cross-sectional investigations.

4.1 Partner studies

Early data on genital wart infection provided clinical evidence of a sexual route of HPV transmission. In 1954, Barrett el al. (1954) reported 24 cases of genital warts in women whose husbands had recently returned from overseas service. All of the men had recently developed genital warts and had reported sexual contact while overseas. In another investigation, Oriel (1971) noted that genital warts developed in 64 percent of partners of individuals with genital warts.

Evidence of HPV DNA type-specific concordance in couples has also been demonstrated. Using in situ hybridization, Schneider et al. (1988) found that 87 percent of 61 men infected with HPV tested positive for the same types that were detected in the cervical specimens of their female partners. Other studies using PCR-based methods have reported type-specific concordance estimates ranging from 23 to 65 percent (Baken et al., 1995, Castellsague et al., 1997, Hippelainen et al., 1994, Strand et al., 1995). Furthermore, sequence variation analyses have shown some couples to be concordant for the same variant of HPV 16 (Ho et al., 1993, Xi et al., 1993). The transient nature of HPV infections may explain why concordance rates are lower than may be expected (Woodman et al., 2001).

4.2 Numbers of sex partners

Strong and consistent associations between increasing lifetime numbers of sex partners and increasing prevalence of HPV have been documented in cross-sectional studies (review by Xi and Koutsky, 1997). Recent longitudinal studies have reported data to suggest that the risk of HPV acquisition in young women is most strongly associated with reports of new and recent sex partners. Ho et al. (1998c) found that the risk of infection increased with increasing numbers of partners reported within the past 12 months. Moscicki et al. (2001) reported a strong positive correlation between the number of new partners per month and increased HPV acquisition. In another analysis, Winer et al. (2003) observed that report of a new sex partner within the past 12 months was associated with an increased risk of HPV acquisition. Furthermore, similar rates of acquisition were observed in enrolled virgins from the date of their first reported intercourse with a male partner and in enrolled non-virgins from the date of report of a new sex partner. Among the enrolled virgins, 29.4 percent became infected with HPV within the 12 months after sexual debut. Data from these studies suggest that rates of acquisition associated with a new partner are high, and that the critical time for HPV DNA detection is likely to be within 12 months of exposure to the virus.

Characteristics of women's male sex partners have been investigated to further elucidate the risk factors related to HPV transmission. Several case-control studies have observed that male partners of women with cervical cancer report higher numbers of female sex partners than do male partners of control women (Bosch et al., 1996, Brinton et al., 1989, Buckley et al., 1981, Castellsague et al., 1997, Kjaer et al., 1991, Munoz et al., 1996a, Zunzunegui et al., 1986). In a cross-sectional study, Burk et al. (1996a) asked university women detailed information about their male sex partners. Increasing lifetime numbers of partners of women's male sex partners, short duration of the sexual relationship, and having a male partner not currently in school were positively associated with HPV detection. Data from longitudinal studies have supported these observations. Ho et al. (1998c) reported that increased rates of HPV detection were associated with increasing lifetime numbers of sex partners of women's current male partners and with having a male partner who was not currently in school. Winer et al. (2003) reported that compared to women reporting a new male partner with no previous sex partners, the rate of HPV infection was 5 times greater among women who reported that their new male partners had had one or more previous sex partners, and 8 times greater among women who did not know how many previous sex partners their new male partners had had. Furthermore, having known a partner for more than 8 months before engaging in sexual intercourse was associated with a decreased rate of detection of HPV. Data from these studies suggest that the better and longer a women knows her partner before engaging in intercourse, the lower her risk of HPV infection.

Another male partner characteristic that has received attention as a risk factor for female HPV infection is circumcision status. In a handful of investigations, report of circumcised male partners did not appear to be more or less common among women with cervical cancer than among control women (Brinton et al., 1989, Kjaer et al., 1991), nor was circumcision status related to a woman's chances of acquiring an incident HPV infection (Winer et al., 2003). In a recent case-control study of cervical cancer in 5 countries, however, Castellsague et al. (2002) reported that in monogamous women whose male partners had multiple sex partners, there was a significant inverse association between male circumcision and the risk of cervical cancer. Furthermore, penile HPV was detected more frequently in uncircumcised men than in circumcised men. Svare et al. (2002) also observed that the risk of HPV DNA positivity was significantly elevated in uncircumcised men attending an STD clinic. More data are needed to determine whether or not male circumcision affects the transmissibility of HPV to female partners.

4.3   Other forms of sexual contact

HPV infection in women who report no history of vaginal intercourse is rare, but has been documented. In studies reporting HPV DNA detection in virgin women, prevalence estimates have ranged from 2 to 21 percent (Bauer et al., 1991, Jochmus-Kudielka et al., 1989, Ley et al., 1991, Pao et al., 1993, Karlsson et al., 1995, Rylander et al., 1994). While most of these infections have been detected in samples from vulvar swabs only, Wheeler et al. (1993) reported that 4 of 13 (31 percent) cervical samples from virgin women contained HPV DNA. Other studies have failed to detect any HPV DNA in virgin women (Andersson-Ellstrom et al., 1996, Fairley et al., 1992, Kjaer et al., 2001).

There is some evidence that HPV can be transmitted through other forms of skin-to-skin contact in women who report no history of vaginal intercourse. In an investigation of men and women with genital warts, HPV DNA was detected in the finger brush samples of 3 of 13 (38 percent) women and 9 of 14 (64 percent) men. Twenty-seven percent of subjects had the same HPV type detected in both genital and finger samples, supporting the possibility that HPV could be transmitted by finger-genital contact (Sonnex et al., 1999). Moscicki et al. (1995) reported that on further interview, all self-reported virgin women who tested positive for HPV revealed vulvar-penile contact or finger penetration. Furthermore, in a recent investigation, the cumulative incidence of HPV infection in virgin women was found to be 7.9 percent, and report of any type of non-penetrative sexual contact (including vulvar-penile, vulvar-finger, or oral-penile) was associated with an increased risk of HPV infection (Winer et al., 2003). Moreover, genital HPV infections and SIL have been detected among women who have had sex only with other women (Marrazzo et al., 1998).

Although oral HPV infection has been clearly documented (Chang et al., 1991), oral-penile contact does not appear to be a significant route of transmission. Kellokoski et al. (1992a, b) found that in women, concordance of HPV types in samples collected from genital and oral sites was rare. Furthermore, there were no cases in which an oral infection in a woman and an anogenital infection in her male partner were positive for the same HPV type. In another study reporting a high frequency of oral-penile contact (60 percent) among a cohort of sexually active female university students, only 5 of 2,619 oral samples (0.02 percent) were positive for HPV DNA (Winer et al., 2003).

4.4   Perinatal transmission

As discussed above, perinatal HPV infection is rare, but has been documented. Neonatal exposure may occur by aspiration of contaminated cervical, vaginal, or vulvar material during birth (Watts and Brunham, 1999). While cesarean delivery might be expected to reduce the risk of transmission from mother to infant, the data have been inconsistent (De Jong et al., 1982, Summersgill et al., 2001, Tseng et al., 1998).

4.5   Condom use

While condoms have been shown to be an effective barrier against HIV transmission in both men and women (Davis and Weller, 1999, de Vincenzi, 1994, Deschamps et al., 1996, Saracco et al., 1993), their ability to protect against other sexually transmitted infections is largely unknown (Zenilman et al., 1995). Data from most studies suggest that condoms are not effective in preventing genital HPV infection (Burk et al., 1996a, Davidson et al., 1994, Ho et al., 1998c, Jamison et al., 1995, Kjaer et al., 1997, Lazcano-Ponce et al., 2001a, Ludicke et al., 2001, Moscicki et al., 2001, Winer et al., 2003, Young et al., 1997). Only three studies have been designed to temporally examine the relationship between condom use and acquisition of new HPV infection (Ho et al., 1998a, Moscicki et al., 2001, Winer et al., 2003), and all of these studies reported a lack of a significant protective effect. Furthermore, for the most part, studies to date have not been designed to capture precise measures of consistency and correctness of condom usage. Improper or inconsistent usage could potentially account for the lack of an observed protective effect in most studies. The one study that did report a significant protective effect of condoms was conducted among a population of Danish female sex workers. When used consistently with private partners, condoms were associated with a decreased risk of HPV infection (Kjaer et al., 2000). Since these sex workers reported always using condoms with clients, it could be inferred that these women had more experience with using condoms and were therefore able to better ensure that their partners were using them consistently and correctly. It is also possible that since HPV is transmitted presumably through skin-to-skin contact, the virus could be transmitted through non-penetrative sexual contact occurring before the male partner puts on the condom. Additionally, condoms may be more effective in preventing female-to-male transmission than male-to-female transmission (Manhart and Koutsky, 2002).

Figure 3 summarizes the results of a meta-analysis of the relationship between condoms and genital warts, cervical HPV DNA infection, cervical SIL and CIN, and invasive cervical cancer. While condoms do not appear to be effective in protecting against initial HPV infection or SIL, the results of this meta-analysis suggest a potential protective effect against the development of genital warts, CIN II/III, and invasive cervical cancer (Manhart and Koutsky, 2002).

4.6   Smoking

Data linking cigarette smoking to HPV infection are inconclusive. The majority of studies have reported no association between smoking and the detection of HPV DNA (Bauer et al., 1993, Burk et al., 1996a, Fisher et al., 1991, Hildesheim et al., 1993, Karlsson et al., 1995, Kjaer et al., 1990, Kjaer et al., 1997, Marrero et al., 1994, Meekin et al., 1992, Moscicki et al., 1990, Reed et al., 1993, Rohan et al., 1991, Silins et al., 2000, Venuti et al., 1994, Villa and Franco, 1989, Wheeler et al., 1993), including a recent prospective study (Moscicki et al., 2001). A handful of studies have found positive associations between smoking and HPV prevalence (Davidson et al., 1994, Fairley et al., 1994b, Ley et al., 1991, Sellors et al., 2000), but these associations tended to diminish after adjustment for sexual behavior variables (Fairley et al., 1994b, Ley et al., 1991). In a recent prospective analysis, a significant association between current smoking and incident HPV infection was detected, even after adjustment for potential confounding variables (including oral contraceptive use, acquisition of a new partner and number of lifetime partners, and condom use with new partners) (Winer et al., 2003). It is unclear whether this positive association is due to residual confounding by unmeasured sexual behaviors, or whether current smoking may actually increase the risk of HPV acquisition.

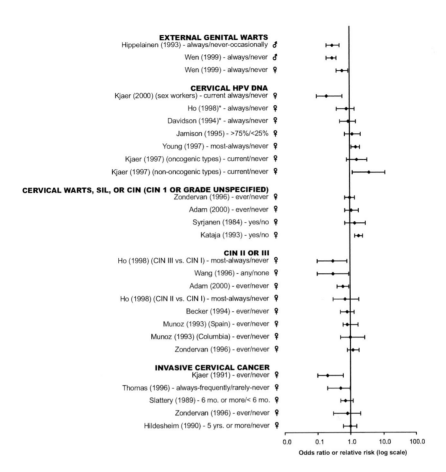

Figure 3. Effect of condom use on prevention of external genital warts; detection of HPV DNA in cervical samples; cervical SIL, cervical warts, or CIN (grade I or unspecified); and CIN II/III and invasive cervical cancer. Asterisk indicates studies reporting relative risk estimates (Adam et al., 2000, Becker et al., 1994b, Davidson et al., 1994, Hildesheim et al., 1990, Hippelainen et al., 1993, Ho et al., 1998a, Ho et al., 1998c, Jamison et al., 1995, Kataja et al., 1993, Kjaer et al., 1990, Kjaer et al., 2000, Kjaer et al., 1997, Munoz et al., 1993, Slattery et al., 1989, Syrjanen et al., 1984, Thomas et al., 1996, Wang and Lin, 1996, Wen et al., 1999, Young et al., 1997, Zondervan et al., 1996). (Figure adapted from Manhart and Koutsky, 2002)

4.7 Host Susceptibility

4.7.1 Hormonal Factors

There is evidence to suggest that HPV infection may be influenced by hormonal factors. Estrogen stimulation enhances expression of the E6 and

E7 genes in SiHa cervical carcinoma cells (Mitrani-Rosenbaum et al., 1989), and progesterone has been shown to increase HPV 16 and HPV 18 gene expression at the messenger RNA level (Chen et al., 1996, Mittal et al., 1993, Yuan et al., 1999). There have also been associations between oral contraceptive use and condylomata acuminata (Schneider and Koutsky, 1992). Furthermore, during pregnancy, when hormone levels are raised, anecdotal reports suggest that condyloma acuminatum increases in size in some women (Fife et al., 1987).

4.7.1.1 Oral Contraceptives. Data on the association between oral contraceptive use and detection of HPV DNA have been inconsistent. While most studies have reported no association between use of oral contraceptives and detection of HPV DNA (Bauer et al., 1993, Burk et al., 1996a, Davidson et al., 1994, Fairley et al., 1994b, Hildesheim et al., 1993, Karlsson et al., 1995, Meekin et al., 1992, Reed et al., 1993, Rohan et al., 1991, Wheeler et al., 1993), a couple of studies found a protective effect (Giuliano et al., 1999, Moscicki et al., 2001), and a handful of other studies have reported a positive relationship between oral contraceptive use and HPV infection (Kjaer et al., 1997, Ley et al., 1991, Lorincz et al., 1990, Negrini and et al., 1990, Sikstrom et al., 1995, Winer et al., 2003), even after adjustment for sexual behavior variables such as lifetime and recent numbers of sex partners. In addition, one study reported a positive relationship between hormonal contraceptive use and increased detection of HPV 16 non-prototype-like variants (Xi et al., 2002). While it is possible that hormonal contraceptives may influence host susceptibility to HPV infection, another possibility is that oral contraceptive use is a surrogate marker for other risky sexual behaviors that were not measured.

4.7.1.2 Pregnancy. Most studies have failed to demonstrate an association between increased HPV prevalence and pregnancy (Basta et al., 1994, Chang-Claude et al., 1996, Csango et al., 1992, de Roda Husman et al., 1995, Delvenne et al., 1992, Freitag et al., 1996, Kataja et al., 1993, Kemp et al., 1992, Kuhler-Obbarius et al., 1994, Nishikawa et al., 1991, Peng et al., 1990, Smith et al., 1991, Soares et al., 1990). Some studies, however, have observed an increased prevalence in pregnant as compared to non-pregnant women (Czegledy et al., 1989, Saito et al., 1992, Schneider et al., 1987, Villa and Franco, 1989), and decreasing prevalence postpartum (Czegledy et al., 1989, Rando et al., 1989, Schneider et al., 1987). Two other studies have reported an association between increasing number of pregnancies and increasing prevalence of HPV infection (Gopalkrishna et al., 1995, Hildesheim et al., 1993). It is possible that fluctuations in hormone levels or changes in immune tolerance or local physiologic change during pregnancy could account for these observations. A methodological issue common to these studies, however, is lack of a comparable control group (Koutsky and Kiviat, 1999).

4.7.2 Immunosuppression

As discussed above, immunosuppressed individuals demonstrate an increased prevalence of HPV infection as compared to otherwise healthy individuals. This observation could be attributed to an increased risk of infection in immunosuppressed individuals or to impairment of the body's ability to suppress a latent infection. The finding that immunosuppressed individuals with HPV infection tend to have higher HPV DNA levels than nonimmunosuppressed individuals supports the latter theory (Ho et al., 1994).

5   NATURAL HISTORY OF HPV INFECTION

Most genital HPV infections do not manifest with clinically visible signs or symptoms (Mao et al., 2003). Nevertheless, genital HPV infections can cause pre-cancerous and cancerous lesions, as well as condylomata, laryngeal papillomas, and papillomas at non-anogenital epithelial sites.

5.1   Duration of genital warts

ecause genital warts tend to be treated, little is known about their natural history. Data from randomized clinical trials show that without treatment, genital warts may disappear, increase in size or number, or remain unchanged (Eron et al., 1986, Condylomata International Collaborative Study Group, 1991, Kirby et al., 1988, Monsonego et al., 1996). With treatment, clearance rates have ranged from 32 to 88 percent (Buck et al., 2002, Edwards et al., 1998, Stone, 1995). The number of warts in the first episode may be associated with time to clearance, with fewer warts predicting faster clearance rates (Wilson et al., 2001).

5.2   Duration of squamous intraepithelial lesions

Woodman et al. (2001) reported that in young women followed up at 6-month intervals, the median duration of an initial episode of cytologic abnormality was 8.7 months. Regression of low-grade lesions is common (Kadish et al., 2002, Ostor, 1993), with several studies reporting that over half of low-grade lesions will regress within several years of observation (Ostor, 1993, Syrjanen et al., 1992). Rates of regression are lower in HIV-infected women (Belafsky et al., 1996, Delmas et al., 2000, Six et al., 1998) and high-grade lesions are less likely to regress than low-grade lesions (Flannelly et al., 1994, Holowaty et al., 1999, Ostor, 1993).

5.3   Persistent detection of HPV infection

Viral persistence refers to an infection that persists in the body for an extended period of time, but not necessarily in a fully infectious form (Mims et al., 1995). It is likely that a portion of HPV infected women have low-level, persistent infections that are undetectable using current testing methods. Therefore, it is important to clarify that the term "persistence," when used in epidemiologic studies of HPV infection, actually refers to persistent detection of HPV infection.

Data from these studies suggest that the majority of HPV infections are detected transiently, with most new infections becoming undetectable within one to two years (Evander et al., 1995, Hildesheim et al., 1994, Ho et al., 1998c, Moscicki et al., 1993, Moscicki et al., 1998, Reeves et al., 1989, Rosenfeld et al., 1992, Schneider et al., 1992, Wheeler et al., 1993). Among cohorts of young women, Ho et al. (1998c) reported that the median duration of initial HPV infection was 8 months, and Woodman et al. (2001) reported a median duration of 13.7 months. Persistent detection of infection is associated with an increased risk of cervical dysplasia (Chua and Hjerpe, 1996, Hildesheim et al., 1994, Ho et al., 1995, Ho et al., 1998c, Koutsky et al., 1992, Moscicki et al., 1998, Nobbenhuis et al., 1999, Schlecht et al., 2001), and HPV 16 has generally been shown to persist longer than other types (Brisson et al., 1996, Elfgren et al., 2000, Giuliano et al., 2002, Munoz and Bosch, 1992). Data on the effect of viral load on HPV persistence or the risk of dysplasia have been inconsistent (Beskow and Gyllensten, 2002, Flannelly et al., 1995, Ho et al., 1998b, Josefsson et al., 2000, Lorincz et al., 2002, van Duin et al., 2002, Woodman et al., 2001, Ylitalo et al., 2000).

In longitudinal studies of HPV persistence, it may not be possible to determine whether re-detection of HPV DNA represents reactivation of a latent infection, intermittent false-negative testing, or a new exposure. Data from a study by Xi et al. (1995), however, showed that in 100 percent of cases, samples obtained from an individual woman at different points in time contained the same HPV 16 variant. This was true even after an intercurrent negative result, and adds to the body of data illustrating the persistent nature of HPV 16 infection.

Rousseau et al. (2001) reported that among a cohort of Brazilian women, persistent detection of HPV DNA was independent of coinfection with other HPV types. Liaw et al. (2001) observed that HPV 16 positivity did not have an effect on the persistence of other type-specific infections. These results suggest that type-specific persistence is independent of other infections.

Other questions arise concerning the natural history of multiple infections. Ho et al. (1998c) found that in a cohort of university women, detection of multiple HPV types was a greater predictor of persistent infection than detection of a high-risk type at a prior visit. Whether coinfection with multiple HPV types confers a greater risk of developing subsequent CIN is unclear (Herrero et al., 2000, Schiffman et al., 1993, Luostarinen et al., 1999, Silins et al., 1999).

Susceptibility to HPV infection and carcinogenic progression may be influenced by genetic variations in major histocompatibility complex (MHC) genes. These genes encode for human leukocyte antigen (HLA) class I and class II alleles. In domestic rabbits, the ability to clear HPV infection over time has been correlated with certain MHC haplotypes (Salmon et al., 2000). A recent longitudinal study explored whether HLA polymorphisms were related to differences in rates of HPV positivity and persistence, and the authors concluded that HLA class II polymorphisms seem to be involved in the clearance and maintenance of infection (Maciag et al., 2002). Certain polymorphisms may alter an HPV-infected woman's risk of developing CIN or cervical cancer. Numerous studies have demonstrated a protective effect of DRB1*13 on the development of CIN or cervical cancer (Apple et al., 1995, Apple et al., 1994, Hildesheim et al., 1998, Krul et al., 1999, Lin et al., 2001, Maciag et al., 2000, Odunsi et al., 1996, Sanjeevi et al., 1996, Sastre-Garau et al., 1996, Wang et al., 2001). Studies evaluating the effects of other polymorphisms have reported varied results (Allen et al., 1996, Brady et al., 1999, Cuzick et al., 2000, Helland et al., 1994, Wank and Thomssen, 1991).

Detection of HPV DNA and serum antibodies do not always coincide, with studies demonstrating that 20 to 50 percent of women with detectable HPV DNA or associated lesions do not have detectable antibodies (Carter et al., 2000, Carter et al., 1996, Carter et al., 1995, Dillner et al., 1995, Eisemann et al., 1996, Kirnbauer et al., 1994, Wikstrom et al., 1997). Persistence of HPV 16 DNA is associated with an increased likelihood of HPV 16 seroconversion (Carter et al., 2000, Carter et al., 1996, de Gruijl et al., 1999, Wideroff et al., 1995). Carter et al. (1996) showed that the median time to seroconversion among university women with incident HPV 16 infections was 8.3 months.

Hildesheim et al. (1994) reported that women ≥30 years of age had a significantly higher percentage of persistent detection of infection at a follow-up visit than women ≤24 years of age. It is likely, however, that baseline infections detected in older women tend to represent persistent infections acquired at a young age, whereas infections detected in younger women are more likely to represent new and more transient infections. Ho et al. (1998c) also noted an association between older age and an increased risk of HPV persistence, but the cohort under study was restricted to university-aged women. Ahdieh et al. (2001) reported that HPV persistence was more common in HIV-positive women >35 years of age than in younger HIV-positive women. In contrast to these trends, Brisson et al. (1996) observed an opposite age-related pattern of persistence. In general, it is difficult to compare results from studies of persistent HPV infection. Different definitions of persistence (for example, HPV positivity on two samples collected six months apart or one year apart) and of older versus younger women have been used. Longitudinal studies following up a wide age-range of women with type-specific (and preferably variant specific) incident infections would help to clarify this phenomenon. However, even in those studies, measures would be of persistent detection rather than persistent infection.

Immunosuppression is associated with increased likelihood and duration of HPV infection. Several studies have found that persistence is more common in HIV-positive women than in HIV-negative women, and that lower CD4 counts are associated with longer duration of detection of HPV infection (Ahdieh et al., 2001, Sun et al., 1997, Vernon et al., 1994) (Minkoff et al., 1998).

The impact of factors such as smoking, oral contraceptive use, and nutrition has not yet been thoroughly investigated. While the risk of cervical dysplasia tends to be increased among smokers (Coker et al., 2002), a couple of studies have reported that smoking was protective against persistent HPV infection (Hildesheim et al., 1994, Ho et al., 1998c). Some studies have reported that oral contraceptive use is associated with an increased likelihood of HPV persistence (Brisson et al., 1996, Vandenvelde and Van Beers, 1992), while another study reported no association (Ho et al., 1998c). Another recent study examined the relationship between HPV persistence and dietary intake and circulating levels of folate, methionine, and B vitamins. Higher circulating levels of vitamin B_{12} were associated with decreased persistence (Sedjo et al., 2002a). In another investigation, higher levels of vegetable consumption and circulating cis-lycopene concentrations were associated with a reduction in HPV persistence (Sedjo et al., 2002b).

CONCLUSION

Genital HPV infections are prevalent among sexually active young adults and the year following sexual debut is a time of high risk among females. Far less is known about risk of infection in men, although current evidence suggests that the rate of acquisition, the duration of infection, or both may be lower among heterosexual men than among women. Anal HPV infection is prevalent among men who have sex with men and peri-anal infection is common among women, regardless of whether they report receptive anal intercourse (Mao et al., 2003). Although receptive oral intercourse is commonly practiced among sexually active women, oral HPV infection is rare and not clearly linked with report of oral-penile contact. Some reports indicate that digital-genital contact or other forms of skin-to-skin contact occasionally transmit genital HPV types. Male condoms, which provide little if any protection against HPV acquisition, may offer some protection against the development of external genital warts, carcinoma in situ, and anogenital cancers. While HPV types 6 and 11 cause most external genital warts, the majority of HPV infections (including oncogenic types HPV 16, 18 and others) are asymptomatic and clinically unremarkable. Regardless of type, the majority of all genital HPV infections are transient and detectable by PCR-based methods for less than 12 months. Immune responses to HPV develop relatively slowly (median of 6 months or longer), and are largely type-specific. Most individuals eventually develop effective, albeit low titer responses that appear to provide protection against infection by the same type. It is not known whether some, or most individuals retain copies of HPV genomes several years after viral DNA can no longer be detected. Furthermore, the rate at which "latent" or undetectable HPV infections in immunocompetent adults become detectable and neoplastic over the course of 10 to 40 years remains to be determined.

Much has been learned about the epidemiology of genital HPV infections in the pre-vaccine era. As we move into the era of prophylactic HPV vaccines, it will be important to monitor how such vaccines impact rates of infection, external genital warts, SIL, and anogenital cancers.

REFERENCES

Adam E, Berkova Z, Daxnerova Z, et al. Papillomavirus detection: demographic and behavioral characteristics influencing the identification of cervical disease. Am J Obstet Gynecol 2000;182:257-64.

af Geijersstam V, Eklund C, Wang Z, et al. A survey of seroprevalence of human papillomavirus types 16, 18 and 33 among children. Int J Cancer 1999;80:489-93.

af Geijersstam V, Wang Z, Lewensohn-Fuchs I, et al. Trends in seroprevalence of human papillomavirus type 16 among pregnant women in Stockholm, Sweden, during 1969-1989. Int J Cancer 1998;76:341-4.

Ahdieh L, Klein RS, Burk R, et al. Prevalence, incidence, and type-specific persistence of human papillomavirus in human immunodeficiency virus (HIV)-positive and HIV-negative women. J Infect Dis 2001;184:682-90.

Allen M, Kalantari M, Ylitalo N, et al. HLA DQ-DR haplotype and susceptibility to cervical carcinoma: indications of increased risk for development of cervical carcinoma in individuals infected with HPV 18. Tissue Antigens 1996;48:32-7.

Alloub MI, Barr BB, McLaren KM, et al. Human papillomavirus infection and cervical intraepithelial neoplasia in women with renal allografts. BMJ 1989;298:153-6.

Andersson-Ellstrom A, Hagmar BM, Johansson B, et al. Human papillomavirus deoxyribonucleic acid in cervix only detected in girls after coitus. Int J STD AIDS 1996; 7:333-6.

Apple RJ, Becker TM, Wheeler CM, et al. Comparison of human leukocyte antigen DR-DQ disease associations found with cervical dysplasia and invasive cervical carcinoma. J Natl Cancer Inst 1995;87:427-36.

Apple RJ, Erlich HA, Klitz W, et al. HLA DR-DQ associations with cervical carcinoma show papillomavirus-type specificity. Nat Genet 1994;6:157-62.

Aral SO, Holmes KK. Epidemiology of sexual behavior and sexually transmitted diseases. In: Holmes KK, Sparling PF, Mardh P-A, et al., eds. Sexually transmitted diseases, third edition. New York: McGraw-Hill. 1999:39-76.

Baken LA, Koutsky LA, Kuypers J, et al. Genital human papillomavirus infection among male and female sex partners: prevalence and type-specific concordance. J Infect Dis 1995;171: 429-32.

Barrett TJ, Silbar JD, McGinley JP. Genital warts -- a venereal disease. JAMA 1954;154:333-334.

Basta A, Strama M, Pitynski K, et al. [Human papilloma virus (HPV) infections of the uterine cervix, vagina and vulva in women of childbearing age]. Ginekol Pol 1994;65:563-9.

Bauer HM, Hildesheim A, Schiffman MH, et al. Determinants of genital human papillomavirus infection in low-risk women in Portland, Oregon. Sex Transm Dis 1993; 20:274-8.

Bauer HM, Ting Y, Greer CE, et al. Genital human papillomavirus infection in female university students as determined by a PCR-based method. JAMA 1991;265:472-7.

Becker TM, Stone KM, Alexander ER. Genital human papillomavirus infection. A growing concern. Obstet Gynecol Clin North Am 1987;14:389-96.

Becker TM, Wheeler CM, McGough NS, et al. Sexually transmitted diseases and other risk factors for cervical dysplasia among southwestern Hispanic and non-Hispanic white women. JAMA 1994a;271:1181-8.

Becker TM, Wheeler CM, McGough NS, et al. Contraceptive and reproductive risks for cervical dysplasia in southwestern Hispanic and non-Hispanic white women. Int J Epidemiol 1994b;23:913-22.

Belafsky P, Clark RA, Kissinger P, et al. Natural history of low-grade squamous intraepithelial lesions in women infected with human immunodeficiency virus. J Acquir Immune Defic Syndr Hum Retrovirol 1996;11:511-2.

Berumen J, Ordonez RM, Lazcano E, et al. Asian-American variants of human papillomavirus 16 and risk for cervical cancer: a case-control study. J Natl Cancer Inst 2001;93:1325-30.

Beskow AH, Gyllensten UB. Host genetic control of HPV 16 titer in carcinoma in situ of the cervix uteri. Int J Cancer 2002;101:526-31.

Bjorge T, Gunbjorud AB, Langmark F, et al. Cervical mass screening in Norway--510,000 smears a year. Cancer Detect Prev 1994;18:463-70.

Bosch FX, Castellsague X, Munoz N, et al. Male sexual behavior and human papillomavirus DNA: key risk factors for cervical cancer in Spain. J Natl Cancer Inst 1996;88:1060-7.

Bosch FX, Manos MM, Munoz N, et al. Prevalence of human papillomavirus in cervical cancer: a worldwide perspective. International biological study on cervical cancer (IBSCC) Study Group. J Natl Cancer Inst 1995;87:796-802.

Bosch FX, Munoz N, de Sanjose S, et al. Human papillomavirus and cervical intraepithelial neoplasia grade III/carcinoma in situ: a case-control study in Spain and Colombia. Cancer Epidemiol Biomarkers Prev 1993;2:415-22.

Brady CS, Duggan-Keen MF, Davidson JA, et al. Human papillomavirus type 16 E6 variants in cervical carcinoma: relationship to host genetic factors and clinical parameters. J Gen Virol 1999;80:3233-40.

Breese PL, Judson FN, Penley KA, et al. Anal human papillomavirus infection among homosexual and bisexual men: prevalence of type-specific infection and association with human immunodeficiency virus. Sex Transm Dis 1995;22:7-14.

Brinton LA, Reeves WC, Brenes MM, et al. The male factor in the etiology of cervical cancer among sexually monogamous women. Int J Cancer 1989;44:199-203.

Brisson J, Bairati I, Morin C, et al. Determinants of persistent detection of human papillomavirus DNA in the uterine cervix. J Infect Dis 1996;173:794-9.

British Cooperative Clinical Group. Cervical cytology screening in sexually transmitted diseases clinics in the United Kingdom. Genitourin Med 1987;63:40-3.

Brown DR, Schroeder JM, Bryan JT, et al. Detection of multiple human papillomavirus types in Condylomata acuminata lesions from otherwise healthy and immunosuppressed patients. J Clin Microbiol 1999;37:3316-22.

Buck HW, Fortier M, Knudsen J, et al. Imiquimod 5% cream in the treatment of anogenital warts in female patients. Int J Gynaecol Obstet 2002;77:231-8.

Buckley JD, Harris RW, Doll R, et al. Case-control study of the husbands of women with dysplasia or carcinoma of the cervix uteri. Lancet 1981;2:1010-5.

Burk RD, Ho GYF, Beardsley L, et al. Sexual behavior and partner characteristics are the predominant risk factors for genital human papillomavirus infection in young women. J Infect Dis 1996a;174:679-689.

Burk RD, Kelly P, Feldman J, et al. Declining prevalence of cervicovaginal human papillomavirus infection with age is independent of other risk factors. Sex Transm Dis 1996b; 23:333-41.

Byrne MA, Taylor-Robinson D, Munday PE, et al. The common occurrence of human papillomavirus infection and intraepithelial neoplasia in women infected by HIV. AIDS 1989;3:379-82.

Carter JJ, Koutsky LA, Hughes JP, et al. Comparison of human papillomavirus types 16, 18, and 6 capsid antibody responses following incident infection. J Infect Dis 2000;181:1911-9.

Carter JJ, Koutsky LA, Wipf GC, et al. The natural history of human papillomavirus type 16 capsid antibodies among a cohort of university women. J Infect Dis 1996;174:927-36.

Carter JJ, Wipf GC, Hagensee ME, et al. Use of human papillomavirus type 6 capsids to detect antibodies in people with genital warts. J Infect Dis 1995;172:11-8.

Cason J, Kaye JN, Jewers RJ, et al. Perinatal infection and persistence of human papillomavirus types 16 and 18 in infants. J Med Virol 1995;47:209-18.

Castellsague X, Bosch FX, Munoz N, et al. Male circumcision, penile human papillomavirus infection, and cervical cancer in female partners. N Engl J Med 2002;346:1105-12.

Castellsague X, Ghaffari A, Daniel RW, et al. Prevalence of penile human papillomavirus DNA in husbands of women with and without cervical neoplasia: a study in Spain and Colombia. J Infect Dis 1997;176:353-61.

Chan SY, Ho L, Ong CK, et al. Molecular variants of human papillomavirus type 16 from four continents suggest ancient pandemic spread of the virus and its coevolution with humankind. J Virol 1992;66:2057-66.

Chang DY, Chen RJ, Lee SC, et al. Prevalence of single and multiple infection with human papillomaviruses in various grades of cervical neoplasia. J Med Microbiol 1997;46:54-60.

Chang F, Syrjanen S, Kellokoski J, et al. Human papillomavirus (HPV) infections and their associations with oral disease. J Oral Pathol Med 1991;20:305-17.

Chang-Claude J, Schneider A, Smith E, et al. Longitudinal study of the effects of pregnancy and other factors on detection of HPV. Gynecol Oncol 1996;60:355-62.

Chen YH, Huang LH, Chen TM. Differential effects of progestins and estrogens on long control regions of human papillomavirus types 16 and 18. Biochem Biophys Res Commun 1996;224:651-9.

Chiasson MA, Ellerbrock TV, Bush TJ, et al. Increased prevalence of vulvovaginal condyloma and vulvar intraepithelial neoplasia in women infected with the human immunodeficiency virus. Obstet Gynecol 1997;89:690-4.

Chirgwin KD, Feldman J, Augenbraun M, et al. Incidence of venereal warts in human immunodeficiency virus-infected and uninfected women. J Infect Dis 1995;172:235-8.

Chua KL, Hjerpe A. Persistence of human papillomavirus (HPV) infections preceding cervical carcinoma. Cancer 1996;77:121-7.

Chuang TY, Perry HO, Kurland LT, et al. Condyloma acuminatum in Rochester, Minn., 1950-1978. I. Epidemiology and clinical features. Arch Dermatol 1984;120:469-75.

Coker AL, Bond SM, Williams A, et al. Active and passive smoking, high-risk human papillomaviruses and cervical neoplasia. Cancer Detect Prev 2002;26:121-8.

Coker AL, Jenkins GR, Busnardo MS, et al. Human papillomaviruses and cervical neoplasia in South Carolina. Cancer Epidemiol Biomarkers Prev 1993;2:207-12.

Coleman N, Birley HD, Renton AM, et al. Immunological events in regressing genital warts. Am J Clin Pathol 1994;102:768-74.

Combita AL, Bravo MM, Touze A, et al. Serologic response to human oncogenic papillomavirus types 16, 18, 31, 33, 39, 58 and 59 virus-like particles in colombian women with invasive cervical cancer. Int J Cancer 2002;97:796-803.

Condylomata International Collaborative Study Group. Recurrent condylomata acuminata treated with recombinant interferon alfa-2a. A multicenter double-blind placebo-controlled clinical trial. JAMA 1991;265:2684-7.

Conley LJ, Ellerbrock TV, Bush TJ, et al. HIV-1 infection and risk of vulvovaginal and perianal condylomata acuminata and intraepithelial neoplasia: a prospective cohort study. Lancet 2002;359:108-13.

Critchlow CW, Holmes KK, Wood R, et al. Association of human immunodeficiency virus and anal human papillomavirus infection among homosexual men. Arch Intern Med 1992; 152:1673-6.

Critchlow CW, Koutsky LA. Epidemiology of human papillomavirus infection. In: Mindel A, ed. Genital Warts: Human Papillomavirus Infection. London: Edward Arnold. 1995:53-81.

Csango PA, Skuland J, Nilsen A, et al. Papillomavirus infection among abortion applicants and patients at a sexually transmitted disease clinic. Sex Transm Dis 1992;19:149-53.

Cubie HA, Plumstead M, Zhang W, et al. Presence of antibodies to human papillomavirus virus-like particles (VLPs) in 11-13-year-old schoolgirls. J Med Virol 1998;56:210-6.

Cui MH, Liu YQ, Li HL, et al. Human papillomavirus in condyloma acuminata and other benign lesions of the female genital tract. Chin Med J (Engl) 1994;107:703-8.

Cuzick J, Terry G, Ho L, et al. Association between high-risk HPV types, HLA DRB1* and DQB1* alleles and cervical cancer in British women. Br J Cancer 2000;82:1348-52.

Czegledy J, Gergely L, Endrodi I. Detection of human papillomavirus deoxyribonucleic acid by filter in situ hybridization during pregnancy. J Med Virol 1989;28:250-4.

Czegledy J, Rogo KO, Evander M, et al. High-risk human papillomavirus types in cytologically normal cervical scrapes from Kenya. Med Microbiol Immunol (Berl) 1992; 180:321-6.

Davidson M, Schnitzer PG, Bulkow LR, et al. The prevalence of cervical infection with human papillomaviruses and cervical dysplasia in Alaska Native women. J Infect Dis 1994; 169:792-800.

Davis KR, Weller SC. The effectiveness of condoms in reducing heterosexual transmission of HIV. Fam Plann Perspect 1999;31:272-9.

de Gruijl TD, Bontkes HJ, Walboomers JM, et al. Immune responses against human papillomavirus (HPV) type 16 virus-like particles in a cohort study of women with cervical intraepithelial neoplasia. I. Differential T-helper and IgG responses in relation to HPV infection and disease outcome. J Gen Virol 1999;80:399-408.

De Jong AR, Weiss JC, Brent RL. Condyloma acuminata in children. Am J Dis Child 1982; 136:704-6.

de Roda Husman AM, Walboomers JM, Hopman E, et al. HPV prevalence in cytomorphologically normal cervical scrapes of pregnant women as determined by PCR: the age-related pattern. J Med Virol 1995;46:97-102.

de Villiers EM. Heterogeneity of the human papillomavirus group. J Virol 1989;63:4898-903.

de Vincenzi I. A longitudinal study of human immunodeficiency virus transmission by heterosexual partners. European Study Group on Heterosexual Transmission of HIV. N Engl J Med 1994;331:341-346.

Delmas MC, Larsen C, van Benthem B, et al. Cervical squamous intraepithelial lesions in HIV-infected women: prevalence, incidence and regression. European Study Group on Natural History of HIV Infection in Women. AIDS 2000;14:1775-84.

Delvenne P, Engellenner WJ, Ma SF, et al. Detection of human papillomavirus DNA in biopsy-proven cervical squamous intraepithelial lesions in pregnant women. J Reprod Med 1992;37:829-33.

Deschamps MM, Pape JW, Hafner A, et al. Heterosexual transmission of HIV in Haiti. Ann Intern Med 1996;125:324-330.

Dillner J, Lehtinen M, Bjorge T, et al. Prospective seroepidemiologic study of human papillomavirus infection as a risk factor for invasive cervical cancer. J Natl Cancer Inst 1997; 89:1293-9.

Dillner J, Wiklund F, Lenner P, et al. Antibodies against linear and conformational epitopes of human papillomavirus type 16 that independently associate with incident cervical cancer. Int J Cancer 1995;60:377-82.

Edelman M, Fox AS, Alderman EM, et al. Cervical Papanicolaou smear abnormalities in inner city Bronx adolescents: prevalence, progression, and immune modifiers. Cancer 1999; 87: 184-9.

Edwards L, Ferenczy A, Eron L, et al. Self-administered topical 5% imiquimod cream for external anogenital warts. HPV Study Group. Human PapillomaVirus. Arch Dermatol 1998;134:25-30.

Eisemann C, Fisher SG, Gross G, et al. Antibodies to human papillomavirus type 11 virus-like particles in sera of patients with genital warts and in control groups. J Gen Virol 1996; 77:1799-803.

Elfgren K, Kalantari M, Moberger B, et al. A population-based five-year follow-up study of cervical human papillomavirus infection. Am J Obstet Gynecol 2000;183:561-7.

Ellerbrock TV, Chiasson MA, Bush TJ, et al. Incidence of cervical squamous intraepithelial lesions in HIV-infected women. JAMA 2000;283:1031-7.

Engels H, Nyongo A, Temmerman M, et al. Cervical cancer screening and detection of genital HPV-infection and chlamydial infection by PCR in different groups of Kenyan women. Ann Soc Belg Med Trop 1992;72:53-62.

Eron LJ, Judson F, Tucker S, et al. Interferon therapy for condylomata acuminata. N Engl J Med 1986;315:1059-64.

Evander M, Edlund K, Gustafsson A, et al. Human papillomavirus infection is transient in young women: a population-based cohort study. J Infect Dis 1995;171:1026-30.

Fairley CK, Chen S, Tabrizi SN, et al. The absence of genital human papillomavirus DNA in virginal women. Int J STD AIDS 1992;3:414-7.

Fairley CK, Chen S, Tabrizi SN, et al. Prevalence of HPV DNA in cervical specimens in women with renal transplants: a comparison with dialysis-dependent patients and patients with renal impairment. Nephrol Dial Transplant 1994a;9:416-20.

Fairley CK, Chen S, Ugoni A, et al. Human papillomavirus infection and its relationship to recent and distant sexual partners. Obstet Gynecol 1994b;84:755-759.

Fife KH, Rogers RE, Zwickl BW. Symptomatic and asymptomatic cervical infections with human papillomavirus during pregnancy. J Infect Dis 1987;156:904-11.

Fisher M, Rosenfeld WD, Burk RD. Cervicovaginal human papillomavirus infection in suburban adolescents and young adults. J Pediatr 1991;119:837-838.

Flannelly G, Anderson D, Kitchener HC, et al. Management of women with mild and moderate cervical dyskaryosis. Bmj 1994;308:1399-403.

Flannelly G, Jiang G, Anderson D, et al. Serial quantitation of HPV-16 in the smears of women with mild and moderate dyskaryosis. J Med Virol 1995;47:6-9.

Fonn S, Bloch B, Mabina M, et al. Prevalence of pre-cancerous lesions and cervical cancer in South Africa -- a multicentre study. S Afr Med J 2002;92:148-56.

Franceschi S, Castellsague X, Dal Maso L, et al. Prevalence and determinants of human papillomavirus genital infection in men. Br J Cancer 2002;86:705-11.

Franco EL, Villa LL, Sobrinho JP, et al. Epidemiology of acquisition and clearance of cervical human papillomavirus infection in women from a high-risk area for cervical cancer. J Infect Dis 1999;180:1415-23.

Fredericks BD, Balkin A, Daniel HW, et al. Transmission of human papillomaviruses from mother to child. Aust N Z J Obstet Gynaecol 1993;33:30-2.

Freitag P, Drazd'akova M, Zivny J. [Prevalence of HPV infection and histologic correlations]. Ceska Gynekol 1996;61:150-3.

Giuliano AR, Harris R, Sedjo RL, et al. Incidence, prevalence, and clearance of type-specific human papillomavirus infections: The Young Women's Health Study. J Infect Dis 2002; 186:462-9.

Giuliano AR, Papenfuss M, Schneider A, et al. Risk factors for high-risk type human papillomavirus infection among Mexican-American women. Cancer Epidemiol Biomarkers Prev 1999;8:615-20.

Goldberg GL, Vermund SH, Schiffman MH, et al. Comparison of Cytobrush and cervicovaginal lavage sampling methods for the detection of genital human papillomavirus. Am J Obstet Gynecol 1989;161:1669-72.

Gopalkrishna V, Murthy NS, Sharma JK, et al. Increased human papillomavirus infection with the increasing number of pregnancies in Indian women. J Infect Dis 1995;171:254-5.

Greer CE, Wheeler CM, Ladner MB, et al. Human papillomavirus (HPV) type distribution and serological response to HPV type 6 virus-like particles in patients with genital warts. J Clin Microbiol 1995;33:2058-63.

Hagensee ME, Kiviat N, Critchlow CW, et al. Seroprevalence of human papillomavirus types 6 and 16 capsid antibodies in homosexual men. J Infect Dis 1997;176:625-31.

Hagensee ME, Slavinsky J, 3rd, Gaffga CM, et al. Seroprevalence of human papillomavirus type 16 in pregnant women. Obstet Gynecol 1999;94:653-8.

Hankins C, Coutlee F, Lapointe N, et al. Prevalence of risk factors associated with human papillomavirus infection in women living with HIV. Canadian Women's HIV Study Group. Canad Med Assoc J 1999;160:185-91.

Healey SM, Aronson KJ, Mao Y, et al. Oncogenic human papillomavirus infection and cervical lesions in aboriginal women of Nunavut, Canada. Sex Transm Dis 2001;28:694-700.

Heim K, Christensen ND, Hoepfl R, et al. Serum IgG, IgM, and IgA reactivity to human papillomavirus types 11 and 6 virus-like particles in different gynecologic patient groups. J Infect Dis 1995;172:395-402.

Helland A, Borresen AL, Kristensen G, et al. DQA1 and DQB1 genes in patients with squamous cell carcinoma of the cervix: relationship to human papillomavirus infection and prognosis. Cancer Epidemiol Biomarkers Prev 1994;3:479-86.

Herrero R, Hildesheim A, Bratti C, et al. Population-based study of human papillomavirus infection and cervical neoplasia in rural Costa Rica. J Natl Cancer Inst 2000;92:464-74.

Herrero R, Schiffman MH, Bratti C, et al. Design and methods of a population-based natural history study of cervical neoplasia in a rural province of Costa Rica: the Guanacaste Project. Rev Panam Salud Publica 1997;1:362-75.

Heystek MJ, de Jonge ET, Meyer HP, et al. Screening for cervical neoplasia in Mamelodi--lessons from an unscreened population. S Afr Med J 1995;85:1180-2.

Hildesheim A, Brinton LA, Mallin K, et al. Barrier and spermicidal contraceptive methods and risk of invasive cervical cancer. Epidemiology 1990;1:266-72.

Hildesheim A, Gravitt P, Schiffman MH, et al. Determinants of genital human papillomavirus infection in low-income women in Washington, D.C. Sex Transm Dis 1993;20:279-85.

Hildesheim A, Schiffman M, Scott DR, et al. Human leukocyte antigen class I/II alleles and development of human papillomavirus-related cervical neoplasia: results from a case-control study conducted in the United States. Cancer Epidemiol Biomarkers Prev 1998;7:1035-41.

Hildesheim A, Schiffman MH, Gravitt PE, et al. Persistence of type-specific human papillomavirus infection among cytologically normal women. J Infect Dis 1994;169:235-240.

Hinchliffe SA, van Velzen D, Korporaal H, et al. Transience of cervical HPV infection in sexually active, young women with normal cervicovaginal cytology. Br J Cancer 1995; 72:943-5.

Hippelainen M, Syrjanen S, Koskela H, et al. Prevalence and risk factors of genital human papillomavirus (HPV) infections in healthy males: a study on Finnish conscripts. Sex Transm Dis 1993;20:321-8.

Hippelainen MI, Yliskoski M, Syrjanen S, et al. Low concordance of genital human papillomavirus (HPV) lesions and viral types in HPV-infected women and their male sexual partners. Sex Transm Dis 1994;21:76-82.

Ho GY, Burk RD, Fleming I, Klein RS. Risk of genital human papillomavirus infection in women with human immunodeficiency virus-induced immunosuppression. Int J Cancer 1994; 56:788-92.

Ho GY, Burk RD, Klein S, et al. Persistent genital human papillomavirus infection as a risk factor for persistent cervical dysplasia. J Natl Cancer Inst 1995;87:1365-71.

Ho GY, Kadish AS, Burk RD, et al. HPV 16 and cigarette smoking as risk factors for high-grade cervical intra-epithelial neoplasia. Int J Cancer 1998a;78:281-5.

Ho GY, Palan PR, Basu J, et al. Viral characteristics of human papillomavirus infection and antioxidant levels as risk factors for cervical dysplasia. Int J Cancer 1998b;78:594-9.

Ho GY, Studentsov Y, Hall CB, et al. Risk factors for subsequent cervicovaginal human papillomavirus (HPV) infection and the protective role of antibodies to HPV-16 virus-like particles. J Infect Dis 2002;186:737-42.

Ho GYF, Bierman R, Beardsley L, et al. Natural history of cervicovaginal papillomavirus infection in young women. N Engl J Med 1998c;338:423-428.

Ho L, Tay SK, Chan SY, et al. Sequence variants of human papillomavirus type 16 from couples suggest sexual transmission with low infectivity and polyclonality in genital neoplasia. J Infect Dis 1993;168:803-9.

Holowaty P, Miller AB, Rohan T, et al. Natural history of dysplasia of the uterine cervix. J Natl Cancer Inst 1999;91:252-8.

Hurley SL, Cason Z, Lemos LB, et al. Abnormal cervical lesions in young adults. Biomed Sci Instrum 1997;33:292-7.

Insinga R, Dasbach E. Clinical incidence of condyloma acuminatum in a set of private U.S. health plans. Abstract presented at the 20th International Papillomavirus Conference, Paris, France, October 4-9, 2002.

Jacobs MV, Walboomers JM, Snijders PJ, et al. Distribution of 37 mucosotropic HPV types in women with cytologically normal cervical smears: the age-related patterns for high-risk and low-risk types. Int J Cancer 2000;87:221-7.

Jamison JH, Kaplan DW, Hamman R, et al. Spectrum of genital human papillomavirus infection in a female adolescent population. Sex Transm Dis 1995;22:236-243.

Jenison SA, Yu XP, Valentine JM, et al. Evidence of prevalent genital-type human papillomavirus infections in adults and children. J Infect Dis 1990;162:60-9.

Jochmus-Kudielka I, Schneider A, Braun R, et al. Antibodies against the human papillomavirus type 16 early proteins in human sera: correlation of anti-E7 reactivity with cervical cancer. J Natl Cancer Inst 1989;81:1698-704.

Josefsson AM, Magnusson PK, Ylitalo N, et al. Viral load of human papilloma virus 16 as a determinant for development of cervical carcinoma in situ: a nested case-control study. Lancet 2000;355:2189-93.

Kadish AS, Timmins P, Wang Y, et al. Regression of cervical intraepithelial neoplasia and loss of human papillomavirus (HPV) infection is associated with cell-mediated immune responses to an HPV type 16 E7 peptide. Cancer Epidemiol Biomarkers Prev 2002;11:483-8.

Kamb ML. Cervical cancer screening of women attending sexually transmitted disease clinics. Clin Infect Dis 1995;20 (Suppl 1):S98-103.

Karlsson R, Jonsson M, Edlund K, et al. Lifetime number of partners as the only independent risk factor for human papillomavirus infection: a population-based study. Sex Transm Dis 1995; 22:119-27.

Kataja V, Syrjanen S, Yliskoski M, et al. Risk factors associated with cervical human papillomavirus infections: a case-control study. Am J Epidemiol 1993;138:735-45.

Kataoka A, Claesson U, Hansson BG, et al. Human papillomavirus infection of the male diagnosed by Southern-blot hybridization and polymerase chain reaction: comparison between urethra samples and penile biopsy samples. J Med Virol 1991;33:159-64.

Kellokoski J, Syrjanen S, Yliskoski M, et al. Dot blot hybridization in detection of human papillomavirus (HPV) infections in the oral cavity of women with genital HPV infections. Oral Microbiol Immunol 1992a;7:19-23.

Kellokoski JK, Syrjanen SM, Chang F, et al. Southern blot hybridization and PCR in detection of oral human papillomavirus (HPV) infections in women with genital HPV infections. J Oral Pathol Med 1992b;21:459-64.

Kemp EA, Hakenewerth AM, Laurent SL, et al. Human papillomavirus prevalence in pregnancy. Obstet Gynecol 1992;79:649-56.

Kirby PK, Kiviat N, Beckman A, et al. Tolerance and efficacy of recombinant human interferon gamma in the treatment of refractory genital warts. Am J Med 1988;85:183-8.

Kirnbauer R, Hubbert NL, Wheeler CM, et al. A virus-like particle enzyme-linked immunosorbent assay detects serum antibodies in a majority of women infected with human papillomavirus type 16. J Natl Cancer Inst 1994;86:494-9.

Kiviat N, Koutsky L, Paavonen J. Cervical neoplasia and other STD related genital and anal neoplasias. In: Holmes KK, Sparling PF, Mardh P-A, et al., eds. Sexually Transmitted Diseases, 3rd ed. New York: McGraw-Hill. 1999:811-831.

Kiviat NB, Critchlow CW, Holmes KK, et al. Association of anal dysplasia and human papillomavirus with immunosuppression and HIV infection among homosexual men. AIDS 1993;7:43-9.

Kiviat NB, Koutsky LA, Paavonen JA, et al. Prevalence of genital papillomavirus infection among women attending a college student health clinic or a sexually transmitted disease clinic. J Infect Dis 1989;159:293-302.

Kjaer SK, Chackerian B, van den Brule AJ, et al. High-risk human papillomavirus is sexually transmitted: evidence from a follow-up study of virgins starting sexual activity (intercourse). Cancer Epidemiol Biomarkers Prev 2001;10:101-6.

Kjaer SK, de Villiers EM, Dahl C, et al. Case-control study of risk factors for cervical neoplasia in Denmark. I: Role of the "male factor" in women with one lifetime sexual partner. Int J Cancer 1991;48:39-44.

Kjaer SK, Engholm G, Teisen C, et al. Risk factors for cervical human papillomavirus and herpes simplex virus infections in Greenland and Denmark: a population-based study. Am J Epidemiol 1990;131:669-82.

Kjaer SK, Svare EI, Worm AM, et al. Human papillomavirus infection in Danish female sex workers. Decreasing prevalence with age despite continuously high sexual activity. Sex Transm Dis 2000;27:438-45.

Kjaer SK, van den Brule AJ, Bock JE, et al. Determinants for genital human papillomavirus (HPV) infection in 1000 randomly chosen young Danish women with normal Pap smear: are there different risk profiles for oncogenic and nononcogenic HPV types? Cancer Epidemiol Biomarkers Prev 1997;6:799-805.

Koch A, Hansen SV, Nielsen NM, et al. HPV detection in children prior to sexual debut. Int J Cancer 1997;73:621-4.

Koutsky L. Epidemiology of genital human papillomavirus infection. Am J Med 1997;102(5A):3-8.

Koutsky LA, Galloway DA, Holmes KK. Epidemiology of genital human papillomavirus infection. Epidemiol Rev 1988;10:122-63.

Koutsky LA, Holmes KK, Critchlow CW, et al. A cohort study of the risk of cervical intraepithelial neoplasia grade 2 or 3 in relation to papillomavirus infection. N Engl J Med 1992; 327:1272-8.

Koutsky LA, Kiviat NB. Human papillomavirus infections. In: Holmes KK, Sparling PF, Mardh P-A, et al., eds. Sexually Transmitted Diseases, 3rd ed. New York: McGraw-Hill. 1999:347-360.

Krul EJ, Schipper RF, Schreuder GM, et al. HLA and susceptibility to cervical neoplasia. Hum Immunol 1999;60:337-42.

Kuhler-Obbarius C, Milde-Langosch K, Helling-Giese G, et al. Polymerase chain reaction-assisted papillomavirus detection in cervicovaginal smears: stratification by clinical risk and cytology reports. Virchows Arch 1994;425:157-63.

Lambropoulos AF, Agorastos T, Frangoulides E, et al. Detection of human papillomavirus using the polymerase chain reaction and typing for HPV16 and 18 in the cervical smears of Greek women. J Med Virol 1994;43:228-30.

Langenberg A, Cone RW, McDougall J, et al. Dual infection with human papillomavirus in a population with overt genital condylomas. J Am Acad Dermatol 1993;28:434-42.

Langley CL, Benga-De E, Critchlow CW, et al. HIV-1, HIV-2, human papillomavirus infection and cervical neoplasia in high-risk African women. AIDS 1996;10:413-7.

Law CL, Qassim M, Thompson CH, et al. Factors associated with clinical and sub-clinical anal human papillomavirus infection in homosexual men. Genitourin Med 1991;67:92-8.

Lazcano-Ponce E, Herrero R, Munoz N, et al. Epidemiology of HPV infection among Mexican women with normal cervical cytology. Int J Cancer 2001a;91:412-20.

Lazcano-Ponce E, Herrero R, Munoz N, et al. High prevalence of human papillomavirus infection in Mexican males: comparative study of penile-urethral swabs and urine samples. Sex Transm Dis 2001b;28:277-80.

Lehtinen M, Dillner J, Knekt P, et al. Serologically diagnosed infection with human papillomavirus type 16 and risk for subsequent development of cervical carcinoma: nested case-control study. Brit Med J 1996;312:537-9.

Ley C, Bauer HM, Reingold A, et al. Determinants of genital human papillomavirus infection in young women. J Natl Cancer Inst 1991;83:997-1003.

Li HX, Zhu WY, Xia MY. Detection with the polymerase chain reaction of human papillomavirus DNA in condylomata acuminata treated with CO2 laser and microwave. Int J Dermatol 1995;34:209-11.

Liaw KL, Hildesheim A, Burk RD, et al. A prospective study of human papillomavirus (HPV) type 16 DNA detection by polymerase chain reaction and its association with acquisition and persistence of other HPV types. J Infect Dis 2001;183:8-15.

Lin P, Koutsky LA, Critchlow CW, et al. HLA class II DR-DQ and increased risk of cervical cancer among Senegalese women. Cancer Epidemiol Biomarkers Prev 2001;10:1037-45.

Lorincz AT, Castle PE, Sherman ME, et al. Viral load of human papillomavirus and risk of CIN3 or cervical cancer. Lancet 2002;360:228-9.

Lorincz AT, Schiffman MH, Jaffurs WJ, et al. Temporal associations of human papillomavirus infection with cervical cytologic abnormalities. Am J Obstet Gynecol 1990;162:645-51.

Ludicke F, Stalberg A, Vassilakos P, et al. High- and intermediate-risk human papillomavirus infection in sexually active adolescent females. J Pediatr Adolesc Gynecol 2001;14:171-4.

Luostarinen T, af Geijersstam V, Bjorge T, et al. No excess risk of cervical carcinoma among women seropositive for both HPV16 and HPV6/11. Int J Cancer 1999;80:818-22.

Maciag PC, Schlecht NF, Souza PS, et al. Major histocompatibility complex class II polymorphisms and risk of cervical cancer and human papillomavirus infection in Brazilian women. Cancer Epidemiol Biomarkers Prev 2000;9:1183-91.

Maciag PC, Schlecht NF, Souza PS, et al. Polymorphisms of the human leukocyte antigen DRB1 and DQB1 genes and the natural history of human papillomavirus infection. J Infect Dis 2002;186:164-72.

Maehama T, Asato T, Kanazawa K. Prevalence of HPV infection in cervical cytology-normal women in Okinawa, Japan, as determined by a polymerase chain reaction. Int J Gynaecol Obstet 2000;69:175-6.

Maiman M, Fruchter RG, Sedlis A, et al. Prevalence, risk factors, and accuracy of cytologic screening for cervical intraepithelial neoplasia in women with the human immunodeficiency virus. Gynecol Oncol 1998;68:233-9.

Manhart LE, Koutsky LA. Do condoms prevent genital HPV infection, external genital warts or cervical neoplasia? A meta-analysis. Sex Transm Dis 2002;29:725-735.

Manns A, Strickler HD, Wikktor SZ, et al. Low incidence of human papillomavirus type 16 antibody seroconversion in young children. Pediatr Infect Dis J 1999;18:833-5.

Mao C, Hughes J, Kiviat N, et al. Clinical findings among young women with genital human papilloma virus infection. Am J Obstet Gynecol. 2003; 188:677-84.

Marais D, Rose RC, Williamson AL. Age distribution of antibodies to human papillomavirus in children, women with cervical intraepithelial neoplasia and blood donors from South Africa. J Med Virol 1997;51:126-31.

Marais DJ, Rose RC, Lane C, et al. Seroresponses to human papillomavirus types 16, 18, 31, 33, and 45 virus-like particles in South African women with cervical cancer and cervical intraepithelial neoplasia. J Med Virol 2000;60:403-10.

Marrazzo JM, Koutsky LA, Stine KL, et al. Genital human papillomavirus infection in women who have sex with women. J Infect Dis 1998;178:1604-9.

Marrero M, Valdes O, Alvarez M, et al. Detection of human papillomavirus by nonradioactive hybridization. Diagn Microbiol Dis 1994;18:95-100.

Martinez J, Smith R, Farmer M, et al. High prevalence of genital tract papillomavirus infection in female adolescents. Pediatrics 1988;82:604-8.

Massad LS, Riester KA, Anastos KM, et al. Prevalence and predictors of squamous cell abnormalities in Papanicolaou smears from women infected with HIV-1. Women's Interagency HIV Study Group. J Acquir Immune Defic Syndr 1999;21:33-41.

Matsumoto K, Yoshikawa H, Taketani Y, et al. Antibodies to human papillomavirus 16, 18, 58, and 6b major capsid proteins among Japanese females. Jpn J Cancer Res 1997;88:369-75.

McKinnon KJ, Ford RM, Hunter JC. High prevalence of human papillomavirus and cervical intraepithelial neoplasia in a young Australian STD population. Int J STD AIDS 1999; 2: 276-9.

Meekin GE, Sparrow MJ, Fenwicke RJ, et al. Prevalence of genital human papillomavirus infection in Wellington women. Genitournin Med 1992;68:228-232.

Melkert PW, Hopman E, van den Brule AJ, et al. Prevalence of HPV in cytomorphologically normal cervical smears, as determined by the polymerase chain reaction, is age-dependent. Int J Cancer 1993;53:919-23.

Mims CA, Dimmock NJ, Nash A, Stephen J. Pathogenesis of Infectious Disease, 4th ed. London: Academic Press. 1995;395.

Minkoff H, Feldman J, DeHovitz J, et al. A longitudinal study of human papillomavirus carriage in human immunodeficiency virus-infected and human immunodeficiency virus-uninfected women. Am J Obstet Gynecol 1998;178:982-6.

Mitrani-Rosenbaum S, Tsvieli R, Tur-Kaspa R. Oestrogen stimulates differential transcription of human papillomavirus type 16 in SiHa cervical carcinoma cells. J Gen Virol 1989;70: 2227-32.

Mittal R, Pater A, Pater MM. Multiple human papillomavirus type 16 glucocorticoid response elements functional for transformation, transient expression, and DNA-protein interactions. J Virol 1993;67:5656-9.

Monsonego J, Cessot G, Ince SE, et al. Randomised double-blind trial of recombinant interferon-beta for condyloma acuminatum. Genitourin Med 1996;72:111-4.

Moscicki AB. Genital HPV infections in children and adolescents. Obstet Gynecol Clin North Am 1996;23:675-97.

Moscicki AB, Ellenberg JH, Vermund SH, et al. Prevalence of and risks for cervical human papillomavirus infection and squamous intraepithelial lesions in adolescent girls: impact of infection with human immunodeficiency virus. Arch Pediatr Adolesc Med 2000;154:127-34.

Moscicki AB, Hills N, Shiboski S, et al. Risks for incident human papillomavirus infection and low-grade squamous intraepithelial lesion development in young females. JAMA 2001; 285:2995-3002.

Moscicki AB, Palefsky J, Gonzales J, et al. Human papillomavirus infection in sexually active adolescent females: prevalence and risk factors. Pediatr Res 1990;28:507-13.

Moscicki AB, Palefsky J, Smith G, et al. Variability of human papillomavirus DNA testing in a longitudinal cohort of young women. Obstet Gynecol 1993;82:578-85.

Moscicki AB, Ramirez JE, Ramos DM. Association between perception of risk and actual risk for HPV infection in young women. Abstract presented at the 14th International Papillomavirus Conference, Quebec City, Canada, July 1995.

Moscicki AB, Shiboski S, Broering J, et al. The natural history of human papillomavirus infection as measured by repeated DNA testing in adolescent and young women. J Pediatr 1998;132:277-84.

Mount SL, Papillo JL. A study of 10,296 pediatric and adolescent Papanicolaou smear diagnoses in northern New England. Pediatrics 1999;103:539-45.

Muller M, Viscidi RP, Ulken V, et al. Antibodies to the E4, E6, and E7 proteins of human papillomavirus (HPV) type 16 in patients with HPV-associated diseases and in the normal population. J Invest Dermatol 1995;104:138-41.

Mund K, Han C, Daum R, et al. Detection of human papillomavirus type 16 DNA and of antibodies to human papillomavirus type 16 proteins in children. Intervirology 1997;40:232-7.

Munoz N, Bosch FX. HPV and cervical neoplasia: review of case-control and cohort studies. IARC Sci Publ 1992:251-61.

Munoz N, Bosch FX, de Sanjose S, et al. The causal link between human papillomavirus and invasive cervical cancer: a population-based case-control study in Colombia and Spain. Int J Cancer 1992;52:743-9.

Munoz N, Bosch FX, de Sanjose S, et al. Risk factors for cervical intraepithelial neoplasia grade III/carcinoma in situ in Spain and Colombia. Cancer Epidemiol Biomarkers Prev 1993;2:423-31.

Munoz N, Castellsague X, Bosch FX, et al. Difficulty in elucidating the male role in cervical cancer in Colombia, a high-risk area for the disease. J Natl Cancer Inst 1996a;88:1068-75.

Munoz N, Kato I, Bosch FX, et al. Risk factors for HPV DNA detection in middle-aged women. Sex Transm Dis 1996b;23:504-10.

Negrini BP, et al. Oral contraceptive use, human papillomavirus infection and risk of early cytological abnormalities of the cervix. Cancer Res 1990;50:4670-4675.

Nishikawa A, Fukushima M, Shimada M, et al. Relatively low prevalence of human papillomavirus 16, 18 and 33 DNA in the normal cervices of Japanese women shown by polymerase chain reaction. Jpn J Cancer Res 1991;82:532-8.

Nobbenhuis MA, Walboomers JM, Helmerhorst TJ, et al. Relation of human papillomavirus status to cervical lesions and consequences for cervical-cancer screening: a prospective study. Lancet 1999;354:20-5.

Nonnenmacher B, Hubbert NL, Kirnbauer R, et al. Serologic response to human papillomavirus type 16 (HPV-16) virus-like particles in HPV-16 DNA-positive invasive cervical cancer and cervical intraepithelial neoplasia grade III patients and controls from Colombia and Spain. J Infect Dis 1995;172:19-24.

Nonnenmacher B, Kruger Kjaer S, Svare EI, et al. Seroreactivity to HPV16 virus-like particles as a marker for cervical cancer risk in high-risk populations. Int J Cancer 1996;68:704-9.

Odunsi K, Terry G, Ho L, et al. Susceptibility to human papillomavirus-associated cervical intra-epithelial neoplasia is determined by specific HLA DR-DQ alleles. Int J Cancer 1996; 67:595-602.

Ogunbiyi OA, Scholefield JH, Raftery AT, et al. Prevalence of anal human papillomavirus infection and intraepithelial neoplasia in renal allograft recipients. Br J Surg 1994;81:365-7.

Oriel JD. Natural history of genital warts. Br J Vener Dis 1971;47:1-13.

Ostor AG. Natural history of cervical intraepithelial neoplasia: a critical review. Int J Gynecol Pathol 1993;12:186-92.

Paavonen J, Koutsky L, Kiviat N. Cervical neoplasia and other STD related genital and anal neoplasias. In: Holmes KK, Mardh P-A, Sparling PF, Wiesner PJ, eds. Sexually Transmitted Diseases, 2nd ed. New York: McGraw-Hill. 1990:561-592.

Pakarian F, Kaye J, Cason J, et al. Cancer associated human papillomaviruses: perinatal transmission and persistence. Br J Obstet Gynaecol 1994;101:514-7.

Palefsky JM, Minkoff H, Kalish LA, et al. Cervicovaginal human papillomavirus infection in human immunodeficiency virus-1 (HIV)-positive and high-risk HIV-negative women. J Natl Cancer Inst 1999;91:226-36.

Palefsky JM, Shiboski S, Moss A. Risk factors for anal human papillomavirus infection and anal cytologic abnormalities in HIV-positive and HIV-negative homosexual men. J Acquir Immune Defic Syndr 1994;7:599-606.

Pao CC, Lin CY, Maa JS, et al. Detection of human papillomaviruses in cervicovaginal cells using polymerase chain reaction. J Infect Dis 1990;161:113-5.

Pao CC, Tsai PL, Chang YL, et al. Possible non-sexual transmission of genital human papillomavirus infections in young women. Eur J Clin Microbiol Infect Dis 1993;12:221-223.

Park JS, Park DC, Kim CJ, et al. HPV-16-related proteins as the serologic markers in cervical neoplasia. Gynecol Oncol 1998;69:47-55.

Pasetto N, Sesti F, De Santis L, et al. The prevalence of HPV16DNA in normal and pathological cervical scrapes using the polymerase chain reaction. Gynecol Oncol 1992; 46: 33-6.

Peng TC, Searle CP, 3rd, Shah KV, et al. Prevalence of human papillomavirus infections in term pregnancy. Am J Perinatol 1990;7:189-92.

Persson G, Andersson K, Krantz I. Symptomatic genital papillomavirus infection in a community. Incidence and clinical picture. Acta Obstet Gynecol Scand 1996;75:287-90.

Petter A, Heim K, Guger M, et al. Specific serum IgG, IgM and IgA antibodies to human papillomavirus types 6, 11, 16, 18 and 31 virus-like particles in human immunodeficiency virus-seropositive women. J Gen Virol 2000;81:701-8.

Peyton CL, Gravitt PE, Hunt WC, et al. Determinants of genital human papillomavirus detection in a US population. J Infect Dis 2001;183:1554-64.

Rando RF, Lindheim S, Hasty L, et al. Increased frequency of detection of human papillomavirus deoxyribonucleic acid in exfoliated cervical cells during pregnancy. Am J Obstet Gynecol 1989;161:50-5.

Reed BD, Zazove P, Gregoire L, et al. Factors associated with human papillomavirus infection in women encountered in community-based offices. Arch Fam Med 1993;2:1227-1228.

Reeves WC, Brinton LA, Garcia M, et al. Human papillomavirus infection and cervical cancer in Latin America. N Engl J Med 1989;320:1437-41.

Rezza G, Giuliani M, Branca M, et al. Determinants of squamous intraepithelial lesions (SIL) on Pap smear: the role of HPV infection and of HIV-1-induced immunosuppression. DIANAIDS Collaborative Study Group. Eur J Epidemiol 1997;13:937-43.

Rice PS, Mant C, Cason J, et al. High prevalence of human papillomavirus type 16 infection among children. J Med Virol 2000;61:70-5.

Robertson DI, Megran DW, Duggan MA, et al. Cervico-vaginal screening in an STD clinic. Can J Public Health 1991;82:264-6.

Rohan T, Mann V, McLaughlin J, et al. PCR-detected genital papillomavirus infection: prevalence and association with risk factors for cervical cancer. Int J Cancer 1991;49:856-860.

Rosenfeld WD, Rose E, Vermund SH, et al. Follow-up evaluation of cervicovaginal human papillomavirus infection in adolescents. J Pediatr 1992;121:307-11.

Rosenfeld WD, Vermund SH, Wentz SJ, et al. High prevalence rate of human papillomavirus infection and association with abnormal Papanicolaou smears in sexually active adolescents. Am J Dis Child 1989;143:1443-7.

Rousseau MC, Pereira JS, Prado JC, et al. Cervical coinfection with human papillomavirus (HPV) types as a predictor of acquisition and persistence of HPV infection. J Infect Dis 2001;184:1508-17.

Rylander E, Ruusuvaara L, Almstromer MW, et al. The absence of vaginal human papillomavirus 16 DNA in women who have not experienced sexual intercourse. Obstet Gynecol 1994;83:735-737.

Sadeghi SB, Sadeghi A, Cosby M, et al. Human papillomavirus infection. Frequency and association with cervical neoplasia in a young population. Acta Cytol 1989;33:319-23.

Saiki RK, Gelfand DH, Stoffel S, et al. Primer-directed enzymatic amplification of DNA with a thermostable DNA polymerase. Science 1988;239:487-91.

Saito J, Fukuda T, Nakatani H, et al. Detection of human papillomavirus DNA in the normal cervices of Japanese women by the dot-blot (Vira Pap) method. Asia Oceania J Obstet Gynaecol 1992;18:283-7.

Salmon J, Nonnenmacher M, Caze S, et al. Variation in the nucleotide sequence of cottontail rabbit papillomavirus a and b subtypes affects wart regression and malignant transformation and level of viral replication in domestic rabbits. J Virol 2000;74:10766-77.

Sanjeevi CB, Hjelmstrom P, Hallmans G, et al. Different HLA-DR-DQ haplotypes are associated with cervical intraepithelial neoplasia among human papillomavirus type-16 seropositive and seronegative Swedish women. Int J Cancer 1996;68:409-14.

Saracco A, Musicco M, Nicolosi A, et al. Man-to-woman sexual transmission of HIV: longitudinal study of 343 steady partners of infected men. J Acquir Immune Defic Syndr 1993;6:497-502.

Sastre-Garau X, Loste MN, Vincent-Salomon A, et al. Decreased frequency of HLA-DRB1 13 alleles in French women with HPV-positive carcinoma of the cervix. Int J Cancer 1996; 69:159-64.

Schafer A, Friedmann W, Mielke M, et al. The increased frequency of cervical dysplasia-neoplasia in women infected with the human immunodeficiency virus is related to the degree of immunosuppression. Am J Obstet Gynecol 1991;164:593-9.

Schiffman MH. Recent progress in defining the epidemiology of human papillomavirus infection and cervical neoplasia. J Natl Cancer Inst 1992;84:394-8.

Schiffman MH, Bauer HM, Hoover RN, et al. Epidemiologic evidence showing that human papillomavirus infection causes most cervical intraepithelial neoplasia. J Natl Cancer Inst 1993; 85:958-64.

Schiffman MH, Kiviat NB, Burk RD, et al. Accuracy and interlaboratory reliability of human papillomavirus DNA testing by hybrid capture. J Clin Microbiol 1995;33:545-50.

Schlecht NF, Kulaga S, Robitaille J, et al. Persistent human papillomavirus infection as a predictor of cervical intraepithelial neoplasia. JAMA 2001;286:3106-14.

Schneider A, Hotz M, Gissmann L. Increased prevalence of human papillomaviruses in the lower genital tract of pregnant women. Int J Cancer 1987;40:198-201.

Schneider A, Kirchhoff T, Meinhardt G, et al. Repeated evaluation of human papillomavirus 16 status in cervical swabs on young women with a history of normal papanicolaou smears. Obstet Gynecol 1992;79:683-688.

Schneider A, Kirchmayr R, De Villiers EM, et al. Subclinical human papillomavirus infections in male sexual partners of female carriers. J Urol 1988;140:1431-4.

Schneider A, Koutsky LA. Natural history and epidemiological features of genital HPV infection. IARC Sci Publ 1992:25-52.

Schrager LK, Friedland GH, Maude D, et al. Cervical and vaginal squamous cell abnormalities in women infected with human immunodeficiency virus. J Acquir Immune Defic Syndr 1989;2:570-5.

Seck AC, Faye MA, Critchlow CW, et al. Cervical intraepithelial neoplasia and human papillomavirus infection among Senegalese women seropositive for HIV-1 or HIV-2 or seronegative for HIV. Int J STD AIDS 1994;5:189-93.

Sedjo RL, Inserra P, Abrahamsen M, et al. Human papillomavirus persistence and nutrients involved in the methylation pathway among a cohort of young women. Cancer Epidemiol Biomarkers Prev 2002a;11:353-9.

Sedjo RL, Roe DJ, Abrahamsen M, et al. Vitamin A, carotenoids, and risk of persistent oncogenic human papillomavirus infection. Cancer Epidemiol Biomarkers Prev 2002b; 11:876-84.

Sedlacek TV, Lindheim S, Eder C, et al. Mechanism for human papillomavirus transmission at birth. Am J Obstet Gynecol 1989;161:55-9.

Sellors JW, Karwalajtys TL, Kaczorowski JA, et al. Prevalence of infection with carcinogenic human papillomavirus among older women. Canad Med Assoc J 2002; 167:871-873.

Sellors JW, Mahony JB, Kaczorowski J, et al. Prevalence and predictors of human papillomavirus infection in women in Ontario, Canada. Survey of HPV in Ontario Women (SHOW) Group. Canad Med Assoc J 2000;163:503-8.

Shah KV, Viscidi RP, Alberg AJ, et al. Antibodies to human papillomavirus 16 and subsequent in situ or invasive cancer of the cervix. Cancer Epidemiol Biomarkers Prev 1997; 6:233-7.

Sikstrom B, Hellberg D, Nilsson S, et al. Contraceptive use and reproductive history in women with cervical human papillomavirus infection. Adv Contracept 1995;11:273-84.

Silins I, Kallings I, Dillner J. Correlates of the spread of human papillomavirus infection. Cancer Epidemiol Biomarkers Prev 2000;9:953-9.

Silins I, Wang Z, Avall-Lundqvist E, et al. Serological evidence for protection by human papillomavirus (HPV) type 6 infection against HPV type 16 cervical carcinogenesis. J Gen Virol 1999;80:2931-6.

Silverberg MJ, Ahdieh L, Munoz A, et al. The impact of HIV infection and immunodeficiency on human papillomavirus type 6 or 11 infection and on genital warts. Sex Transm Dis 2002; 29:427-435.

Simsir A, Brooks S, Cochran L, et al. Cervicovaginal smear abnormalities in sexually active adolescents. Implications for management. Acta Cytol 2002;46:271-6.

Six C, Heard I, Bergeron C, et al. Comparative prevalence, incidence and short-term prognosis of cervical squamous intraepithelial lesions amongst HIV-positive and HIV-negative women. AIDS 1998;12:1047-56.

Slattery ML, Overall JC, Jr., Abbott TM, et al. Sexual activity, contraception, genital infections, and cervical cancer: support for a sexually transmitted disease hypothesis. Am J Epidemiol 1989;130:248-58.

Slavinsky J, 3rd, Kissinger P, Burger L, et al. Seroepidemiology of low and high oncogenic risk types of human papillomavirus in a predominantly male cohort of STD clinic patients. Int J STD AIDS 2001;12:516-23.

Smith EM, Johnson SR, Cripe T, et al. Perinatal transmission and maternal risks of human papillomavirus infection. Cancer Detect Prev 1995;19:196-205.

Smith EM, Johnson SR, Jiang D, et al. The association between pregnancy and human papilloma virus prevalence. Cancer Detect Prev 1991;15:397-402.

Soares VR, Nieminen P, Aho M, et al. Human papillomavirus DNA in unselected pregnant and non-pregnant women. Int J STD AIDS 1990;1:276-8.

Sonnex C, Strauss S, Gray JJ. Detection of human papillomavirus DNA on the fingers of patients with genital warts. Sex Transm Infect 1999;75:317-9.

Stone KM. Human papillomavirus infection and genital warts: update on epidemiology and treatment. Clin Infect Dis 1995;20 (Suppl 1):S91-7.

Stone KM, Karem KL, Sternberg MR, et al. Seroprevalence of human papillomavirus type 16 infection in the United States. J Infect Dis 2002;186:1396-1402.

Strand A, Rylander E, Wilander E, et al. HPV infection in male partners of women with squamous intraepithelial neoplasia and/or high-risk HPV. Acta Derm Venereol 1995;75:312-6.

Strickler HD, Kirk GD, Figueroa JP, et al. HPV 16 antibody prevalence in Jamaica and the United States reflects differences in cervical cancer rates. Int J Cancer 1999;80:339-44.

Sugase M, Moriyama S, Matsukura T. Human papillomavirus in exophytic condylomatous lesions on different female genital regions. J Med Virol 1991;34:1-6.

Summersgill KF, Smith EM, Levy BT, et al. Human papillomavirus in the oral cavities of children and adolescents. Oral Surg Oral Med Oral Pathol Oral Radiol Endod 2001;91:62-9.

Sun XW, Ellerbrock TV, Lungu O, et al. Human papillomavirus infection in human immunodeficiency virus-seropositive women. Obstet Gynecol 1995;85:680-6.

Sun XW, Kuhn L, Ellerbrock TV, et al. Human papillomavirus infection in women infected with the human immunodeficiency virus. N Engl J Med 1997;337:1343-9.

Svare EI, Kjaer SK, Nonnenmacher B, et al. Seroreactivity to human papillomavirus type 16 virus-like particles is lower in high-risk men than in high-risk women. J Infect Dis 1997; 176:876-83.

Svare EI, Kjaer SK, Worm AM, et al. Risk factors for genital HPV DNA in men resemble those found in women: a study of male attendees at a Danish STD clinic. Sex Transm Infect 2002; 78:215-8.

Syrjanen K, Hakama M, Saarikoski S, et al. Prevalence, incidence, and estimated life-time risk of cervical human papillomavirus infections in a nonselected Finnish female population. Sex Transm Dis 1990;17:15-9.

Syrjanen K, Kataja V, Yliskoski M, et al. Natural history of cervical human papillomavirus lesions does not substantiate the biologic relevance of the Bethesda System. Obstet Gynecol 1992;79:675-82.

Syrjanen K, Vayrynen M, Castren O, et al. Sexual behaviour of women with human papillomavirus (HPV) lesions of the uterine cervix. Br J Vener Dis 1984;60:243-8.

Tachezy R, Hamsikova E, Hajek T, et al. Human papillomavirus genotype spectrum in Czech women: correlation of HPV DNA presence with antibodies against HPV-16, 18, and 33 virus-like particles. J Med Virol 1999;58:378-86.

Temmerman M, Kidula N, Tyndall M, et al. The supermarket for women's reproductive health: the burden of genital infections in a family planning clinic in Nairobi, Kenya. Sex Transm Infect 1998;74:202-4.

Temmerman M, Tyndall MW, Kidula N, et al. Risk factors for human papillomavirus and cervical precancerous lesions, and the role of concurrent HIV-1 infection. Int J Gynaecol Obstet 1999;65:171-81.

Thomas DB, Ray RM, Pardthaisong T, et al. Prostitution, condom use, and invasive squamous cell cervical cancer in Thailand. Am J Epidemiol 1996;143:779-86.

Thomas KK, Hughes JP, Kuypers JM, et al. Concurrent and sequential acquisition of different genital human papillomavirus types. J Infect Dis 2000;182:1097-1102.

Tortolero-Luna G. Epidemiology of genital human papillomavirus. Hematol Oncol Clin North Am 1999;13:245-57.

Tsao YP, Yang KY, Han CP, et al. Genital human papillomavirus infections in Taiwan. Int J Gynaecol Obstet 1994;44:39-45.

Tseng CJ, Liang CC, Soong YK, et al. Perinatal transmission of human papillomavirus in infants: relationship between infection rate and mode of delivery. Obstet Gynecol 1998; 91: 92-6.

Turpin J, Liaw KL, Overness T, et al. The incidence and prevalence of genital warts and HPV infection in young sexually active Norwegian women. Abstract presented at the 20th International Papillomavirus Conference, Paris, France, October 4-9, 2002.

Utagawa ML, Pereira SM, Cavaliere MJ, et al. Cervical intraepithelial neoplasia in adolescents: study of cytological findings between 1987 and 1995 in Sao Paulo State-Brazil. Arch Gynecol Obstet 1998;262:59-64.

van Doornum G, Prins M, Andersson-Ellstrom A, et al. Immunoglobulin A, G, and M responses to L1 and L2 capsids of human papillomavirus types 6, 11, 16, 18, and 33 L1 after newly acquired infection. Sex Transm Infect 1998;74:354-60.

van Doornum GJ, Hooykaas C, Juffermans LH, et al. Prevalence of human papillomavirus infections among heterosexual men and women with multiple sexual partners. J Med Virol 1992;37:13-21.

van Duin M, Snijders PJ, Schrijnemakers HF, et al. Human papillomavirus 16 load in normal and abnormal cervical scrapes: an indicator of CIN II/III and viral clearance. Int J Cancer 2002; 98:590-5.

Vandenvelde C, Scheen R, Van Pachterbeke C, et al. Prevalence of high risk genital papillomaviruses in the Belgian female population determined by fast multiplex polymerase chain reaction. J Med Virol 1992;36:279-82.

Vandenvelde C, Van Beers D. Risk factors inducing the persistence of high-risk genital papillomaviruses in the normal cervix. J Med Virol 1992;38:226-32.

Venuti A, Badaracco G, Sedati A, et al. Determinants of human papillomavirus types 16 and 18 infections in the lower female genital tract in an Italian population. Eur J Gynaec Oncol 1994;15:205-210.

Vernon SD, Reeves WC, Clancy KA, et al. A longitudinal study of human papillomavirus DNA detection in human immunodeficiency virus type 1-seropositive and -seronegative women. J Infect Dis 1994;169:1108-12.

Villa LL. Human papillomaviruses and cervical cancer. Adv Cancer Res 1997;71:321-41.

Villa LL, Franco EL. Epidemiologic correlates of cervical neoplasia and risk of human papillomavirus infection in asymptomatic women in Brazil. J Natl Cancer Inst 1989;81:332-340.

Viscidi RP, Kotloff KL, Clayman B, et al. Prevalence of antibodies to human papilloma-virus (HPV) type 16 virus-like particles in relation to cervical HPV infection among college women. Clin Diagn Lab Immunol 1997;4:122-6.

Walboomers JM, Jacobs MV, Manos MM, et al. Human papillomavirus is a necessary cause of invasive cervical cancer worldwide. J Pathol 1999;189:12-9.

Walboomers JM, Meijer CJ. Do HPV-negative cervical carcinomas exist? J Pathol 1997; 181:253-4.

Wallin KL, van Doornum GJ, Andersson-Ellstrom A, et al. Seroepidemiology of human papillomavirus type 73: a sexually transmitted low-risk virus. Int J Cancer 2000;85:353-7.

Wang PD, Lin RS. Risk factors for cervical intraepithelial neoplasia in Taiwan. Gynecol Oncol 1996;62:10-8.

Wang SS, Wheeler CM, Hildesheim A, et al. Human leukocyte antigen class I and II alleles and risk of cervical neoplasia: results from a population-based study in Costa Rica. J Infect Dis 2001;184:1310-4.

Wang Z, Konya J, Avall-Lundkvist E, et al. Human papillomavirus antibody responses among patients with incident cervical carcinoma. J Med Virol 1997;52:436-40.

Wank R, Thomssen C. High risk of squamous cell carcinoma of the cervix for women with HLA-DQw3. Nature 1991;352:723-5.

Watts DH, Brunham RC. Sexually transmitted diseases, including HIV infection in pregnancy. In: Holmes KK, Sparling PF, Mardh P-A, et al., eds. Sexually Transmitted Diseases, 3rd ed. New York: McGraw-Hill. 1999:1089-1132.

Watts DH, Koutsky LA, Holmes KK, et al. Low risk of perinatal transmission of human papillomavirus: results from a prospective cohort study. Am J Obstet Gynecol 1998;178: 365-73.

Watts KJ, Thompson CH, Cossart YE, et al. Sequence variation and physical state of human papillomavirus type 16 cervical cancer isolates from Australia and New Caledonia. Int J Cancer 2002;97:868-74.

Weaver B, Feng Q, Kiviat N, et al. Evaluation of genital sampling techniques for HPV DNA detection in men. Abstract presented at the 20th International Papillomavirus Conference, Paris, France, October 4-9, 2002.

Wen LM, Estcourt CS, Simpson JM, et al. Risk factors for the acquisition of genital warts: are condoms protective? Sex Transm Infect 1999;75:312-6.

Wheeler CM. Clinical aspects and epidemiology of human papillomavirus infections. In: Zuckerman AJ, Mushahwar LK, eds. Human Papillomaviruses (McCance, DJ, ed.), Perspectives in Medical Virology, 8. Amsterdam, The Netherlands: Elselvier Science. 2002: 1-29.

Wheeler CM, Parmenter CA, Hunt WC, et al. Determinants of genital human papillomavirus infection among cytologically normal women attending the University of New Mexico student health center. Sex Transm Dis 1993;20:286-9.

Wideroff L, Schiffman MH, Nonnenmacher B, et al. Evaluation of seroreactivity to human papillomavirus type 16 virus-like particles in an incident case-control study of cervical neoplasia. J Infect Dis 1995;172:1425-30.

Wikstrom A, Eklund C, von Krogh G, et al. Antibodies against human papillomavirus type 6 capsids are elevated in men with previous condylomas. Apmis 1997;105:884-8.

Wikstrom A, Lidbrink P, Johansson B, et al. Penile human papillomavirus carriage among men attending Swedish STD clinics. Int J STD AIDS 1991;2:105-9.

Wilson JD, Brown CB, Walker PP. Factors involved in clearance of genital warts. Int J STD AIDS 2001;12:789-92.

Winer RL, Lee SK, Hughes JP, et al. Genital human papillomavirus infection: incidence and risk factors among a cohort of female university students. Am J Epidemiol 2003; 157: 218-26.

Woodman CB, Collins S, Winter H, et al. Natural history of cervical human papillomavirus infection in young women: a longitudinal cohort study. Lancet 2001;357:1831-6.

Wright TC, Jr., Ellerbrock TV, Chiasson MA, et al. Cervical intraepithelial neoplasia in women infected with human immunodeficiency virus: prevalence, risk factors, and validity of Papanicolaou smears. New York Cervical Disease Study. Obstet Gynecol 1994a;84:591-7.

Wright TC, Kurman R, Ferenczy A. Precancerous lesions of the cervix. In: Kurman R ed., Blaustein's Pathology of the Female Genital Tract, 4th ed. Springer-Verlag, New York, Inc. 1994b:229-278.

Xi LF, Carter JJ, Galloway DA, et al. Acquisition and natural history of human papillomavirus type 16 variant infection among a cohort of female university students. Cancer Epidemiol Biomarkers Prev 2002;11:343-51.

Xi LF, Critchlow CW, Wheeler CM, et al. Risk of anal carcinoma in situ in relation to human papillomavirus type 16 variants. Cancer Res 1998;58:3839-44.

Xi LF, Demers GW, Koutsky LA, et al. Analysis of human papillomavirus type 16 variants indicates establishment of persistent infection. J Infect Dis 1995;172:747-755.

Xi LF, Demers W, Kiviat NB, et al. Sequence variation in the noncoding region of human papillomavirus type 16 detected by single-strand conformation polymorphism analysis. J Infect Dis 1993;168:610-7.

Xi LF, Koutsky LA. Epidemiology of genital human papillomavirus infections. Bull Inst Pasteur 1997;95:161-178.

Xi LF, Koutsky LA, Galloway DA, et al. Genomic variation of human papillomavirus type 16 and risk for high grade cervical intraepithelial neoplasia. J Natl Cancer Inst 1997;89:796-802.

Yamada T, Manos MM, Peto J, et al. Human papillomavirus type 16 sequence variation in cervical cancers: a worldwide perspective. J Virol 1997;71:2463-72.

Yamada T, Wheeler CM, Halpern AL, et al. Human papillomavirus type 16 variant lineages in United States populations characterized by nucleotide sequence analysis of the E6, L2, and L1 coding segments. J Virol 1995;69:7743-53.

Ylitalo N, Sorensen P, Josefsson AM, et al. Consistent high viral load of human papillomavirus 16 and risk of cervical carcinoma in situ: a nested case-control study. Lancet 2000; 355:2194-8.

Young TK, McNicol P, Beauvais J. Factors associated with human papillomavirus infection detected by polymerase chain reaction among urban Canadian aboriginal and non-aboriginal women. Sex Transm Dis 1997;24:293-8.

Yuan F, Auborn K, James C. Altered growth and viral gene expression in human papillomavirus type 16-containing cancer cell lines treated with progesterone. Cancer Invest 1999; 17:19-29.

Zenilman JM, Weisman CS, Rompalo AM, et al. Condom use to prevent incident STDs: the validity of self-reported condom use. Sex Transm Dis 1995;22:15-21.

Zondervan KT, Carpenter LM, Painter R, et al. Oral contraceptives and cervical cancer--further findings from the Oxford Family Planning Association contraceptive study. Br J Cancer 1996;73:1291-7.

Zunzunegui MV, King MC, Coria CF, et al. Male influences on cervical cancer risk. Am J Epidemiol 1986;123:302-7.

zur Hausen H. Genital papillomavirus infections. In: Rigby PWJ, Wilkie NM, eds. Viruses and Cancer. Cambridge: Cambridge University Press. 1985:83-90.

Section 3

ETIOLOGY

Chapter 7

The Etiology of Squamous Cell Cervical Cancer

F. Xavier Bosch, M.D., M.P.H.
Servei d'Epidemiologia I Registre del Cancer Institut Catalia d'Oncologia

INTRODUCTION

Cervical cancer is singular in many aspects. It is a major cause of cancer-related deaths in many developing countries yet it is a preventable and treatable cancer in populations with adequate cytology-based screening programs and health services. It is viral in origin and a few human papillomavirus (HPV) types are involved in the origin of the largest fraction of cases worldwide. This recognition is leading the field to explore HPV vaccines as one of the promising preventive options for the future. The relevant risk factors for exposure to HPV and for progression to cancer include deeply rooted behavioral traits such as some aspects of sexual behavior, some reproductive and contraceptive practices, and smoking patterns. These are complex behaviors, difficult to understand and modify in any meaningful way.

The challenges are now to use efficiently the wealth of acquired knowledge. Additional research in the natural history and the epidemiology of the infection is required and the information has to be transferred to health professionals and to the general population. There is still a need to define the best use of HPV tests in clinical and screening protocols and much work remains to be done in developing novel treatments of the viral infections. Finally, a major challenge ahead lies in the development of HPV vaccines and of the strategies to make them available to the underserved populations represented by women in most of the third world countries.

1   DESCRIPTIVE EPIDEMIOLOGY

1.1   The incidence of cervical cancer

Table 1 shows recent estimates of the incidence of invasive cervical cancer extracted from systematic sources, and compiled by IARC for the year 2000 (Ferlay et al. 2001).   The table includes the estimated number of new cases per year by geographical region, the crude incidence rates, the age-adjusted (world standard) rates and the age-specific incidence rates for four age groups.   These estimates are based upon available incidence data, mortality statistics and additional miscellaneous information. Whenever information is missing, estimates based upon comparable populations according to pre-defined rules are presented.

The number of cases and the crude rates provide an estimate of the impact of cervical cancer in the relevant population. Age-adjusted incidence rates are useful to broadly compare populations in terms of risk, however this is an abstract parameter calculated to reduce the effect of the different age structures of the world's populations. The table clearly shows the impact of the adjustment procedure, which tends to reduce adjusted rates in developed countries and increase the rates in the developing parts of the world. This phenomenon is entirely due to the choice of a world standard population which averages the distribution of the age groups and to the strong relation between cancer incidence and age. Developed countries have older populations than the standard population whereas developing countries have younger populations.

In terms of the number of cases, Asia contributes nearly a quarter of a million new cases per year, followed by countries in Central and South America. Africa and Europe each contribute some 65,000 to 70,000 new cases per year. In terms of risk, the Caribbean, Central and South American countries rank first along with Eastern and Southern African countries. In Europe, Eastern countries are distinctively at high risk. The lowest rates registered are observed in South Eastern and Western regions in Asia, Australia, New Zealand and the Northern countries in America.

Age-specific incidence rates are useful in showing the important geographic differences in incidence, without the limitations of the all-ages crude rates and the artifacts introduced by the adjustment procedure. For example, in the 55-64 age range, where the incidence of the disease is the highest in most populations,

Table 1. Estimated incidence of cervical cancer in

	Estimated number of cases in 2000	INCIDENCE RATE		AGE SPECIFIC INCIDENCE RATE/10^5			
		Crude	Standardized	15-44	45-54	55-64	65+
World	470,606	15.7	16.1	9.5	44.9	51.8	41.9
More Developed	91,451	15	11.3	11.9	22.4	23.8	26.3
Less Developed	379,153	15.8	18.7	9.0	53.6	65.0	53.8
Africa	67,078	17.1	27.3	11.0	71.5	100.5	95.4
Eastern	30,206	24.4	44.3	16.1	1114.8	174.4	153.9
Middle	6,947	14.4	25.1	8.5	54.0	73.3	137.4
Northern	10,479	12.2	16.8	6.2	49.0	68.5	45.9
Southern	5,541	23.2	30.3	15.5	67.8	98.5	118.2
Western	13,903	12.5	20.3	9.5	57.4	70.6	60.3
America	92,136	22	21	15.1	55.2	57.8	55.0
Caribbean	6,670	34.8	35.8	17.7	82.7	102.1	155.6
Central	21,596	31.7	40.3	22.5	111.7	109.9	136.1
South	49,025	28.1	30.9	16.8	85.5	90.2	101.4
Northern	14,845	9.5	7.9	9.0	15.4	16.8	14.2
United States	13,230	9.4	7.8	8.8	15.5	17.2	13.8
Europe	64,928	17.2	13	14.1	26.3	26.5	28.1
Eastern	35,482	21.9	16.8	17.8	34.5	34.9	36.6
Northern	6,049	12.6	9.8	12.0	17.6	16.7	20.2
Southern	10,116	13.7	10.2	10.5	20.8	23.7	20.9
Western	13,282	14.2	10.4	11.3	20.5	19.6	25.1

Table 1. Estimated incidence of cervical cancer in the world, continued

Asia	245,670	13.6	14.9	14.9	44.0	52.8	39.6
Eastern	51,266	7.1	6.4	6.4	18.4	18.9	25.4
South-Eastern	39,648	15.3	18.3	18.3	59.0	58.2	45.9
South-Central	151,297	20.9	26.5	26.5	79.2	100.8	65.6
Western	3,458	3.8	4.8	4.8	13.1	15.3	14.1
Japan	11,681	18.1	11.1	11.1	21.2	25.6	42.2
Asia (excluding Japan)	234,335	13.5	15.2	15.2	45.4	55.1	39.4
Oceania	2,156	14.2	12.6	12.6	27.4	28.2	29.0
Pacific Islands*	1,078	29.1	40.3	40.3	91.2	107.1	167.8
Australia & N. Zealand	1,077	9.4	7.7	7.7	15.5	14.8	16.6

Melanesia, Micronesia and Polinesia. Adapted from Ferlay et al., 2001 the Caribbean countries show rates above 100 per 100 000, whereas in the United States or Canada, these do not reach the level of 20 per 100 000. In those aged 65 and over, the difference is 10 times higher in the Caribbean countries.

Figure 1 shows the estimated age-specific incidence rates of invasive cancer in the world by grossly defined level of development. The figure clearly shows that cervical cancer is rare in the young age groups (<45 years) and only small differences are observed between developed and developing populations. However, there is a striking difference in the advanced age groups, which is largely attributable to the impact of screening and early treatment. Figure 2 shows the age-specific incidence rates based on well-developed cancer registries in the US and Canada. The figure shows strong differences across ethnic groups. Data on white populations from the SEER and Canadian registries shows that incidence rises steeply between ages 20 and 35 and stays stable in the middle age groups, with some slight increase after 55-60. For blacks, Hispanic and Chinese, the incidence rates increase steadily throughout lifetime, reaching 2 to 3 times the incidence rate among whites in the most advanced age groups. In a number of registries, including several in Europe, a second mode in incidence rates occurs in the age groups 60 and above, perhaps in relation to some decrease in screening coverage.

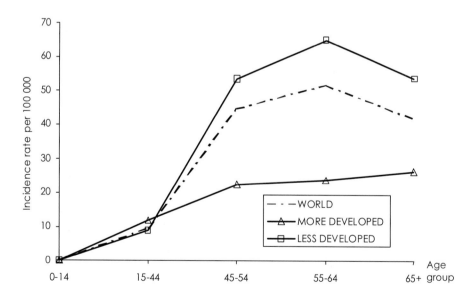

Figure 1. Age specific incidence of cervical cancer by level of development (Cancer Incidence in Five Continents, 1997).

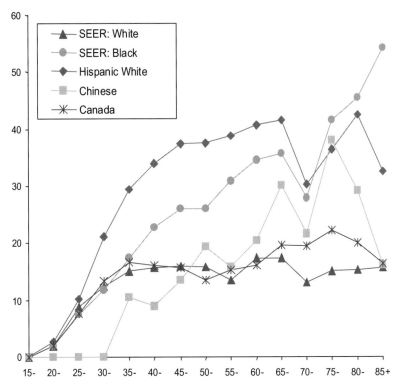

US SEER program includes nine participants: 5 states & 4 metropolitan areas. This represents about 10% of the total population of the US. States: Connecticut, Iowa, New Mexico, Utah and Hawaii. Metropolitan Areas: San Francisco Bay Area (California), Detroit (Michigan), Atlanta (Georgia) and Seattle (Washington).
Hispanic White: Los Angeles, San Francisco, New Mexico, and Central California
Chinese: Los Angeles, San Francisco, Hawaii

Figure 2. Age specific incidence rates of cervical cancer in the US by ethnic group
(Cancer Incidence in Five Continents, 1997)

1.2   The incidence of cervical cancer precursors

Some cancer registries provide information on the incidence of pre-neoplasic cervical lesions (CIN3, carcinoma in-situ). Figure 3 shows the age specific estimates of incidence of CIN 3 and invasive cancer in two population-based registries (Mallorca and Tarragona) in Spain, a country at low risk of cervical cancer.

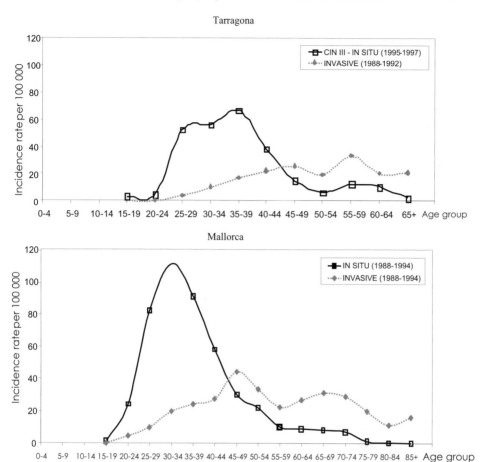

Reference: Cancer Incidence in Five Continents, 1997 and personal communication

Figure 3. Age specific incidence rates of CIN III and invasive cancer in two
population-based cancer registries in Tarragona and Majorca, Spain.

The striking relative proportion of CIN3 to invasive cancer is similar to observations in other registries. The data indicate that the development of CIN3 is a very common event in the young age groups (rates for CIN3 reached values of 70 and 110 per 100 000 in the age groups 30 to 40) and strongly suggest that an important proportion of the CIN3 lesions diagnosed in the younger age groups are not true precursors of invasive cancer. The inclusion of CIN 2 cases in the group of CIN3/carcinoma in situ cases may explain a fraction of the high incidence observed in these registries.

The Spanish data also show a slight increase of CIN 3 lesions and of cervical cancer in the age group 55 and above; this observation is consistent with a second mode in the HPV DNA prevalence as reported in some populations, for example in Mexico and Costa Rica (Herrero et al., 2000; Lazcano et al. 2001).

1.3   Some limitations of the descriptive data

Cancer registration is a well-developed discipline that has achieved remarkable progress over the last decades. Likewise, reasonable estimates of mortality are available from a number of regions in the world, largely in developed countries. These form the bases of the estimates presented in Table 1 and Figures 1-3. However, some important difficulties limit the interpretation of the available estimates. In brief, these include: a) the marked reduction of cervical cancer incidence and mortality achieved by screening, either in organized programs or, to a lesser extent, in spontaneous case-finding settings; b) the dependence of cancer registries on the quality of the health services in the population, the availability of diagnostic and registration resources and the accessibility of these services to the population at large; c) the absence of cancer registries and mortality statistics in extensive areas of the world, notably in developing countries at high risk of cervical cancer; d) the lack of registries of pre-invasive cervical lesions in most countries and e) the limited number of surveys reporting on the cervical prevalence of HPV DNA in representative samples of the female population and in males.

2   HUMAN PAPILLOMAVIRUS AND OTHER RISK FACTORS FOR CERVICAL CANCER AND ITS PRECURSORS

The evidence relating HPV infections to cervical cancer includes a large and consistent body of studies indicating a strong and specific role of the presence of HPV DNA in all settings where investigations have taken place. The association has been recognized as causal in nature by a number of international review panels since the early 1990s (reviewed in Bosch et al., 2002). A brief summary of some key studies and results is presented below.

2.1   The prevalence of HPV-DNA in cervical cancer

State-of-the art amplification techniques used in case-control studies, case-series and prevalence surveys have unequivocally shown that in adequate specimens of cervical cancer, HPV-DNA can be detected in 90 to 100% of cases. This compares to a prevalence of some 5-20% from cervical specimens of women identified as suitable epidemiological controls. Detailed investigations of the few cervical cancer specimens that appear initially as HPV DNA negatives in every series suggest that these are largely false negatives. As a consequence, the claim has been made that this is the first *necessary cause* of a human cancer ever identified, and provides a strong rationale for the use of HPV tests in screening programs and for the development of HPV vaccines (Bosch et al., 1995; Walboomers et al., 1999).

2.1.1 HPV type distribution in cervical cancer

Of the more than 35 HPV types found in the genital tract, HPV 16 accounts for some 50% to 60% of the cervical cancer cases in most countries, followed by HPV 18 (10-12%) and HPV 31 and 45 (4-5% each). Cervical adenocarcinomas show a slightly different distribution with a predominance of HPV 18 (see Chapter 8). Figure 4 shows the cumulative distribution of the most common HPV types by histology. Among cases, HPV 16, 18, 45 and 31 or 59 accounted for 80% of the distribution in squamous cell cancers and for 94% in adenocarcinomas. In the remaining 20% of cervical cancers, many additional types are found in frequency ranging from 0.1% to 3%.

For the purpose of HPV testing in clinical practice and the preparation of HPV vaccines, the wide range of types found in invasive cancers poses a formidable challenge. HPV testing for the most common 10-15 high-risk types would safely cover the vast majority of the cancer-associated HPVs. In this regard, Hybrid Capture II probe B contains a cocktail of 13 high-risk types. However, vaccine preparation with multiple antigens is proving to be difficult and costly and the currently available prototypes may only offer protection for just a fraction of the high-risk HPV types. It is thus anticipated that even when vaccination products are available covering 2 to 5 high-risk types, combined strategies of screening and vaccination will be required for the prevention of most cervical cancer cases.

HPV 16, 18, 45 and 31 or 59 also account for 43% of the prevalence observed in women with normal cervical smears, corresponding to controls in most case control studies or *ad hoc* HPV prevalence surveys from the general

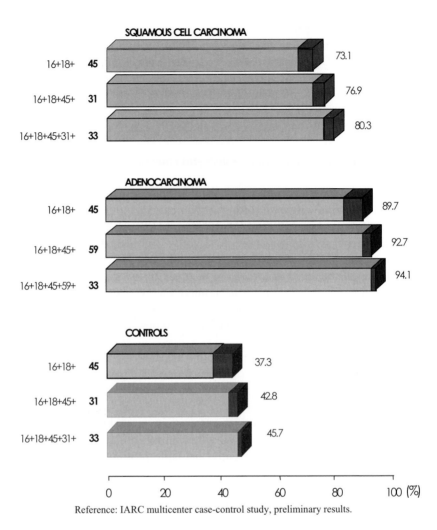

Reference: IARC multicenter case-control study, preliminary results.

Figure 4. Cumulative prevalence of HPV types in cervical cancer cases by histology and in HPV positive controls.

population. In series of women without cervical lesions, the HPV type distribution embraces a much larger series of viral types. HPV 16 remains again the most common type (some 23% of the HPV DNA positive) followed by HPV 18 (10% of the HPV DNA positive), HPV 45 (8% of the HPV DNA positive), HPV 31 (5 % of the HPV DNA positive), and smaller proportions of up to 30 additional HPV types. In most studies, HPV 18 predominates in adenocarcinomas in absolute or relative terms. The reasons for such specificity are unknown.

2.2   Risk estimates from case control studies

Table 2 shows the summary results of some of the best case-control studies completed to date, including the preliminary results of the IARC's research program on HPV and cervical cancer. To date, this is the largest data set available on invasive cancer and a major source of reference data. Table 2 shows very high ORs with most estimates in the range of 50 to 150, and several estimates much higher. The table also shows consistent findings for pre-invasive lesions, for squamous cell carcinomas and adeno-carcinomas, for studies that tested once or twice for HPV DNA, for studies that tested for HPV as a cocktail of several types or for studies that restricted the analyses to high-risk HPV types.

Table 2. Odds ratios and 95% confidence intervals
found in case-control studies published after 2000

AUTHOR / YEAR	OR	(95% CI)	COMMENTS
Herrero et al. 2000	320	(97-1000)	HSIL / CIS (HPV 16)
	46	(14-150)	CX (any HPV type)
	710	(110-4500)	CX (HPV 16)
Munoz et al. 2000	86.7	(68.3-110.0)	SCC (any HPV type)
	188.3	(134.5-63.6)	SCC (HPV 16)
Bosch et al. 2000	47.5	(27.0-83.7)	ADC (all HPV types)
	179.5	(81.2-396.7)	ADC (HPV 18)
Thomas et al. 2000	155	(72-385)	SCC (oncogenic HPV types)
	106	(41-317)	ADC (oncogenic HPV types)
	83	(39-232)	SCC (HPV 16)
	24	(8.7-76)	ADC (HPV 16)
Ylitalo et al. 2000	31.2	(10.6-918)	CIS / HPV 16
			Two consecutive HPV + smears
Josefsson et al. 2000	68.8	(5.8-299.6)	CIS / HPV 16 high viral load

CX: cervical cancer
SCC: Squamous cell carcinomas
ADC: adenocarcinoma

CIS: carcinoma in situ
HSIL: high grade squamous
     intraepithelial lesion

2.2.1   Do all high-risk HPV types predict equivalent risk of cervical cancer?

The pool of IARC studies is large enough to provide, for the first time, type-specific risk estimates for over 14 HPV types. The preliminary results are based on 2288 invasive squamous cell carcinomas, 141 adenocarcinomas and 2513 matched controls in nine countries. The adjusted odds ratios (OR) for HPV DNA detection (the factor by which the reference risk of cervical cancer is multiplied if HPV DNA is detected) was for squamous cell carcinomas OR (any type) = 83.3 (95% CI: 54.9-105.3). Type specific risk estimates were as follows: HPV 16, OR= 182; HPV 18, OR= 231; HPV 45, OR=148; HPV 31, OR=71.5; HPV 33, OR=77.6; HPV 35, OR=34.8; HPV51, OR= 42.7; HPV 52, OR=145.7; HPV 58, OR=78.9; HPV 59, OR=347.3. The corresponding risk estimates for cervical adenocarcinoma were OR (all types) = 47.5 (95% CI 27.0-83.7) and type specific risk estimates were for HPV 16, OR=95.4 and for HPV 18, OR=179.5. According to these results, the types that have to be considered of high risk for cervical cancer are, at least, the following 14 HPV types: HPV 16, 18, 45, 31, 52, 33, 58, 35, 59, 51, 56, 39, 73, 82. The risk for any given high-risk type was not statistically different from the risk reported for HPV 16 (Bosch et al., 2000; Muñoz et al., 2000). The standard estimates of the attributable fraction (the proportion of disease that is related to HPV DNA) derived from these and most other studies range from 90 to 98%. Several studies in both developed and developing countries have shown that HPV and HPV type distribution are related to cervical cancer precursor lesions with the same strength as with the more advanced invasive cancers (Bosch et al., 1993; Kjaer et al., 1996; Liaw et al., 1995; Moreno et al., 1995; Olsen et al., 1995) .

These results provide a strong rationale for including at least these 14 HPV types in testing systems for clinical purposes and for accepting HPV DNA group-testing as a risk predictor in screening or triage programs.

2.3   Risk estimates from follow-up studies

Follow-up or cohort studies are designed to monitor women from cytological normalcy to the stage of high-grade cervical intraepithelial neoplasia (HSIL or CIN 2/3). Studies that have included repeated cervical sampling for viral persistence and cervical abnormalities have shown that the median duration of infection with HPV is around 8 months for high risk HPV types as compared to 4.8 months for the low risk HPV types (Franco et al., 1999; Ho et al., 1998; Woodman et al., 2001). These time intervals, although fairly constant across studies, still suffer from imprecision in the estimates of time at first exposure, from the variability in the end-point definition, and from censoring due to treatment of the early lesions.

Follow-up studies of women with and without cervical abnormalities have indicated that the continuous presence of HR-HPV is necessary for the development, maintenance and progression of CIN (Ho et al., 1998; Nobbenhuis et al., 2001). A substantial fraction (i.e., 15-30%) of women with HR-HPV DNA who are cytomorphologically normal at recruitment will develop CIN 2 or CIN 3 within the subsequent 4-year interval (Rozendaal et al., 1996; Rozendaal et al., 2000). Conversely, among women found to be HR-HPV DNA negative and cytologically identified as either ASCUS, borderline or mild dysplasia, CIN 2/3 is unlikely to develop during a follow-up of at least two years and their cytology is likely to return to normal (Nobbenhuis et al., 2001; Zielinski et al., 2001). Women found positive for low risk HPVs rarely become persistent carriers and their probability of progression to CIN 2/3 is extremely low (Rozendaal et al., 1996).

As ongoing cohorts expand their follow up time, more precise estimates are being provided on the predictive value of viral persistence as defined by repeated measurements of viral types and variants. One such cohort, in Sao Paulo, Brazil, has shown that the incidence rate of cervical lesions in women who were HPV negative twice was 0.73 per 1000 women-months. The corresponding incidence rate among women with repeated HPV 16 or HPV-18 positive results was 8.68 per 1000 women-months, a 12-fold increased incidence rate. The OR for HPV persistence among women who were twice HPV positive for the same oncogenic type was 41.2 (95% CI=10.7-158.3) (Schlecht et al., 2001). Retrospective assessment of HPV status using archival smears from cases of cervical cancer and controls has provided evidence that HPV DNA preceded the development of invasive disease, and showed its value in identifying false-negatives smears (Zielinski et al., 2001). An interesting observation from a research group in Amsterdam suggests that clearance of HR-HPV in otherwise established cytological lesions is a marker associated with regression of CIN lesions (Nobbenhuis et al., 2001; Zielinski et al., 2001). Finally, persistence of HPV-DNA detection after treatment for CIN 2/3 is an accurate predictor of relapse, and is at least as sensitive as repeated vaginal cytology (Nobbenhuis et al., 2001).

These results are useful in defining the clinical role of HPV testing. However most observations on pre-invasive disease have limitations for making inferences about cervical cancer causality. This is because even in controlled settings, observations are not allowed to continue beyond the stage of high-grade squamous intraepithelial lesions (HSIL/CIN 3) or carcinoma in situ. Lack of follow up and censoring of women at high risk may explain the relatively lower risk estimates obtained from cohort studies as compared to case-control studies.

Retrospective cohort studies have documented the existence of HPV exposure years before the development of invasive cervical cancer, thus reproducing the conditions of a longitudinal study. With this approach, a relative risk estimate of 16.4 (95%CI 4.4-75.1) was observed for invasive cervical cancer in Sweden using DNA extracted from stored Pap smears (Wallin et al., 1999) and of 32 (95% CI 6.8-153) in the Netherlands (Zielisnki et al., 2001), and a relative risk of about 5 was observed in Sweden for carcinoma in situ of the cervix (Ylitalo et al., 2000). In a similar study design, an OR of 2.4 (95% CI 1.6-3.7) was obtained using serologic markers of HPV exposure (Hakim et al., 2000).

2.4   Other risk factors for cervical cancer

Soon after the introduction of HPV testing in research protocols, it became clear that most of the key risk factors that described sexual behavior, such as the number of sexual partners, merely reflected the probability of HPV exposure. Other factors, such as the estimates of age at first exposure (as indicated by age at first sexual intercourse or age at first marriage) are still under evaluation for independency. In addition, a number of environmental factors that had historically been related to cervical cancer are currently being re-assessed. These include hormonal factors (use of oral contraceptives and multiparity), cigarette smoking, other STDs (herpes simplex virus type 2 (HSV-2), Chlamydia trachomatis (CT) and occasionally any other STD), and dietary factors. Special consideration should be given to exposure to HIV and to other situations of immunosuppression, but these will not be addressed in detail in this discussion.

Because of the growing evidence that HPV infection is necessary for the development of cervical cancer, it soon became a standard procedure in the reports of case-control studies to include analyses restricted to HPV positive cases and controls. Table 3 presents a current view on the factors that may increase the risk of progression to CIN3/invasive cancer among HPV DNA positive women. The table is largely based on the IARC studies, which are consistent with several other reports.

Table 3. Risk factors for cervical cancer among human papillomavirus positive women. Results of the IARC multicenter study.

RISK FACTOR	RISK EXPOSURE	REFERENCE
HPV DNA in cervical exfoliates	Positive for high risk types	Bosch et al. 1992
Use of Oral Contraceptives	5 or more years of use	Moreno et al 2002
Smoking	Ever	Plummer et al., submitted
Parity	5 or more pregnancies	Muñoz et al. 2002
Clamydia trachomatis	Ab. Positive	Smith et al. 2002a
HSV – 2	Ab. Positive	Smith et al., 2002b
Sexual partner	□ Uncircumcised with 6+ add'l partners □ Multiple additional partners	Castellsagué et al. 2002

2.4.1. Oral contraceptives

In the IARC studies, ever use of OCs was associated with a statistically significant increase in risk of cervical cancer (OR=1.47, 95% CI=1.02-2.12). Use of OCs for less than 5 years was not related to cervical cancer (OR = 0.77, 95% CI=0.46-1.29) but the risk increased significantly for 5-9 years of use (OR = 2.72, 95% CI=1.36-5.46) and for 10+ years (OR=4.48, 95% CI=2.24-9.36) (Moreno et al., 2002). A meta-analysis of the literature, including some of the early studies that used modestly sensitive HPV testing systems, also found a 2 to 3 fold increased risk among long term users (Beral et al., personal communication).

The evidence for an association of cervical cancer with the use of hormonal contraceptives is not entirely consistent. A number of studies that investigated HPV positive women found no associations or only weak associations in subgroup analyses. These apparently conflicting results may reflect the increased cytological surveillance of women that are taking OCs in developed countries and the use of different "case" definition (from ASCUS up to HSIL/CIN3 as opposed to cervical cancer) in cohort studies. Because of the potential public health importance of confirming an interaction between long-term use of OCs and HPV infections in the development of cervical cancer, efforts are now being devoted to verify the results in different populations. If confirmed, this interaction would support the introduction of HPV tests in the screening protocols of long-term users of OCs.

2.4.2 Smoking

The pooled results of the IARC's study found that "ever smoking" was associated with a two-fold, statistically significant, increased risk of cervical cancer with a significant dose response (Plummer et al., personal communication). These findings are consistent with other studies examining different aspects of smoking such as "current vs. never smoking" among HPV positive women in the Costa Rica study (OR=2.3) (Hildesheim et al., 2001), the Portland study (OR=2.7 for CIN 2-3) (Schiffman et al., 1993), the Copenhagen study (OR=1.9), (Kjaer 1998) and the Manchester study (OR= 2.2) (Deacon et al., 2000). These recent studies are providing growing evidence on the carcinogenic effect of cigarette smoking in women with HPV infection.

An extensive review of the relation between smoking and cervical cancer was published in 1998 (Szarewsky and Cuzick, 1998). It included eight cohort and 44 case-control studies. The report concluded that the association was largely consistent in studies that adjusted for HPV DNA or restricted analyses to HPV positive women. The magnitude of the increase in risk for current smokers was of the order of 1- to 3-fold. The ORs tended to be higher in more advanced pre-invasive neoplasms and in several studies a dose-response relationship was observed with the amount of tobacco consumed. A review of the evidence, conducted by the Surgeon General in the US, concluded that the hypothesis claiming a causal association between cigarette smoking and cervical cancer was plausible. However, the report indicated that the extent to which cigarette smoking could be considered independent of HPV could not be definitively assessed (Surgeon General's Advisory Committee on Women and Smoking, 2001). The Monograph program at IARC reviewed the evidence in 2002 and concluded that smoking was an independent risk factor for cervical cancer (IARC 2003, in preparation).

The mechanisms by which cigarette smoking may affect cervical cancer remain elusive. Several hypotheses backed up by some evidence have been proposed, for example a direct effect of the tobacco metabolites, an indirect effect related to tobacco-induced immunosupression, or even an effect related to reduced dietary antioxidants induced by smoking (Szarewski et al., 1998). This is certainly an area where further studies are warranted.

2.4.3   Parity

HPV positive women who reported seven or more full term pregnancies had a four-fold increased risk of cervical cancer as compared to HPV positive women that were nulliparous (OR=3.8, 95% CI=2.7-5.5) after adjustment for socioeconomic and sexual behavior factors. There was still a two-fold increased risk when women reporting 7 or more pregnancies were compared to HPV positive women who reported 1-2 full term pregnancies (Muñoz et al., 2002). Similar results were obtained in Costa Rica (Hildesheim et al., 2001) and Thailand (Thomas et al., 2001). In populations with low parity the effects are less visible. The effect of parity, perhaps related to the hormonal changes occurring during pregnancy, along with the results of studies of OCs, strongly argue in favor of a genuine interaction between the HPV life cycle and the host's hormonal environment. Some authors have suggested that part of the international reduction in cervical cancer incidence observed in developed countries may be related to the general reduction in the number of pregnancies.

2.4.4   Other sexually transmitted agents (STA) and cervical inflammation

Markers of exposure to other STAs have been repeatedly found to be associated with cervical cancer. Results from the IARC´s multicenter study found a 2-fold increased risk for the presence of antibodies to Chlamydia trachomatis (OR = 2.1, 95% CI=1.1-4.0) (Smith et al., 2002a) and to herpes simplex type 2 viruses (OR = 2.0, 95% CI=1.3-3.0) (Smith et al., 2002b; de Sanjosé et al., 1994). Non-specific inflammatory changes have also been related to modest increases in risk among HPV-positive women (Castle et al., 2001). The difficulties with the evaluations of such factors lie in the strong colinearity observed among all STDs and the limitations of some of the biomarkers currently used to assess ever exposure or persistent exposure.

2.4.5   Husband's circumcision

As with any STD, the role of males as vectors of HPV has been established for some time (Bosch et al., 1996; Castellsagué et al., 1997; Franceschi et al., 2002). A recent report also confirmed a long-term epidemiological hypothesis claiming that male circumcision was protective against penile cancer and against cervical cancer in wives (Castellsagué et al., 2002). This study reported a significant reduction in HPV prevalence among circumcised males, all other factors being constant. The wives of circumcised males also had a significantly lower prevalence of HPV DNA and, most importantly, of cervical cancer. The protection against HPV and HPV-related neoplasia was more clearly observed among women whose husbands reported 6 or more additional sexual partners than among spouses of males with 5 or fewer number of lifetime sexual partners.

2.4.6   Other factors

Other environmental risk factors with potential impact in defining preventive strategies are currently under evaluation. Early age at exposure has been proven to be a strong determinant of the prognosis of carcinogenic viral infections in relation to cancer development, for example for HBV induced liver cancer or for EBV infection in relation to Burkitt's lymphoma. Likewise, most studies have shown that the risk of cervical cancer is related to age at first sexual intercourse. Definite evidence that cervical cancer progression is linked to age at first HPV exposure has not been provided. Low socio-economic level among cervical cancer cases is a consistent finding in descriptive and case-control studies with still a poorly understood interpretation. Likewise, nutritional factors are probably relevant and some intervention trials with selected nutrients have been initiated (Potischman et al., 1996). However, few studies have been designed so far to fully explore nutritional issues.

The interpretation of the risk estimates for co-factors should consider that, as far as we understand them today, these are conditional effects that apply if, and probably only if, HPV DNA is persistently present in the cervical cells. Moreover, these factors have not generally been found related to HPV DNA prevalence (with perhaps the exception of husband's circumcision). In conjunction with the risk analyses of HPV prevalence, some authors view these results as indicative of a promoter effect of OC use, smoking or multiparity from HPV infections to HPV-related neoplasia and cancer.

2.5   Some limitations of the epidemiological evidence

One limitation of the available studies is the crudeness of information available on variables that may indeed modulate the effect. This makes it difficult to explain to the finer details the geographic variation in cervical cancer incidence and the variability in risk estimates reported in different populations. For example, the inconsistencies in finding associations of cervical cancer with the use of OCs may be explained by factors related to the intensity, duration or the chemical composition of the exposure. Factors which are largely country-specific, like the variability in time since widespread introduction, availability of combined vs. sequential products, estrogen/progesterone doses, etc., could be important determinants yet these are difficult to estimate from questionnaire-based studies and, as a consequence, would be only partially accounted for in the analyses of the available studies.

A second general limitation is that many studies did not consider host factors in relation to HPV. HLA types and p53 polymorphisms are being actively investigated because of the indication that they may play a role in the natural history of HPV infections (Stern et al., 1994; Storey et al., 1998). The putative effect of such individual susceptibility factors is not adjusted for in the risk analyses of the environmental factors. However, at this stage, there is limited information to substantiate an effect of these host factors as independent of HPV (Mankni et al., 2000; Zehbe et al., 2001) .

There is a clear need to pursue research in understanding the factors that determine whether a woman with an HPV infection will clear the infection or become a persistent carrier. Further, studies are still needed to explore if additional factors play a role in determining neoplastic progression and how to best use this information in screening and patient management.

3   CAUSALITY EVALUATION – CURRENT CONCEPTS AND IMPLICATIONS

The evaluation of the evidence relating HPV to cervical neoplasia in terms of the established considerations of causality has been done on several occasions. Of the classical Hill criteria, largely adopted by review institutions, HPV DNA as detected in cervical cells satisfies most of them, notably the ones of greater significance such as *temporality, strength of the association, biologic plausibility and coherence with current knowledge.* Table 4 summarizes the HPV DNA and cervical cancer evidence as recently evaluated (Bosch et al., 2002).

Table 4. Compliance of the HPV and cervical cancer association with the most relevant of the criteria used to asses causality

CRITERIA	CONCEPT	EVALUATION	MOST RELEVANT CONTRIBUTION
Time sequence	Exposure must precede disease	Strong evidence	▫ Cohort studies ▫ Cross-sectional prevalence surveys ▫ Screened populations
Strength and consistency	High OR/RR Robust association in different settings	Strong evidence	▫ Cohort studies ▫ Case-control studies ▫ Nested case-control studies
Biological plausibility	Understanding the carcinogenic mechanisms	Strong evidence	▫ Viral-host interaction studies
Coherence	Consistent with previous knowledge	Strong evidence	▫ Epidemiology of HPV and Cervix
Dose-response	Risk of disease is related to level of exposure	Inconsistent	▫ Studies of viral-load
Experimental (prevention)	Reduction of disease following reductions in exposure	Not available	▫ HPV vaccination studies

Temporality. Temporality, or time-sequence, refers to the necessity that the cause precedes the effect in time. The temporality of an association is probably the only "sine qua non" condition: If the "cause" does not precede the effect that indeed is indisputable evidence that the association is not causal. This criterion is fulfilled by the follow-up studies documenting HPV exposure (using either HPV DNA or serum antibodies) years before the development of cervical cancer. Additional evidence is provided by cross-sectional prevalence surveys showing that the bulk of HPV infection precedes the bulk of cervical cancer cases and by screening trials showing that the viral presence predicts by several months the occurrence of neoplasia.

Strength. Strength of the association is typically measured by the magnitude of the ratio of incidence rates between exposed and unexposed individuals. The argument claims that strong associations are more likely to be causal and weak associations are more vulnerable to undetected biases. Nevertheless, the fact that an association is weak does not rule out a causal connection. The level and the consistency of the associations shown in Table

2 is one of the strongest ever reported for a human cancer, only matched by some studies of HBV or HCV and liver cancer.

Biologic Plausibility and Coherence. Taken from the Surgeon General's report on Smoking and Heath (1964) (Surgeon General's Advisory Committee on Women and Smoking, 2001), the term coherence implies that a cause and effect interpretation for an association does not conflict with what is known of the natural history and biology of the disease. In the HPV example, the mechanisms by which HPV induces cancer in humans and the molecular genetics of the process are being intensively investigated. Excellent reviews are readily available (Shah et al., 1996; zur Hausen et al., 2000) and a discussion is presented in other sections of this book (see Chapters 3 and 4). Accordingly, the causal nature of this association is indicated by: 1) Regular presence of HPV-DNA in the neoplastic cells of respective tumor biopsy specimens; 2) Demonstration of viral oncogene expression (E6 and E7) in tumor material but not in stromal cells; 3) Transforming properties of these E6 and E7 genes; 4) Requirement for E6 and E7 expression for maintaining the malignant phenotype of cervical carcinoma cell lines; 5) Interaction of viral oncoproteins with growth-regulating host-cell proteins; and 6) Epidemiological studies pointing at these HPV infections as the major risk factors for cervical cancer development (zur Hausen et al., 2000).

Experimental Evidence. In human data, the experimental criterion takes the form of preventive interventions and explores whether there is evidence that reduction in exposure to the agent is associated with a reduction in risk. Evidence for this important criterion will only be available when vaccination trials achieve a reduced incidence of cervical cancer among vaccinated women.

4   THE CONCEPT OF HPV AS A NECESSARY CAUSE OF CERVICAL CANCER

Most results from individual clinical or epidemiological studies are compatible with the hypothesis that a fraction of cases of cervical cancer (some 5 to 10%) is independent of HPV. This hypothesis should be retained as a scientific and research option, and attempts should be made to evaluate this possibility. The theoretical grounds for proposing the existence of HPV negative cervical cancer cases lie in: 1) Epithelial cells are capable of developing into cancer cells and cancer growth in all human tissues regardless of a known, viral or non viral, cause. Thus, cells in the human cervix might do so too. 2) Cellular genetic changes that underlie HPV-related carcinogenesis could occur spontaneously in the absence of HPV. Available evidence suggests that this event is extremely rare within the lifespan expectation of the human population. 3) Relatively few cases of cervical cancer in very old women have been investigated. It is likely that the non-HPV related cancers, because they occur very rarely, cluster among very old women. 4) Non-epithelial cancers (lymphomas and sarcomas) do occur in the cervix at a low frequency.

To explain the HPV negative cases, two alternatives could be considered. It is conceivable that some cervical cancer cases truly occur unrelated to the viral exposure. Some previous analyses that have compared the epidemiological profile of "HPV-positive" and "HPV-negative" women with cervical cancer did not find significant differences in their sexual or reproductive behavior. Therefore, the HPV-unrelated hypothesis would argue in favor of a role for one or several other STDs. Current results of some major studies found modest and inconsistent effects from previous exposures to Chlamydia trachomatis (Koskela et al., 2000; Smith et al., 2002a; van den Brule et al., 2002) and/or type 2 herpes simplex virus infections (Smith et al., 2002b). However, these effects are mostly seen in the presence of HPV DNA. The effect of some putative but yet unidentified, sexually transmitted, viral factor has not been substantiated.

Conversely, the fraction of HPV negative cases regularly reported by field studies may still suffer from under-detection and misclassification of the HPV DNA status. In this regard, a particularly relevant exercise was undertaken to verify HPV misclassification in the cases included in a large survey of cases conducted by IARC in the early 1990's (IBSCC study). In brief, the project included over 1000 cervical cancer cases from 22 countries. Biopsies were analyzed using the MY 09/11 PCR system and serum samples were analyzed using VLP antibodies. The first results were published reporting an HPV DNA prevalence of 93.0% (Bosch et al., 1995). Subsequently, the apparently HPV-negative cases were further investigated. The second level evaluation included: a) a comparison of the serological and epidemiological profiles of the "HPV DNA negatives" and the "HPV DNA positives"; b) a review of the pathology of the specimen. Serial cuts from the paraffin blocks were used to ensure that the specimen used for HPV DNA testing included neoplastic tissue; and c) a different technology was used for HPV DNA testing using shorter primers in the E7 region and two sets of consensus primers (CP I/II and GP5+/6+). The final results of the study indicated that the majority of the HPV-negative cases were in fact HPV-positive and that the HPV types newly identified were the common types with an overrepresentation of HPV 18. The reasons for non-detection of HPV DNA at first round of testing were poor biopsy preservation or lack of cancer cells in the specimen and differences in sensitivity of the HPV DNA detection methods used. The shorter primers used in the reevaluation were better suited to detect integrated HPV DNA which tends to occur more often in HPV 18-related cancer cases. Based upon the final results of this study and the considerable body of evidence accumulated from other studies it was proposed that HPV DNA is in fact a necessary cause of cervical cancer (Walboomers et al., 1999).

The key consideration from this discussion, however, is that with the current level of understanding, it would be difficult to justify an etiological model that would not include HPV DNA for the vast majority of cervical cancer cases occurring worldwide. On these grounds, HPV fulfils the criteria for a necessary cause of cervical cancer, the only necessary cause identified in cancer epidemiology to date.

5   CLINICAL IMPLICATIONS

Recognition of the central role of HPV in cervical cancer has profound implications for clinical and preventive strategies. On the one hand, the concept of risk groups comes into focus. High-risk women can now be sharply redefined as the group of persistent HPV carriers. For practical purposes this represents substantial progress from previous versions of the definition of the high-risk group that identified women with at least one of a constellation of ill-defined factors (low socioeconomic status, high number of sexual partners, smoking, use of oral contraceptives, history of STDs, ever exposure to a sexually promiscuous male, etc.). Exposure to at least one of these characteristics would nowadays include the vast majority of women in most countries, thus being of little practical interest to discriminate in management protocols. Most of these factors are now viewed either as surrogates of HPV exposure or as relevant co-factors given the presence of HPV DNA.

On the other hand, if indeed HPV is a *necessary cause* of cervical cancer, the implication is that specific preventive practices targeting some putative non-HPV-related cervical cancer cases are no longer justified. Finally, technology is now available to enable HPV DNA positive women to be identified in the general population. In the near future, properly designed HPV vaccines should be able to offer a realistic preventive option to the underserved populations of the world, where most of the cases and deaths due to cervical cancer still occur.

CONCLUSION

Research at the population level has largely accomplished its task by providing an exhaustive body of evidence on the viral etiology of cervical cancer. It is now time for public health institutions to evaluate these achievements, consider the costs and benefits involved, and apply this knowledge to their guidelines, recommendations and policies.

REFERENCES

Cancer Incidence in Five Continents, vol. VII. IARC Scientific Publications No. 143 ed. Lyon: International Agency for Research on Cancer, 1997.

Bosch FX, Castellsagué X, Muñoz N, de Sanjosé S, Ghaffari AM, González LC et al. Male sexual behavior and Human Papillomavirus DNA: key risk factors for cervical cancer in Spain. J Natl Cancer Inst 1996; 88:1060-1067.

Bosch FX, Lorincz A, Munoz N, Meijer CJ, Shah KV. The causal relation between human papillomavirus and cervical cancer. J Clin Pathol 2002; 55:244-265.

Bosch FX, Manos M, Muñoz N, et al. Prevalence of human papillomavirus in cervical cancer: a worldwide perspective. J Natl Cancer Inst 1995; 87:796-802.

Bosch FX, Muñoz N, Chichareon S, et al. HPV and cervical adenocarcinoma: an IARC based multicentric case-control study. In: Castellsagué X, Bosch FX, de Sanjose S, Moreno V, Ribes J, editors. 18th International Papillomavirus Conference - program and abstracts book. Barcelona: Thau, S.L., 2000: 131 (Available on line: http:/www.hpv2000.com).

Bosch FX, Muñoz N, de Sanjosé S, et al. Risk Factors for cervical cancer in Colombia and Spain. Int J Cancer 1992; 52:750-758.

Bosch FX, Muñoz N, de Sanjosé S, et al. Human Papilloma virus and Cervical Intraepithelial Neoplasia Grade III/Carcinoma in situ:a case-control study in Spain and Colombia. Cancer Epidemiol Biomarkers Prev 1993; 2:415-422.

Castellsague X, Bosch FX, Munoz N, et al. Male circumcision, penile human papillomavirus infection, and cervical cancer in female partners. N Engl J Med 2002; 346: 1105-1112.

Castellsagué X, Ghaffari A, Daniel RW, et. al. Prevalence of penile human papillomavirus DNA in husbands of women with and without cervical neoplasia: A study in Spain and Colombia. J Infect Dis 1997; 176:353-361.

Castle PE, Hillier SL, Rabe LK, et al. An Association of cervical inflammation with high-grade cervical neoplasia in women infected with oncogenic human papillomavirus (HPV). Cancer Epidemiol Biomarkers Prev 2001; 10:1021-1027.

de Sanjosé S, Muñoz N, Bosch FX, et al. Sexually transmitted agents and cervical neoplasia in Colombia and Spain. Int J Cancer 1994; 56:358-363.

Deacon J, Peto J, Yule R, et al. Sexual behaviour and smoking as determinants of cervical HPV infection and of CIN3 among those infected: a case-control study nested within the Manchester cohort. Br J Cancer 2000; 88:1565-1572.

Ferlay J, Bray F, Pisani P, Parkin DM. Globocan 2000: Cancer incidence, Mortality and Prevalence Worldwide, Version 1.0. IARC CancerBase No. 5. IARC Press, 2001.

Franceschi S, Castellsague X, dal Maso L, et al. Prevalence and determinants of human papillomavirus genital infection in men. Br J Cancer 2002; 86:705-711.

Franco EL, Villa LL, Sobrinho JP, et al. Epidemiology of acquisition and clearance of cervical human papillomavirus infection in women from a high-risk area for cervical cancer. J Infect Dis 1999; 180:1415-1423.

Hakim IA, Harris RB, Weisgerber UM. Tea Intake and squamous cell carcinoma of the skin: influence of type of tea beverages. Cancer Epidemiol Biomarkers Prev 2000; 9:727-731.

Herrero R, Hildesheim A, Bratti C, et al. Population-based study of human papillomavirus infection and cervical neoplasia in rural Costa Rica. J Natl Cancer Inst 2000; 92:464-474.

Hildesheim A, Herrero R, Castle PE, et al. HPV co-factors related to the development of cervical cancer: results from a population-based study in Costa Rica. Br J Cancer 2001; 84: 1219-1226.

Ho GYF, Bierman R, Beardsley L, et al. Natural history of cervicovaginal papillomavirus infection in young women. N Engl J Med 1998; 338, 423-428.

Josefsson AM, Magnusson PK, Ylitalo N, et al. Viral load of human papilloma virus 16 as a determinant for development of cervical carcinoma in situ: a nested case-control study. Lancet 2000; 355:2189-2193.

Kjaer SK. Risk factors for cervical neoplasia in Denmark. APMIS Suppl 1998; 80:1-41.

Kjaer SK, Van den Brule AJC, Bock JE, et al. Human Papilloma virus - The most significant risk determinant of cervical intraepithelial neoplasia. Int J Cancer 1996; 65:601-606.

Koskela P, Anttila T, Björge T, et al. *Chlamydia Trachomatis* infection as a risk factor for invasive cervical cancer. Int J Cancer 2000; 85:35-39.

Lazcano Ponce E, Herrero R, Muñoz N, et al. Epidemiology on HPV infection among mexican women with normal cervical cytology. Int J Cancer 2001; 91:1-9.

Liaw K, Hsing AW, Chen ChJ, et al. Human papilloma virus and cervical neoplasia: a case-control study in Taiwan. Int J Cancer 1995; 62:565-571.

Makni H, Franco EL, Kaiano J, et al. p53 polymorphism in codon 72 and risk of human papillomavirus-induced cervical neoplasia:Effect of inter-laboratory variation. Int J Cancer 2000; 87:528-533.

Moreno V, Bosch FX, Munoz N, et al. Effect of oral contraceptives on risk of cervical cancer in women with human papillomavirus infection: the IARC multicentric case-control study. Lancet 2002; 359:1085-1092.

Moreno V, Muñoz N, Bosch FX, et al. Risk factors for progression of cervical intraepithelial neoplasm grade III to invasive cervical cancer. Cancer Epidemiol Biomarkers Prev 1995; 4:459-467.

Muñoz N, Bosch FX, Chichareon S, et al. A multinational case-control study on the risk of cervical cancer linked to 25 HPV types: which are the high-risk types? In: Castellsagué X, Bosch FX, de Sanjosé S, Moreno V, Ribes J, eds. International Papillomavirus Conference- Program and abstracts book. Barcelona: Thau S.L., 2000: 125 (Available online: http:/www.hpv2000.com).

Muñoz N, Franceschi S, Bosetti C, et al. Role of parity and human papillomavirus in cervical cancer: the IARC multicentric case-control study. Lancet 2002; 359:1093-1102.

Nobbenhuis MA, Helmerhorst TJ, van Den Brule AJ, et al. Cytological regression and clearance of high-risk human papillomavirus in women with an abnormal cervical smear. Lancet 2001; 358:1782-1783.

Nobbenhuis MA, Walboomers JM, Helmerhorst TJ, et al. Relation of human papillomavirus status to cervical lesions and consequences for cervical-cancer screening: a prospective study. Lancet 1999; 354:20-25.

Nobbenhuis MAE, Meijer CJLM, Van den Brule AJC, et al. Addition of high-risk HPV testing improves the current guidelines on follow-up after treatment for cervical intraepithelial neoplasia. Br J Cancer 2001; 84:796-801.

Olsen AO, Gjoen K, Sauer T, et al. Human papilloma virus and cervical intraepithelial neoplasia grade II-III: A population-based case-control study. Int J Cancer 1995; 61:312-315.

Potischman N, Brinton LA. Nutrition and cervical neoplasia. Cancer Causes Control 1996; 7:113-126.

Public Health Service 2. Surgeon General's Advisory Committee on Women and Smoking. Available online: http:/www.cdc.gov/tobacco. 2001.

Rozendaal L, Walboomers JM, van der Linden JC, et al. PCR-based high-risk HPV test in cervical cancer screening gives objective risk assessment of women with cytomorphologically normal cervical smears. Int J Cancer 1996; 68:766-769.

Rozendaal L, Westerga J, van der Linden JC, et al. PCR based high risk HPV testing is superior to neutral network based screening for predicting incident CIN III in women with normal cytology and borderline changes. J Clin Pathol 2000; 53:606-611.

Schiffman MH, Bauer HM, Hoover RN, et al. Epidemiologic evidence showing that human papillomavirus infection causes most cervical intraepithelial neoplasia. J Natl Cancer Inst 1993; 85:958-964.

Schlecht NF, Kulaga S, Robitaille J, et al. Persistent human papillomavirus infection as a predictor of cervical intraepithelial neoplasia. J Am Med Assoc 2001; 286:3106-3114.

Shah KV, Howley PM. Papillomaviruses. In: Fields BN, Knipe DN, Howley PM, eds. Fields Virology. Philadelphia: Lippincott-Raven Publishers, 1996, pp 2077-2109.

Smith JS, Muñoz N, Herrero R, et al. Evidence for *Chlamydia trachomatis* as a human papillomavirus cofactor in the etiology of invasive cervical cancer in Brazil and the Philippines. J Infect Dis 2002a; 185:324-331.

Smith JS, Herrero R, Bosetti C, et al. Herpes simplex virus-2 as a human papillomavirus cofactor in the etiologyof invasive cervical cancer. J Natl Cancer Inst 2002b; 94:1604-13.

Stern P, Duggan-Keen M. MHC expression in the natural history of cervical cancer. In: Stern PL, Stanley MA, eds. Human papillomaviruses and cervical cancer. Biology and immunology. New York: Oxford University Press, 1994: 162-176.

Storey A, Thomas M, Kalita A, et al. Role of a p53 polymorphism in the development of human papillomavirus-associated cancer. Nature 1998; 393:229-234.

Szarewski A, Cuzick J. Smoking and cervical neoplasia: a review of the evidence. J Epidemiol Biostat 1998; 3(3):229-256.

Thomas DB, Ray RM, Koetsawang A, et al. Human papillomaviruses and cervical cancer in Bangkok. I. Risk Factors for invasive cervical carcinomas with human papillomavirus types 16 and 18 DNA. Am J Epidemiol 2001; 153:723-731.

van den Brule AJC, Kjaer SK, Munk C. Development of HPV induced cervical intraepithelial neoplasias: infection with Chamdya tractomatis as a possible cofactor. In: Castellsagué X, Bosch FX, de Sanjosé S, et al., eds. 18th International Papillomavirus Conference - program and abstracts book. 2002.

Walboomers JMM, Jacobs MV, Manos MM, et al. Human papillomavirus is a necessary cause of invasive cervical cancer worldwide. J Pathol 1999; 189:12-19.

Wallin KL, Wiklund F, Ängström T, et al. Type-specific persistence of human papillomavirus DNA before the developments of invasive Cervical Cancer. N Engl J Med 1999; 341:1633-8.

Woodman CB, Collins S, Winter H, et al. Natural history of cervical human papillomavirus infection in young women: a longitudinal cohort study. Lancet 2001; 357:1831-1836.

Ylitalo N, Josefsson A, Melbye M, et al. A Prospective Study Showing Long-Term Infecton with Human Papillomavirus 16 before the Development of Cervical Carcinoma *in situ*. Cancer Res 2000; 60:6027-6032.

Zehbe I, Voglino G, Wilander E, et al. p53 codon 72 polymorphism and various human papillomavirus 16 E6 genotypes are risk factors for cervical cancer development. Papillomavirus Report 2001; 12:66-66.

Zielinski GD, Snijders PJF, Rozendaal L, et al. High-risk HPV testing in women with borderline and mild dyskaryosis: long-term follow-up data and clinical relevance. J Pathol 2001; 193:1-8.

Zielinski GD, Snijders PJF, Rozendaal L, et al. HPV presence precedes abnormal cytology in women developing cervical cancer and signals false negative smears. Br J Cancer 2001; 85:398-404.

zur Hausen H. Papillomaviruses causing cancer: Evasion from host-cell control in early events in carcinogenesis. Review. J Natl Cancer Inst 2000; 92:690-698.

Chapter 8

The Epidemiology of Adenocarcinoma of the Cervix

Thomas E. Rohan, M.B.B.S., Ph.D.
Department of Epidemiology and Population Health, Albert Einstein College of Medicine

INTRODUCTION

Cancer of the cervix is the second most common malignant neoplasm amongst women worldwide (Parkin et al., 2001). Annually, it accounts for approximately 10% of all new cases of cancer in women (about 470,000 cases) (Parkin et al., 1999) and for about 8.5% of deaths from cancer (about 235,000 deaths) (Pisani et al., 1999). It is particularly common in developing countries, and is the main cancer amongst women in sub-Saharan Africa, Latin America and the Caribbean, and South and South East Asia (Parkin et al., 2001). Histologically, about 75% of cervical cancers are squamous cell carcinomas (Vizcaino et al., 1998), the majority of the remainder being adenocarcinomas and mixed adenosquamous tumors (Schiffman et al., 1996). Given the relative rarity of the other histological types, it is perhaps not surprising that most epidemiological studies of cervical cancer either have focused on squamous cell carcinomas (see Chapter 7) or have not differentiated between squamous and other types (Schiffman et al., 1996). However, recent evidence for the increasing importance of adenocarcinoma of the cervix, both in absolute terms and in terms of its relative contribution to total cervical cancer incidence rates (Smith et al., 2000), highlights the need to elucidate its etiology and natural history, and to develop or refine approaches to its detection and prevention.

217

1   NATURAL HISTORY

In contrast to that of squamous cell cervical carcinoma, little is known about the natural history of adenocarcinoma of the cervix (Kudo, 1992). This may reflect the fact that adenocarcinoma arises in the endocervix, so that its putative precursor lesions are less accessible to sampling than their squamous cell counterparts, and therefore less amenable to study.

By analogy to the natural history of squamous cell carcinoma of the cervix, it might be postulated that adenocarcinoma of the cervix arises by the development of progressively more severe precursor lesions in endocervical tissue leading ultimately to adenocarcinoma *in situ* (AIS), the preinvasive form of adenocarcinoma of the cervix, and then to invasive cancer. However, although so-called "endocervical glandular intraepithelial lesions" have been described (Meisels and Morin, 1997), it is not clear that they are true precursors of adenocarcinoma. Indeed, the identity of the earliest abnormal lesions leading to adenocarcinoma is somewhat uncertain, as is the cellular origin of endocervical adenocarcinoma (Kudo, 1992). With respect to the latter, however, it has been suggested that cervical adenocarcinomas may arise from the subcolumnar reserve cells (Ferenczy, 1997). A critique of the very notion that there are precursors of cervical adenocarcinoma is presented in Chapter 1.

The 2001 Bethesda System for the classification of cervical cytology included three categories for abnormalities of glandular cells less severe than adenocarcinoma: atypical glandular cells, either endocervical, endometrial, or "glandular cells" not otherwise specified; atypical glandular cells, either endocervical or "glandular cells" favor neoplasia; and adenocarcinoma *in situ* (Wright et al., 2002). The presence of atypical glandular cells on a cervical smear may indicate the presence of underlying, concurrent cervical neoplasia, either squamous or glandular (Ronnett et al., 1999; Soofer and Sidawy, 2000; Nasuti et al., 2002). However, it appears that there have not been any well-designed prospective studies in which women with atypical glandular cells have been followed to determine progression and regression rates.

Adenocarcinoma *in situ* is considered to be a precursor of invasive adenocarcinoma because the two conditions have similar cytologic features and are often observed to be contiguous to each other; furthermore, as with invasive adenocarcinoma, *in situ* lesions are commonly infected with human papillomavirus (HPV), especially HPV type 18 (Franco and Ferenczy, 2002). On the basis of the mean ages of patients with AIS and adenocarcinoma registered in the SEER program, it has been estimated that it may take about 13 years to progress from the former to the latter (Plaxe and Saltzstein, 1999).

2   DESCRIPTIVE EPIDEMIOLOGY

2.1   Incidence rates

As with those of squamous cell carcinoma of the cervix, the age-specific incidence rates of adenocarcinoma of the cervix increase progressively to a peak at about age 40 or so, after which they either hold steady or decrease slightly (Schiffman et al., 1996; Hemminki et al., 2001). These are unusual patterns for epithelial tumors, for most of which incidence rates usually continue to increase progressively with age. However, similar patterns for cervical cancer have been observed in different parts of the world, suggesting a similar underlying biological process for cervical cancer development, regardless of ethnicity (Gustafsson et al., 1997). A number of explanations have been proposed for the pattern for cervical cancers, including the cessation of relevant etiological exposures after a certain age, the existence of a susceptible subpopulation at risk, or the disappearance of target cells, for example because they are rendered quiescent or because they are induced to undergo terminal differentiation (Gustafsson et al., 1997; Hemminki et al., 2001).

2.2   Time trends

Several reports in the last few years have documented recent increases in the age-adjusted incidence rates of adenocarcinoma of the cervix in many developed and some developing countries (Zheng et al., 1996; Stockton et al., 1997; Vizcaino et al., 1998; Bergstrom et al., 1999; Sasieni and Adams, 2001; Liu et al., 2001), and concomitantly, a decrease in the age-adjusted incidence rates of squamous cell carcinomas (Stockton et al., 1997; Bergstrom et al., 1999; Vizcaino et al., 2000; Liu et al., 2001). The increase in adenocarcinoma rates appears to have occurred primarily in women born after the 1930s and in those younger than 55 years of age. For example, in the United Kingdom, the incidence rate of adenocarcinoma in women aged 30-34 years increased from less than 0.5 per 100,000 in 1971 to more than 4.5 per 100,000 in the late 1980s, whereas the rate in women aged 60-64 years remained steady between 1971 and 1992; further analysis of these data showed that the rapid increase in rates was due to a cohort effect (Figure 1) (Sasieni and Adams, 2001).

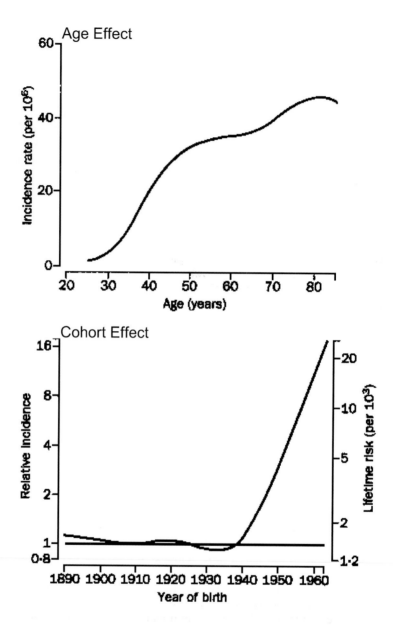

Figure 1. Age and cohort effects estimated from data for England 1971-87. Age effect is for a cohort born in 1924. Relative incidence of cohort effect is relative to that in the 1924 cohort. Lifetime risk is calculated from mortality rates in 1994. [Reprinted with permission from Elsevier Science (The Lancet, 2001, 357, 1490-3)]

It has been suggested that at least part of the recent increase in the incidence rates of adenocarcinoma of the cervix might be due to factors such as changes and improvements in the histological classification of the disease over time, the limited effectiveness of conventional cervical cytology using the Ayre spatula to detect adenocarcinoma, and increased awareness by cytologists of the significance of putative early lesions such as atypical glandular cells, with consequent referral for further investigation (Kjaer and Brinton, 1993; Vizcaino et al., 1998). However, these explanations are unlikely to account fully for the magnitude of the observed increase, suggesting that other factors (e.g., use of oral contraceptives and changes in sexual practice resulting in increased transmission of HPV infection) might be responsible, at least in part (Vizcaino et al., 1998; Liu et al., 2001).

Some limitations of the available descriptive data are described in section 1.3 of Chapter 7.

3   ETIOLOGY

There have been considerably fewer studies of the etiology of cervical adenocarcinoma than of that of squamous cell cervical cancer, due perhaps to the relative rarity of the former and to the related fact that many studies of adenocarcinoma have been hampered by the inclusion of small numbers of cases. Nevertheless, on the basis of the available evidence, it has been suggested that adenocarcinoma of the cervix might have a risk factor profile intermediate between those of squamous cell carcinoma of the cervix and endometrial cancer (Franco and Ferenczy, 2002), because (as reviewed below) it appears to share some, but not all, of the risk factors for both of those conditions. With respect to squamous cell cervical carcinoma, HPV infection is overwhelmingly the most important predictor of increased risk, whereas other putative risk factors such as high parity, oral contraceptive use, cigarette smoking, and possibly some aspects of diet (e.g., a relatively low intake of carotenoids), appear not to have independent effects, but rather to act as cofactors whose effects are conditional upon the presence of HPV infection (Bosch et al., 2002). For endometrial cancer, risk is increased in association with obesity, diabetes, nulliparity, and use of estrogen replacement therapy, and is decreased in association with oral contraceptive use and possibly cigarette smoking (Grady and Ernster, 1996). Essentially, therefore, the former is indicative of an infectious etiology whereas the latter is indicative of an hormonal etiology.

3.1   HPV infection

3.1.1   The prevalence of HPV-DNA in cervical adenocarcinomas

As with squamous cell cervical carcinomas, infection with HPV plays a major role in the etiology of cervical adenocarcinoma. Indeed, numerous studies have demonstrated the presence of HPV in cervical adenocarcinomas (e.g., Andersson et al., 2001; Bosch et al., 1995; Bosch et al., 2000; Hording et al., 1997; Iwasawa et al., 1996; Lee et al., 1998; Tenti et al., 1996), the predominant types being HPV 16 and 18. However, in contrast to the predominance of HPV 16 that has been observed in squamous cell carcinomas (Bosch et al., 1995), all but one (Bosch et al., 2000) of the studies of adenocarcinoma have suggested that the prevalence of HPV 18 may equal or exceed that of HPV 16 in cervical adenocarcinomas. The latter point is demonstrated in Table 1, which shows the prevalence of HPV types 16 and 18 in some of the larger and more recent case series of adenocarcinoma. In these studies, the prevalence of HPV 18 ranged from 16% to 59%, while that of HPV 16 ranged from 18-55%.

3.1.2   The association between HPV infection and risk of adenocarcinoma

There is now a substantial amount of evidence to suggest that infection with HPV is associated with increased risk of cervical adenocarcinoma and its precursor, adenocarcinoma *in situ* of the cervix. In a recent case-control study which employed type-specific serologic assays to detect evidence of HPV infection, risk of adenocarcinoma *in situ* was increased 3-fold in association with infection with HPV 18, but was not increased in association with HPV 16 infection (Madelaine et al., 2001). However, the estimates of risk were relatively weak, which may reflect the limitations of serological assays.

The association between HPV infection and risk of invasive cervical adenocarcinoma has been investigated in several hospital-based case-control studies, the more recent of which used sensitive PCR-based HPV detection assays to detect the presence of HPV in exfoliated cervical cells (Table 2). Although most of these studies (Ngelangel et al., 1998; Chichareon et al., 1998; Bosch et al., 2000; Sasagawa et al., 2001; Thomas et al., 2001) tested for the presence of a wide range of mucosatropic HPV types, the prevalence of all but HPV types 16, 18, and 45 was too low to allow calculation of stable estimates of risk. For infection with these three HPV types, however, the associated odds ratios were extremely high and generally of comparable magnitude to those which have been observed for squamous cell carcinoma of the cervix (Bosch et al., 2002; Chapter 7). As a consequence, the associated attributable fractions are also of comparable magnitude to those for squamous carcinomas (i.e., at least 90%) (see Chapter 7). In those studies in which estimates of risk were presented separately for infection with HPV 16 and HPV 18 (Table 2), odds ratios for the latter were higher than those for the former, perhaps consistent with the known higher transforming ability of HPV 18 (Barnes et al., 1990; Kurman et al., 1988).

Table 1. Prevalence of HPV in studies of adenocarcinoma of the cervix with 50 cases or more.

Reference	Country	HPV detection method*	No.of subjects	HPV prevalence (%)		
				Total	HPV 16	HPV 18
Tenti et al. (1996)	Italy	PCR, SB	138	85	$55^{\perp}$	$57^{\perp}$
Iwasawa et al. (1996)	Finland	PCR	108	75	$20^{\perp}$	$59^{\perp}$
Hording et al. (1997)	Denmark	PCR, DB	50	70	18	52
Lee et al. (1998)	Taiwan	PCR, SB	69	32	$18^{\perp}$	$16^{\perp}$
Bosch et al. (2000)	Multicenter	PCR, SB	141	89	49	38
Andersson et al. (2001)	Sweden	PCR,SSCP	131	71	24	37

* PCR = polymerase chain reaction; DB = dot blot; SB = Southern blot
$\perp$ Combined HPV16/18 infection rates in the studies of Tenti et al. (1996), Iwasawa et al. (1996), and Lee et al. (1998) were 27%, 3%, and 1.5%,respectively

Table 2. Case-control studies of the association between HPV infection and risk of adenocarcinoma of the cervix.

Reference	Country	No. cases/ controls	HPV detection method	Exposure	OR (95% CI)*
Brinton et al., 1993	Costa Rica, Panama, Colombia, Mexico	43/1467	FISH$^{\perp}$	HPV 16/18	5.4 (2.7-11.0)
Ngelangel et al., 1998	Philippines	33‡/381	PCR, Southern blot	HPV 16 HPV 18 HPV 45	549 (44-6912) 948 (97-9240) 259 (26-2618)
Chichareon et al., 1998	Thailand	39‡/261	PCR, Southern blot	HPV 16 HPV 18 HPV 45	63 (17-232) 278 (50-1535) 16 (1.2-228)
Bosch et al., 2000§	Thailand, Peru, Philippines, Brazil,Morocco, Paraguay	141‡/1466	PCR, Southern blot	HPV 16 HPV 18 HPV 45	95 (47-187) 180 (81-397) 41 (12-141)
Sasagawa et al., 2001	Japan	12/1562	PCR	HPV 16 HPV 18	15 (3.2-75) 94 (28-317)
Thomas et al., 2001	Thailand	42‡/ 291	PCR	HPV 16 HPV 18	24 (8.7-76) 4

* OR = odds ratio, CI = confidence interval. All odds ratios indicate risk associated with presence of the specified HPV type and are adjusted for age.$^{\perp}$ FISH = Filter *in situ* hybridisation. ‡ Adenocarcinoma plus adenosquamous carcinoma. § The studies of Ngelangel et al. (1998) and Chichareon et al. (1998) are subsets of this multicenter study.

On the basis of the accumulated biological and epidemiological evidence, the International Agency for Research on Cancer concluded in 1995 that HPV types 16 and 18 are carcinogenic to humans and classified them as group 1 carcinogens (IARC, 1995). More recently, it has been proposed that HPV is a necessary but not sufficient cause of cervical carcinoma (Bosch et al., 2002; also see Chapter 7). Although the evidence that contributed to this proposal derived largely from studies of squamous cell cervical neoplasia, it seems likely (given the data presented here) that HPV has a similar role in the development of cervical adenocarcinoma.

3.2   Other risk factors

There have been a number of studies of risk factors for cervical adenocarcinoma other than infection with HPV (Anton-Culver et al., 1992; Brinton et al., 1987; Brinton et al., 1993; Bjørge and Kravdal,1996; Chicareon et al., 1998; Kvåle et al., 1988; Lacey et al., 2001; Ngelangel et al., 1998; Parazzini et al., 1988; Silcocks et al., 1987; Ursin et al., 1996). Of these, some have involved simultaneous examination of risk factors for adenocarcinomas and squamous cell carcinomas (Anton-Culver et al., 1992; Brinton et al., 1987; Brinton et al., 1993; Bjørge and Kravdal, 1996; Chicareon et al., 1998; Kvåle et al., 1988; Lacey et al., 2001; Ngelangel et al., 1998; Silcocks et al., 1987), based either on the use of data collected routinely by population-based cancer registries (Anton-Culver et al., 1992; Bjørge and Kravdal, 1996; Silcocks et al., 1987) or on data acquired in traditional case-control (Brinton et al., 1987; Brinton et al., 1993; Chicareon et al., 1998; Lacey et al., 2001; Ngelangel et al., 1998) or cohort studies (Kvåle et al., 1988), whereas others have focused on adenocarcinomas only (Parazzini et al., 1988; Ursin et al., 1996).

Using registry data, Silcocks et al. (1987) showed that women with adenocarcinoma were more likely than those with squamous cell carcinoma to be single and nulliparous, and to have a history of hypertension, and Bjørge and Kravdal (1996) showed that the inverse association between age at first birth and risk was stronger for squamous cell carcinoma than for adenocarcinoma. In contrast, the case-control and cohort studies mostly have observed fairly similar patterns of associations for squamous cell carcinomas and adenocarcinomas with respect to factors such as number of sexual partners (generally positively associated), age at first sexual intercourse (generally inversely associated), number of births (positive association), years since last Papanicolou smear (positive association), and ages at menarche and menopause (no association), perhaps the most noticeable differences being evidence for a positive association between body weight and risk of adenocarcinoma but not squamous cell carcinoma in the study of

Brinton et al. (1987) and to a lesser extent in a later study by Brinton (Brinton et al., 1993), and the suggestive associations in opposite directions between cigarette smoking and risk (positive association for squamous cell carcinoma and inverse association for adenocarcinoma) in the study of Lacey et al. (2001). In other case-control studies focusing on adeno-carcinoma only, Parazzini et al. (1988) showed that risk was increased in association with relatively high parity, early age at first birth, a relatively large number of sexual partners, early age at first intercourse, and a relatively high body mass index, and Ursin et al. (1996) showed increases in risk with greater weight change from age 18, number of sexual partners, early age at first pregnancy, and some suggestion of an association with a history of hypertension.

Suspicion of a possible role for oral contraceptives in the etiology of cervical adenocarcinoma arose from early case reports of atypical polypoid endocervical hyperplasia resembling adenocarcinoma occurring only in women taking progestin-like oral contraceptives (interestingly, the possibility of co-existent infection was noted) (Taylor et al., 1967) and of cervical adenocarcinoma occurring in a woman who had used combined oral contraceptives (Czernobilsky et al., 1974), and from the observation that estrogen and progesterone receptors appeared to be detected more frequently in cervical adenocarcinomas than in squamous cell carcinomas (Ford et al., 1983). In light of these observations, the association between use of oral contraceptives and risk of adenocarcinoma has been examined in several case-control studies (Table 3), the majority of which have shown some suggestion of a positive association with prolonged use. Although one study of oral contraceptives and risk of adenocarcinoma suggested that risk was particularly high in women using oral contraceptives with high progestin potency and low estrogen dose (Thomas et al., 1996), another report from the same study (Thomas et al., 1995) showed no association between use of depot-medroxyprogesterone acetate and risk of invasive adenocarcinomas, which led the investigators to suggest that the estrogenic components of oral contraceptives might be responsible for the increased risk. In this regard, a recent case-control study showed a positive association with unopposed estrogen use (OR = 2.7, 95% CI = 1.1-6.8) and a null association with combined estrogen-progestin hormone replacement preparations (Lacey et al., 2000).

Most of the risk factor studies described above were conducted prior to the development and subsequent refinement of assays for HPV detection, and therefore the estimates of association that they presented for other factors were mostly not adjusted for HPV status, which limits interpretation of their findings. Of those studies that did adjust for HPV, two studies of oral

Table 3. Case-control studies of the association between oral contraceptive (OC) use and risk of adenocarcinoma of the cervix.

Reference	Country	No. cases/controls	Measure of OC use			
			Ever use	Ever use	Duration of use	OR (95% CI)
Brinton et al., 1986*	United States	62/789	-	-	≤10 years vs. 0	2.95 (1.1-8.2)
Parazzini et al., 1988	Italy	31/409	Ever vs. never	0.8 (0.2-2.4)	-	-
Brinton et al., 1990*	International[γ]	61/1429	Ever vs. never	2.41 (1.3-4.6)	≤10 years vs. 0	1.79 (0.5-6.5)
Ursin et al., 1994	United States	195/386	Ever vs. never	2.1 (1.1-3.8)	≤12 years vs. 0	4.4 (1.8-10.8)
Thomas et al., 1996*	International[γ]	377/2887	Ever vs. never	1.5 (1.1-1.9)	≤8 years vs. 0	2.2 (1.4-3.5)
Lacey et al., 1999	United States	124/307	Ever vs. never	1.0 (0.5-1.9)	> 6 years vs. 0	1.2 (0.6-2.6)

* Case series included adenocarcinomas and adenosquamous tumors.
[γ] The study by Brinton et al. (1990) was conducted in Panama, Costa Rica, Colombia, and Mexico; the study by Thomas et al. (1996) was conducted in Thailand, Kenya, Mexico, Philippines, Australia, Chile, Israel, and Colombia.

contraceptive use and risk of adenocarcinoma did not show convincing evidence for a positive association (Brinton et al., 1990; Lacey et al., 1999) whereas the inverse association between cigarette smoking and adeno-carcinoma risk observed in one study (Lacey et al., 2001) was stronger after adjustment for HPV.

3.3 Risk factors as cofactors for the effects of HPV infection

As indicated earlier (see section 3.1.2), it was proposed recently that HPV is a necessary but not sufficient cause of cervical carcinoma. This suggests that other factors (so-called cofactors) act in concert with HPV to increase risk of progression to cancer. Identification of cofactors requires examination of their association with cervical cancer risk in analyses restricted to HPV positive women, to allow assessment of the extent to which they contribute to risk independently of HPV exposure. To date, such analyses have been conducted more extensively for squamous cell cervical cancers than for adenocarcinoma. Indeed, in only a few studies (all of which employed the case-control design) have risk factors for adenocarcinoma been examined in HPV positive women (Brinton et al., 1990; Chicareon et al., 1998; Lacey et al., 1999; 2000; 2001; Ngelangel et al., 1998). Of these, one (Brinton et al., 1990) showed a positive association with duration of oral contraceptive use (although an association of similar magnitude was observed in HPV negative women); one (Ngelangel et al., 1998) showed a positive association with number of household amenities, and some suggestion of an increased risk with increasing number of livebirths; one (Chicareon et al., 1998) showed a positive association with the number of sexual partners and with a history of venereal disease, but no association with cigarette smoking; and one (Lacey et al., 1999) showed increased risk with prolonged use of oral contraceptives (Lacey et al., 1999), increased risk with use of hormone replacement therapy (Lacey et al., 2000) and an inverse association with cigarette smoking of more than 20 years' duration (Lacey et al., 2001). Clearly, further analyses of this kind are required before consensus can be reached concerning the roles of cofactors in determining risk of adenocarcinoma.

4 PREVENTION

Disease prevention can be conducted at three levels, primary (involving prevention of disease occurrence), secondary (involving early detection of disease), and tertiary (involving prevention of progression of clinical disease). Primary and secondary prevention are particularly relevant to the present discussion.

4.1   Primary prevention

Approaches to the primary prevention of cervical adenocarcinoma have received little attention. However, given the central role of HPV infection in the etiology of adenocarcinoma, and given that HPV infection is acquired (primarily) through sexual activity, attempts to modify sexual behavior might contribute to the prevention of this cancer. Indeed, some sex and AIDS education programs have been shown to delay the initiation of intercourse, reduce the frequency of intercourse, reduce the number of sexual partners, or increase the use of condoms (Kirby et al., 1994; Rock et al., 2000). However, many studies of sexual health interventions have not been methodologically sound (Oakley et al., 1995), and therefore there is a need for further evaluation of such interventions (see Chapter 9). Perhaps more promising are current attempts to develop vaccines against HPV infection, which may open up new avenues for primary prevention. Indeed, a recent report describing the effect of an HPV 16 vaccine on the incidence of HPV 16 infection and HPV 16-related cervical intraepithelial neoplasia offers much hope in this regard (Koutsky et al., 2002).

4.2   Secondary prevention

Secondary prevention by Pap smear screening has been shown to be very effective in reducing the incidence of and mortality from squamous cell cervical cancer (Franco and Ferenczy, 2002). Screening for squamous cervical cancer is possible because it has defined precursor lesions (squamous intraepithelial lesions) and there is a concomitant identifiable pre-clinical phase. In principle, screening for cervical adenocarcinoma should also be possible, given that it too has an identifiable preclinical phase and a recognized precursor lesion, namely adenocarcinoma in situ (Mathers et al., 2002), which precedes invasive adenocarcinoma by a mean interval of about 13 years (Plaxe and Saltzstein, 1999). However, given their location in the endocervical canal, adenocarcinomas (and their precursors) are not detected readily by screening, presumably due to the difficulty in accessing and sampling them (Sigurdsson, 1993). Indeed, Pap cytology has higher false negative rates for adenocarcinomas than for squamous cell carcinoma of the cervix, an issue of concern given that adenocarcinomas may progress rapidly (Hildesheim et al., 1999).

Evidence concerning the effect of screening on rates of cervical adenocarcinoma is somewhat inconsistent. For example, screening was observed to have no effect on the incidence rates of cervical adenocarcinoma in Iceland (Sigurdsson, 1993), but was associated with a reduction in the mortality rate of the disease in Finland (Nieminen et al., 1995). Also, a case-control study in Latin America showed that screening was associated with a reduction in the risk of cervical adenocarcinoma of similar magnitude to that of squamous cell cervical carcinoma (Herrero et al., 1992), whereas a case-control study in Australia showed that it was less effective in preventing adenocarcinoma than squamous cell carcinoma of the cervix (Mitchell et al., 1995).

As indicated earlier, in addition to adenocarcinoma in situ, the 2001 Bethesda System for the classification of cervical cytology includes two categories for abnormalities of glandular cells less severe than adenocarcinoma: atypical glandular cells, either endocervical, endometrial, or "glandular cells" not otherwise specified; and atypical glandular cells, either endocervical or "glandular cells" favor neoplasia (Wright et al., 2002). (In the original version of the Bethesda system the term "atypical glandular cells of undetermined significance" was used to describe essentially the same lesions (Solomon, 1989)). It has been suggested that patients who demonstrate such changes persistently (that is, on two smears) should be referred for colposcopy and endocervical curettage (Soofer and Sidawy, 2000). HPV testing might have a role in triaging patients with these cytological changes, thereby reducing the number referred for colposcopy (Ronnett et al., 1999).

CONCLUSION

Cervical adenocarcinoma is an increasingly important contributor to the public health burden imposed by cervical cancer. However, research on the etiology of cervical adenocarcinoma lags behind that of squamous cell cancer of the cervix, perhaps due to the relative rarity of the former. In light of this, it is difficult to draw firm conclusions regarding the etiology of cervical adenocarcinoma, with the exception of the clear role for infection with HPV. Therefore, there is much scope for further etiological research, with particular emphasis on the roles of cofactors of HPV infection in influencing risk of progression to cancer, and on the roles of host factors such as HLA type (Cuzick et al., 2000) in modifying the effect of HPV on risk.

Given that infection with HPV occupies a central position in its etiology, strategies designed to reduce the risk of or to prevent HPV infection, or to modify the effects of HPV cofactors, appear to offer the best approach to the primary prevention of cervical adenocarcinoma. At the same time, secondary preventive efforts may be enhanced by the development of new technologies designed to improve the sampling of cells from the endocervical canal, perhaps supplemented by the incorporation of HPV testing into screening algorithms. Overall, there are many reasons to be optimistic that cancer control initiatives will ultimately be successful against cervical adeno-carcinomas.

ACKNOWLEDGEMENT

I am very grateful to Keerti Shah for his careful review of an early draft of this chapter.

REFERENCES

Andersson S, Rylander E, Larsson B, et al. The role of human papillomavirus in cervical adenocarcinoma carcinogenesis. Eur J Cancer 2001;37:246-50.

Anton-Culver H, Bloss, JD, Bringman D, et al. Comparison of adenocarcinoma and squamous cell carcinoma of the uterine cervix: A population-based epidemiologic study. Am J Obstet Gynecol 1992;166:1507-14.

Barnes W, Woodworth C, Waggoner S, et al. Rapid dysplastic transformation of human genital cells by human papillomavirus type 18. Gyencol Oncol 1990;38:343-6.

Bergstrom R, Sparen P, Adami HO. Trends in cancer of the cervix uteri in Sweden following cytological screening. Br J Cancer 1999;81:159-66.

Bjorge T, Kravdal O. Reproductive variables and risk of uterine cervical cancer in Norwegian registry data. Cancer Causes Control 1996;7:351-357.

Bosch FX, Lorincz A, Munoz N, et al. The causal relation between human papillomavirus and cervical cancer. J Clin Pathol 2002;55:244-65.

Bosch FX, Munoz N, Chichareon S, et al. HPV and cervical adenocarcinoma: an IARC based multicentric case-control study. In: Castellsague X, Bosch FX, de Sanjose S, al. e, editors. 18th International Papillomavirus Conference - program and abstracts book.; 2000; Barcelona: Thau SL, 2000, p. 131 (available on line: http://www.hpv2000.com).

Brinton LA, Herrero R, Reeves WC, et al. Risk factors for cervical cancer by histology. Gynecol Oncol 1993;51:301-6.

Brinton LA, Reeves WC, Brenes MM, et al. Oral contraceptive use and risk of invasive cervical cancer. Int J Epidemiol 1990;19:4-11.

Brinton LA, Tashima KT, Lehman HF, et al. Epidemiology of cervical cancer by cell type. Cancer Res 1987;47:1706-11.

Chichareon S, Herrero R, Munoz N, et al. Risk factors for cervical cancer in Thailand: a case-control study. J Natl Cancer Inst 1998;90:50-7.

Cuzick J, Terry G, Ho L, et al. Association between high-risk HPV types, HLA DRB1* and DQB1* alleles and cervical cancer in British women. Br J Cancer 2000;82:1348-52.

Czernobilsky B, Kessler I, Lancet M. Cervical adenocarcinoma in a woman on long-term contraceptives. Obstet Gynecol 1974;43:517-21.

Ferenczy A. Glandular Lesions: An Increasing Problem. In: Franco EL, Monsonego J, eds. New developments in cervical cancer screening and prevention. London: Blackwell, 1997, pp. 122-30.

Ford LC, Berek JS, Lagasse LD, et al. Estrogen and progesterone receptor sites in malignancies of the uterine cervix, vagina, and vulva. Gynecol Oncol 1983;15:27-31.

Franco EL, Ferenczy, A. Cervix. In: Franco EL, Rohan TE, eds. Cancer Precursors: Epidemiology, Detection, and Prevention. New York: Springer, 2002, pp. 249-86.

Grady D, Ernster VL. Endometrial cancer. In: Schottenfeld D, Fraumeni JF Jr, eds. Cancer epidemiology and prevention. New York: Oxford University Press, 1996, pp. 1058-89.

Gustafsson L, Ponten J, Bergstrom R, et al. International incidence rates of invasive cervical cancer before cytological screening. Int J Cancer 1997;71:159-165.

Hemminki K, Li X, Mutanen P. Age-incidence relationships and time trends in cervical cancer in Sweden. Eur J Epidemiol 2001;17:323-8.

Herrero R, Brinton LA, Reeves WC, et al. Screening for cervical cancer in Latin America: a case-control study. Int J Epidemiol 1992;21:1050-6.

Hildesheim A, Hadjimichael O, Schwartz PE, et al. Risk factors for rapid-onset cervical cancer. Am J Obstet Gynecol 1999;180:571-7.

Hording U, Daugaard S, Visfeldt J. Adenocarcinoma of the cervix and adenocarcinoma of the endometrium: distinction with PCR-mediated detection of HPV DNA. Apmis 1997; 105: 313-6.

IARC. Human papillomaviruses. Monogr Eval Carcinog Risks Hum, Lyon: IARC, 1995,64.

Iwasawa A, Nieminen P, Lehtinen M, et al. Human papillomavirus DNA in uterine cervix squamous cell carcinoma and adenocarcinoma detected by polymerase chain reaction. Cancer 1996;77:2275-9.

Kirby D, Short L, Collins J, et al. School-based programs to reduce sexual risk behavior: a review of effectiveness. Public Health Rep 1994;109:339-60.

Kjaer SK, Brinton LA. Adenocarcinomas of the uterine cervix: the epidemiology of an increasing problem. Epidemiol Rev 1993;15:486-98.

Koutsky L, Ault KA, Wheeler CM, et al. A controlled trial of a human papillomavirus type 16 vaccine. N Engl J Med 2002;347:1645-51.

Kudo R. Cervical Adenocarcinoma. In: Sasano N, ed. Current Topics in Pathology. Berlin: Springer-Verlag, 1992, pp. 81-111.

Kurman RJ, Schiffman MH, Lancaster WD, et al. Analysis of individual human papillomavirus types in cervical neoplasia: a possible role for type 18 in rapid progression. Am J Obstet Gynecol 1988;159:293-6.

Kvale G, Heuch I, Nilssen, S. Reproductive factors and risk of cervical cancer by cell type. Br J Cancer 1988;58:820-4.

Lacey JV, Jr., Brinton LA, Abbas FM, et al. Oral contraceptives as risk factors for cervical adenocarcinomas and squamous cell carcinomas. Cancer Epidemiol Biomarkers Prev 1999; 8:1079-85.

Lacey JV, Jr., Brinton LA, Barnes WA, et al. Use of hormone replacement therapy and adenocarcinomas and squamous cell carcinomas of the uterine cervix. Gynecol Oncol 2000; 77:149-54.

Lacey JV Jr., Frisch M, Brinton LA, et al. Associations between smoking and adenocarcinomas and squamous cell carcinomas of the uterine cervix (United States). Cancer Causes Control 2001;12:153-61.

Lee MF, Chang MC, Wu CH. Detection of human papillomavirus types in cervical adenocarcinoma by the polymerase chain reaction. Int J Gynaecol Obstet 1998;63:265-70.

Liu S, Semenciw R, Mao Y. Cervical cancer: the increasing incidence of adenocarcinoma and adenosquamous carcinoma in younger women. CMAJ 2001;164:1151-52.

Madeleine MM, Daling JR, Schwartz SM, et al. Human papillomavirus and long-term oral contraceptive use increase the risk of adenocarcinoma *in situ* of the cervix. Cancer Epidemiol Biomarkers Prev 2001;10:171-7.

Mathers ME, Johnson SJ, Wadehra V. How predictive is a cervical smear suggesting glandular neoplasia? Cytopathology 2002;13:83-91.

Meisels A, Morin C. Lesions of the Endocervix. In: Meisels A, Morin, C., eds. Cytopathology of the Uterus 2nd Edition: ASCP Press; 1997. p. 261.

Mitchell H, Medley G, Gordon I, et al. Cervical cytology reported as negative and risk of adenocarcinoma of the cervix: no strong evidence of benefit. Br J Cancer 1995;71(4):894-7.

Nasuti JF, Fleisher SR, Gupta PK. Atypical glandular cells of undetermined significance (AGUS): clinical considerations and cytohistologic correlation. Diagn Cytopathol 2002; 26:186-90.

Ngelangel C, Munoz N, Bosch FX, et al. Causes of cervical cancer in the Philippines: a case-control study. J Natl Cancer Inst 1998;90:43-9.

Nieminen P, Kallio M, Hakama M. The effect of mass screening on incidence and mortality of squamous and adenocarcinoma of cervix uteri. Obstet Gynecol 1995;85:1017-21.

Oakley A, Fullerton D, Holland J, et al. Sexual health education interventions for young people: a methodological review [see comments]. Br Med J 1995;310:158-62.

Parazzini F, La Vecchia C, Negri E, et al. Risk factors for adenocarcinoma of the cervix: a case-control study. Br J Cancer 1988;57:201-4.

Parkin DM, Bray FI, Devesa SS. Cancer burden in the year 2000. The global picture. Eur J Cancer 2001;37:S4-S66.

Parkin DM, Pisani P, Ferlay J. Estimates of the worldwide incidence of 25 major cancers in 1990. Int J Cancer 1999;80:827-41.

Pisani P, Parkin DM, Bray F, et al. Estimates of the worldwide mortality from 25 cancers in 1990. Int J Cancer 1999;83:18-29.

Plaxe SC, Saltzstein SL. Estimation of the duration of the preclinical phase of cervical adenocarcinoma suggests that there is ample opportunity for screening. Gynecol Oncol 1999; 75:55-61.

Rock CL, Michael CW, Reynolds RK, et al. Prevention of cervix cancer. Crit Rev Oncol Hematol 2000;33:169-85.

Ronnett BM, Manos MM, Ransley JE, et al. Atypical glandular cells of undetermined significance (AGUS): cytopathologic features, histopathologic results, and human papillomavirus DNA detection. Hum Pathol 1999;30:816-25.

Sasagawa T, Basha W, Yamazaki H, et al. High-risk and multiple human papillomavirus infections associated with cervical abnormalities in Japanese women. Cancer Epidemiol Biomarkers Prev 2001;10:45-52.

Sasieni P, Adams J. Changing rates of adenocarcinoma and adenosquamous carcinoma of the cervix in England. Lancet 2001;357:1490-3.

Schiffman MH, Brinton LA, Devesa SS, et al. Cervical Cancer. In: Schottenfeld D, Fraumeni, Jr., J. F., editor. Cancer Epidemiology and Prevention, 2nd ed. New York: Oxford University Press, 1996, pp. 1090-1116.

Sigurdsson K. Effect of organized screening on the risk of cervical cancer. Evaluation of screening activity in Iceland, 1964-1991. Int J Cancer 1993;54:563-70.

Silcocks PBS, Thornton-Jones H, Murphy M. Squamous and adenocarcinoma of the uterine cervix: A comparison using routine data. Br J Cancer 1987;55:321-325.

Smith HO, Tiffany MF, Qualls CR, et al. The rising incidence of adenocarcinoma relative to squamous cell carcinoma of the uterine cervix in the United States--a 24-year population-based study. Gyencol Oncol 2000;78:97-105.

Solomon D. The 1988 Bethesda system for reporting cervical/vaginal cytologic diagnoses. Developed and approved at the National Cancer Institute Workshop, Bethesda, Maryland, USA, December 12-13, 1988. Acta Cytol 1989;33:567-74.

Soofer SB, Sidawy MK. Atypical glandular cells of undetermined significance: clinically significant lesions and means of patient follow-up. Cancer 2000;90:207-14.

Stockton D, Cooper P, Lonsdale RN. Changing incidence of invasive adenocarcinoma of the uterine cervix in East Anglia. J Med Screen 1997;4:40-3.

Taylor HB, Ivey NS, Norris HJ. Atypical endocervical hyperplasia in women taking oral contraceptives. JAMA 1967;202:185-7.

Tenti P, Romagnoli S, Silini E. Human papillomavirus types 16 and 18 infection in infiltrating adenocarcinoma of the cervix. Am J Clin Pathol 1996;106:52-56.

Thomas DB, Ray RM. Depot-medroxyprogesterone acetate (DMPA) and risk of invasive adenocarcinomas and adenosquamous carcinomas of the uterine cervix. WHO Collaborative Study of Neoplasia and Steroid Contraceptives. Contraception 1995;52:307-12.

Thomas DB, Ray RM. Oral contraceptives and invasive adenocarcinomas and adenosquamous carcinomas of the uterine cervix. The World Health Organization Collaborative Study of Neoplasia and Steroid Contraceptives. Am J Epidemiol 1996; 144:281-9.

Thomas DB, Ray RM, Koetsawang A, et al. Human papillomaviruses and cervical cancer in Bangkok. I. Risk factors for invasive cervical carcinomas with human papillomavirus types 16 and 18 DNA. Am J Epidemiol 2001;153:723-31.

Ursin G, Pike MC, Preston-Martin S, et al. Sexual, reproductive, and other risk factors for adenocarcinoma of the cervix: results from a population-based case-control study (California, United States). Cancer Causes Control 1996;7:391-401.

Vizcaino AP, Moreno V, Bosch FX, et al. International trends in the incidence of cervical cancer: I. Adenocarcinoma and adenosquamous cell carcinomas. Int J Cancer 1998;75:536-45.

Vizcaino AP, Moreno V, Bosch FX, et al. International trends in incidence of cervical cancer: II. Squamous-cell carcinoma. Int J Cancer 2000;86:429-35.

Wright TC Jr., Cox JT, Massad LS, et al. 2001 Consensus Guidelines for the management of women with cervical cytological abnormalities. JAMA 2002;287:2120-9.

Zheng T, Holford TR, Ma Z, et al. The continuing increase in adenocarcinoma of the uterine cervix: a birth cohort phenomenon. Int J Epidemiol 1996;25:252-8.

Section 4

PREVENTION

Chapter 9

Educational Strategies for the Prevention of Cervical Cancer

Electra D. Paskett, Ph.D.[1]; Mary Ellen Wewers, Ph.D., R.N.,M.P.H.[1,2]; Mack T. Ruffin IV, M.D., M.P.H.[3]
[1]School of Public Health/Comprehensive Cancer Center, Ohio State University; [2]College of Nursing, Ohio State University; [3]Department of Family Medicine, University of Michigan Medical School.

INTRODUCTION

Cervical cancer is the second leading type of cancer death in women in the world (Parkin et al., 1999). In the United States, and other developed countries, invasive cervical cancer incidence and mortality rates have decreased by 75% since 1950. The success in nearly eliminating this cancer in these countries is attributed mainly to the introduction and adoption of Pap smear screening programs, which occurred in the 1950s in the United States (Ries et al., 2000). Still, in 2002, 13,000 women in the U.S. will be diagnosed with invasive cervical cancer and 4,100 women will die from this cancer – all preventable.

Educational strategies for cervical cancer prevention focus on reducing risky behaviors and on improving cervical cancer screening and follow-up. After a brief review of the risk factors, this chapter discusses the strategies currently being used and examines their success. It also offers suggestions for future work.

1   RISK FACTORS FOR CERVICAL CARCINOMA

Here we review the behavioral, social, and biological risks for cervical carcinoma, which many of the educational strategies target. Some of these are addressed in more detail in Chapter 7 along with additional information about cervical cancer incidence and mortality rates.

1.1   Behavioral risks

The behavioral risk factors for cervical cancer reported in the medical literature include early age of initiating sexual intercourse (Boyd et al., 1964; Hulka, 1982; Rotkin, 1973), multiparity (Bosch et al., 1992; Brinton et al., 1989; Ngelangel et al., 1998), multiple partners (Boyd et al., 1964; Green 1979; Hulka, 1982; Parkin et al., 1985; Vyslouzilova et al., 1997), a sexual partner with multiple partners (Harris et al., 1980; Peters et al., 1986; Terris et al., 1967; Vyslouzilova et al., 1997), frequent sexually transmitted infections, including human papillomavirus (HPV) (Harris et al., 1980; Peters et al., 1986; Terris et al., 1967; Vyslouzilova et al., 1997), and smoking of cigarettes (Clarke et al., 1982; de Vet et al., 1994; Hellberg et al., 1986; La Vecchia et al., 1986; Lyon et al., 1983; Nischan et al., 1988; Sasson et al., 1985; Stellman et al., 1980; Trevathan et al., 1983). Epidemiological data about these risk factors is provided in detail in Chapter 7.

Early epidemiological studies (Boyd et al., 1964; Jones et al., 1958) revealed that the risk of cervical cancer was especially high among women marrying at an early age. Subsequent reports focussed on the importance of sexual activity and the age of onset of the activity (Kessler 1977; Parkin et al., 1985; Terris et al., 1967). From a variety of case-control studies, women who become sexually active before the age of 16 have about a two-fold or greater risk compared with women who start after the age of 20.

High parity has been shown to be a risk factor for cervical cancer in populations where multiparity is common (Brinton et al., 1989; Eluf-Neto 1994; Ngelangel et al., 1998). The risk usually persists after accounting for HPV infection.

The risk of cervical dysplasia and carcinoma are also influenced by the number of sexual partners, often indexed by multiple marriages, separations, and divorce (Boyd et al., 1964; Green 1979; Hulka 1982; Parkin et al., 1985; Vyslouzilova et al., 1997). Within many data sets, the risk appears to increase directly with the number of sexual partners reported.

Investigators often overlook the role of the male partner. Geographic clusters of cervical and penile cancer have been reported (Bosch et al., 1990; Cocks et al., 1980; Li et al., 1982; Macgregor et al., 1980), as well as elevated rates of cervical cancer among wives of men with penile cancer (Graham et al., 1979; Martinez 1969; Smith et al., 1980). The role of the male partner was further supported by the finding that wives of men previously married to cervical cancer patients were found to have elevated rates of cervical cancer compared to control wives (Kessler 1977). The role of the male partner has been primarily linked to the risk of transferring HPV to the woman. (Castellsague et al., 2002)

Various sexually transmitted infections, other than HPV, such as herpes simplex virus 2 (HSV-2) and chlamydia have been suspected to be involved in development of cervical carcinoma. However, after adjustment for HPV infection, the association between HSV-2 and cervical cancer diminished (de Sanjose et al., 1994; Jha et al., 1993). These infections may potentiate the oncogenic effect of HPV by influencing local immune response.

Since the first association between cigarette smoking and cervical cancer was noted, a number of studies have investigated the relationship further, with the majority having concluded that smoking increases the risk of cervical cancer (Daling et al., 1992; Licciardone et al., 1990; Winkelstein 1977). The presence of a tobacco-specific carcinogen in human cervical mucus of women who smoke provides evidence for and lends support to the biologic plausibility of the association between cigarette smoking and cervical cancer (Prokopczyk et al., 1997). Tobacco exposure may also play a role in inadequate immune response to HPV infection (Poppe et al., 1996; Simons et al., 1993; 1994; Szarewski et al., 2001).

1.2   Social risks

Ample evidence exists that the Pap smear has contributed remarkably to the prevention of invasive cervical cancer as reviewed in detail in Chapter 10. Numerous studies clearly document a statistically valid drop in the incidence and mortality rates of this disease (Boyes 1981; Boyes et al., 1982; Boyes et al., 1981; Christopherson 1976; Cramer 1974; Hakama 1978; Hakama et al., 1976; Johannesson et al., 1978; Miller 1986; Morrison et al., 1996). Women with no or limited screening for cervical cancer are at significantly increased risk for invasive cervical cancer and death from the disease (Carmichael et al., 1986; Martin 1972; Morell et al., 1982; van der Graaf et al., 1988). The strongest predictor of being diagnosed with cervical cancer is the lack of a Pap smear being offered in the previous five years (Celentano et al., 1988). The few studies that have examined cervical cancer rates in rural populations have found higher prevalence of more advanced stage of disease (Miller et al., 1996; Rosenfeld 1998), indicating a lack of screening. Screening for cervical cancer represents a microcosm of social development.

Pap smear screening will only be successful in reducing cervical cancer incidence and mortality rates if: 1) regular, ongoing screening is maintained; and 2) abnormalities detected on screening are promptly and properly treated. Rates of non-compliance with follow-up recommendations vary across settings and populations, from 20% to 74% (Khanna et al., 2001; Lavin et al., 1997; Melnikow et al., 1999). Reasons for non-adherence include lack of knowledge about the result and need for treatment, inconvenience, embarrassment, provider influence, and barriers such as cost, access to care, transportation, low socioeconomic status, and lack of time (Laedtke et al., 1992; Paskett et al., 1990). In the United States, the problem of delayed or no follow-up for abnormal findings may be a greater problem among African-American women (Munoz et al., 1989) and Appalachian women (Schootman et al., 1999), which may explain higher mortality rates seen in these women.

1.2.1   Screening test and utilization

The Pap smear test is still the most widely performed screening test for cervical cancer screening available today. While newer technologies, such as liquid-based cytology collection and neural net re-screening procedures have been introduced, the Pap test is still the preferred test. However, three issues raise concerns about the Pap test: accuracy, screening intervals, and upper age limits for testing. These issues are addressed in more detail in Chapter 10.

Behavioral Risk Factor Surveillance System (BRFSS) data from 2000 indicate that 86.8% of women surveyed nationally reported having had a Pap smear within the past 3 years (CDC 1998-2000). These data must be interpreted with caution, however, as several studies have reported that women overestimate the frequency of Pap smear screening and the BRFSS excludes women without telephones, shown in at least one study as a factor in lack of screening (Paskett et al., 1999).

1.2.2   Barriers to screening

Women less likely to receive any or regular Pap smears include:
- younger women (due to lack of knowledge) (Cochran et al., 2001; McPhee et al., 1997; Wilcox et al., 1993);
- older women (due to low estimation of risk, limited mobility, co-morbid conditions, and less frequent contacts with the medical system) (McPhee et al., 1997; Norman et al., 1991) ;
- women with lack of coverage for the test (Potosky et al., 1998), system barriers (Fruchter et al., 1980), or who have cost concerns (Frank-Stromborg et al., 1998);
- women of lower income/social class (Breen et al., 1996);
- minority women (McPhee et al., 1997);
- women with geographic barriers (Blackman et al., 1999);
- women with a lack of knowledge (Rimer et al., 1996), fear (Skaer et al., 1996), embarrassment/pain (Perez-Stable et al., 1994), modesty concerns

(Penn et al., 1995), time constraints/forgetfulness (Lantz et al., 1996), or social support (Skaer et al., 1996); and

- those who lack a provider recommendation (Bastani et al., 2002; Kaplan et al., 2000).

Rural women represent a special population that faces many of these barriers to screening, plus others unique to their environment. For example, rural women face transportation issues due to larger distances to travel to provider sites, lack of mass transit, and poor road conditions (Dignan et al., 1990; Norman et al., 1991), and are less likely to have seen a physician in the past year (Mueller et al., 1999; Mueller et al., 1998). Differences in provider and medical system resources between rural and metropolitan areas also indicate greater barriers to screening for rural women (Gulitz et al., 1998; Mueller et al., 1999; Norton et al., 1989).

1.3   Biological risks

As reviewed in detail in Chapter 7, the epidemiological association between HPV infection and cervical carcinoma fulfills all of the established epidemiological criteria for causality. However, the mere presence of HPV DNA at the cervix does not necessarily establish a clinical manifestation of a squamous intraepithelial lesion (SIL). Cervical infection with HPV requires some type of co-factor before progression to significant disease.

2   EDUCATIONAL STRATEGIES FOR PREVENTION

The possible educational strategies to prevent cervical cancer mortality can be classified into primary, secondary and tertiary prevention. The educational strategies in primary prevention are generally aimed at risk reduction. Therefore, the educational strategies include reducing high-risk sexual behaviors and eliminating the use of tobacco products. The educational strategies in secondary prevention aim to increase the percent of the population of women routinely screened for cervical cancer. Finally, educational strategies in tertiary prevention aim to increase the percent of women who have adequate evaluation for an abnormal screening test, complete treatment for cervical disease, and adhere to surveillance for treatment efficacy. This section of the chapter will address educational strategies in each of these areas.

2.1   Primary prevention – reducing risky behaviors

Of the behavioral risk factors, half are related to sexual behavior. In addition, the biological risk is impacted by the same sexual behaviors. So educational strategies aimed at reducing these risks are of interest. Smoking, another behavioral risk, may also be impacted by educational strategies.

2.1.1   Sexual behavior

The variety and success of various interventions to reduce risky sexual behaviors has been limited. The prevalence of sexual risk behavior is higher among younger women. Therefore, most of the educational strategies focus on this age group. Risk reduction interventions seem to decrease risk adoption, stabilize non-risk behaviors and, possibly, destabilize risk behavior (Stanton et al., 1997). In one study, over 270 published articles on sexual health intervention were evaluated for quality (Oakley et al., 1995). Only two of the 12 studies judged to be methodologically sound were effective in showing an impact on young people's sexual behavior (Oakley et al., 1995). Brief behavioral intervention among high-risk female adolescents was shown to increase condom use by their sexual partners, but incident infection did not appear to be reduced, because condom use remained inconsistent (Orr et al., 1996). Community-based HIV risk-reduction programs that are gender relevant and culturally sensitive and provide social skills training can effectively enhance consistent condom use (DiClemente et al., 1995). An evaluation of school-based programs to reduce sexual risk behaviors examined 23 published studies. Not all sex and AIDS education programs had significant effects on adolescent sexual risk-taking behavior, but specific programs did delay the initiation of intercourse, reduce the frequency of intercourse, reduce the numbers of sexual partners, or increase the use of condoms (Kirby et al., 1994).

2.1.2   Tobacco use

Over forty-six million persons, or 23.3% of the U.S. adult population, are smokers (Trosclair et al., 2002). Smoking prevalence is highest for those aged 18-24 (26.8%) and 25-44 (27%). American Indians/Alaska Natives have the highest prevalence (36.0%), while Asian Americans/Pacific Islanders have the lowest estimates (14.4%).

Smoking is more pronounced in the less educated and poor. With respect to the former, 47.2% of those with a General Education Development (GED)[1] diploma are categorized as current smokers; with respect to the latter, smoking prevalence is highest for those living below the poverty line (31.7%). Knowledge about the consequences of tobacco use is lower among current smokers, especially those of lower educational level (CDC 2001). *Healthy*

---

[1] The General Educational Development (GED) is an international high school equivalency testing program for adults. The GED tests are designed to measure the skills that correspond to those of recent high school graduates.

People 2010 identified people with a high school education or less, who are aged 20 and older, as a special population of tobacco users in need of risk reduction interventions (2000).

In the U.S. and U.K. since the 1970s to present day, the prevalence of tobacco use has significantly increased among lower socioeconomic groups, as compared to privileged persons (Jarvis et al., 2001). A substantial widening in the gap is becoming more evident, since the prevalence of tobacco consumption has diminished dramatically in the more affluent (CDC 1998). While members of both socioeconomic groups initiate tobacco use behavior at similar rates, more affluent smokers are able to quit the behavior, generally before health consequences develop (CDC 1998). Therefore, unless efforts are tailored specifically to disadvantaged or vulnerable smokers, the gap in prevalence between groups will continue to grow.

Among adolescents, smoking prevalence has risen significantly since 1990 with more than 3000 children and adolescents becoming regular smokers daily. For students in grades 6-12, 49.5% reported ever smoking and 18% currently smoke cigarettes (CDC 2000). For adolescent current smokers, 55.8% want to stop smoking and 58.2% tried to stop during the past year (CDC 2000). The factors responsible for an increased prevalence of tobacco use in the United States remain poorly understood.

Among adult women, smoking prevalence is higher in women of reproductive age, compared to the overall population of adult women (25.3% vs. 21%), with 14 million women of reproductive age in the U.S. being current smokers (Trosclair et al., 2002). During the 1990s, past month smoking prevalence among white high school senior girls in the U.S. rose from 31.2% in 1992 to 41% in 1998; for African American girls, the increase was from 7% to 12%. A population-based estimate of continued smoking throughout pregnancy was 12.9% in 1998, with estimates consistently highest among pregnant smokers aged 18-24. Socioeconomic status has a dramatic effect on prenatal smoking behavior, as evidenced by a 12-fold difference in prevalence, based on education. Specifically, 25.5% of women with less than a high school education smoke throughout pregnancy, compared to only 2.2% of mothers with a college degree.

2.1.2.1   *Antecedents of tobacco use.* Understanding the mechanisms responsible for the maintenance of a smoking behavior in vulnerable groups is critical in order to tailor efforts to these groups. Compelling psycho-pharmacological evidence can explain maintenance of the behavior as being due to nicotine dependence (U.S. Department of Health and Human Services, 1988). It has also been noted that poorer smokers are more nicotine dependent (Jarvis and Wardle, 2001), suggesting social structure may influence the continuance of smoking.

Few investigations characterize the mechanisms responsible for increased dependence among smokers that are relatively poor. Engaging in a tobacco use behavior has been referred to as "self-medication," primarily because of the reinforcing effects associated with nicotine (Pomerleau et al., 2000; Pomerleau et al., 1984). These effects include tension reduction, relaxation, and euphoria. Since poorer individuals often experience increased stressors, smoking may serve as an effective strategy for managing the unpleasant symptoms associated with stress (Jarvis et al., 2001). In addition, the relationship between nicotine dependence and exposure to tobacco smoke constituents, as well as genetic factors that influence nicotine metabolism, have only recently been observed as critical variables among special populations (Ahijevych et al., 1996; Caraballo et al., 1998).

Other antecedent determinants of the behavior that deserve consideration include other psychological states, such as depression, material factors (e.g., income, insurance status, access to treatment) and the social environment (e.g., indoor air restrictions, number of co-workers, family and friends who smoke, rural and poor neighborhoods). Finally, while an evidence-based clinical practice cessation guideline (*Treating Tobacco Use and Dependence*) has been developed (Fiore et al., 2000), it has only been tested in vulnerable populations to a limited extent.

2.1.2.2 *Tobacco cessation.* Approximately 41% of adult smokers try to quit each year. In 2000, 15.7 million adult smokers stopped smoking for at least one day during the past year in a serious quit attempt. However, based on U.S. estimates, the annual quit rate is approximately 0.5%, with 4.7% reporting periods of abstinence for periods of 3-12 months in 2000 (Trosclair et al., 2002).

Various approaches to tobacco cessation have been described in the literature (Kelley et al., 2003; Song et al., 2002). Traditional smoking cessation approaches generally include clinic-based (individual and group) and community-based programs. Voluntary health organizations, such as the American Cancer Society, the American Heart Association, and the American Lung Association, are known for their self-help tobacco cessation materials and organized clinic-based approaches (Orleans 1985). Evaluation of these multicomponent clinic-based programs indicated smoking cessation abstinence rates of 20-30% at one-year follow-up among highly motivated individuals (Fiore et al., 1990; Pierce et al., 1989).

Assisted methods of cessation, such as an organized program or course, are techniques commonly used by well-educated individuals (Fiore et al., 1990) but are not usual approaches to cessation for those persons from lower socioeconomic levels. Limited numbers of tobacco users participate in these programs. According to Harris and Leininger (1993), the demand for organized cessation clinics is quite small, and the supply of clinics is uneven, with inadequate numbers of programs present in rural areas.

Community-based approaches to tobacco cessation include efforts to combine cessation services via self-help materials (Cummings 2002), media campaigns (Wewers et al., 1991), and telephone hotlines (Cummings et al., 1993). As compared to clinic programs, community-based initiatives are associated with lower cessation rates (Orleans et al., 1999; Taylor et al., 1998), but are considered effective, since they have the capacity to reach greater numbers of tobacco users. The effective implementation of health promotion projects in community settings has been shown to be related to a variety of factors. Altman and others (Altman 1995; Altman et al., 1991) noted that lack of project success was related to factors such as: 1) low priority of health promotion and prevention issues among community residents; 2) volunteer membership turnover; 3) lack of community commitment; and 4) cultural differences between project staff and the community. In light of these factors, the implementation of health promoting behaviors, such as tobacco cessation, remains a challenge for community health care providers and program planners.

In 1996, the Agency for Health Care Policy and Research (AHCPR) initially produced a Smoking Cessation Guideline (Fiore et al., 1996) that provided recommendations for the management of tobacco users who are seen in a variety of health care settings, including primary-care clinics. An updated guideline, *Treating Tobacco Use and Dependence,* was released from the Agency for Healthcare Research and Quality (AHRQ) in 2000 (Fiore et al., 2000). Evidence-based recommendations for treatment acknowledged a strong dose-response relationship between the intensity of tobacco dependence counseling and its effectiveness. Treatment that included person-to-person contact (counseling) and pharmacotherapy was shown to be highly efficacious. First-line pharmacotherapies were nicotine replacement therapy (NRT) and bupropion. Psychosocial therapies included clinic-based treatment that involved setting a quit date, in-treatment social support, and the use of skill training, or problem solving approaches, to avoid smoking. While the AHRQ guideline suggested that NRT was highly efficacious, its use in special populations (e.g., vulnerable groups) has received little testing. To date, the efficacy of NRT pharmacotherapy remains an understudied area of investigation. The current guideline strongly urged that further investigations be conducted to confirm efficacy of NRT among specific populations (Fiore et al., 2000).

Efforts have, to date, been relatively unsuccessful in promoting cessation and abstinence in the less educated and poor, whether clinic-based programs or community-based programs. Their lack of engagement in preventive health care services may, in part, be due to barriers to access and lack of information about prevention.

2.1.2.3   Cervical cancer screening and smoking cessation. Unfortunately, women who smoke are less likely to receive cervical screenings, as compared to non-smokers. Rakowski et al. (1999) reported that women who consumed at least one pack of cigarettes per day were 50% less likely to have had a Pap smear in the past 3 years. In contrast, former smokers were observed to have significantly higher screening rates than never smokers do. These findings suggest that persons who smoke also participate to a lesser extent in other health-promoting activities.

Investigations of smoking cessation among women seeking cervical cancer screening have been limited. McBride et al. (1998), in a study of 613 current smokers from Group Health Cooperative, the large health maintenance organization in western Washington state, noted that only 30% of smokers were aware of well-established sexual risk factors for cervical cancer. Regarding tobacco use, 49% were aware that smoking increased their risk of cervical cancer, with younger women (< 35 years) significantly more aware than older women (45+ years) (54% versus 40%, respectively). The majority of women sampled endorsed using the risk of cervical cancer as a motivator for quitting smoking. Approximately one-half of sample participants reported that their provider had asked about smoking and had encouraged smoking cessation. In a subsequent study, these investigators evaluated a minimal self-help smoking cessation intervention following cervical cancer screening in the same setting (McBride et al., 1999). Using a randomized controlled design, participants were assigned to a self-help intervention or usual care. Intervention participants received a self-help booklet, smoking and reproductive health information, and three telephone counseling calls. At six months post baseline, cessation rates in the usual care (10.5%) and self-help groups (10.9%) did not differ. Although not significant, at 15 months, rates of quitting were higher for usual care participants (15.5%) as compared to self-help participants (10.6%). Quit rates at six and 15 months were similar for women with an abnormal Pap test, as compared to those with normal Pap findings. These results suggest that a minimal smoking cessation intervention, especially a self-help strategy, may not be sufficient to assist women in quitting smoking and is consistent with a previous meta-analytic finding that self-help smoking cessation interventions are only marginally efficacious (Fiore et al., 2000).

To date, the health-related effects of smoking cessation have yet to be systematically studied with regard to cervical health. One preliminary study has evaluated the effect of smoking cessation on CIN lesion size (grade 1 or less) among 82 women volunteers (Szarewski et al., 2001). Using computer-aided image analysis to assess lesion size, investigators (unaware of the women's smoking status) observed that of the 28 women who stopped or reduced their smoking consumption, 82% demonstrated a reduction in lesion size of at least 20% at 6 months follow-up. For the women who did not quit or reduce their smoking behavior, only 28% demonstrated at least a 20% reduction in lesion size. Adjustment for socioeconomic status and stage of menstrual cycle did not affect the findings. These results provide encouraging preliminary evidence that smoking cessation may offer immediate benefits in reducing minor cervical lesions. Further investigations are warranted to more fully examine the association between smoking cessation and cervical health.

2.2   Secondary prevention — improving cervical cancer screening

Interventions to improve cervical cancer screening have focused on the patient, the physician, and system interventions—each alone or in some combination with one of the others. Studies have evaluated interventions that were behavioral, cognitive, and/or sociologic in design. In general, behavioral reminders address forgetfulness. Theory-based cognitive interventions have been shown to address fears or lack of knowledge about Pap smears (Hillman et al., 1998; Kreuter et al., 1996), and sociologic interventions, using lay health educators, appear to be effective in minority and inner-city populations (Bird et al., 1998; Margolis et al., 1998; Navarro et al., 1998).

2.2.1   Behavioral interventions

Interventions targeting the patient alone have shown an absolute increase in cervical screening of 10%. Patient interventions with the highest level of accrual to screening involved mailing letter invitations. Patient-based reminders are effective strategies for recalling patients who are overdue for screening. The study by Somkin et al. (1997) additionally assessed recruiting never-screened patients to a screening program, which did reveal a small positive effect in the nonutilizer group of 7%. This intervention was done with the use of a computer system and database where patient files could easily be scanned and a letter generated for each outstanding patient.

Interventions involving both the patient and the physician resulted in an absolute increase of cervical screening of 10-30% (Turner et al., 1989). Some studies suggest that patient and physician interventions may have an additive effect (Becker et al., 1989; Turner et al., 1989) with additional gains of 10-15% in screening rates. One explanation may be that the patient acts as a reminder system to the physician.

Interventions targeting physicians alone resulted in absolute increases in cervical screening rates ranging from 9 to 40%. The interventions with the highest success rates included physician reminder systems, both computerized and manual, that provided a reminder on the chart during patient examination that screening was needed or to check the last screening date. The studies reviewed documented that the patient refusal rate for screening was extremely low. Based on the studies by McPhee et al. (McPhee et al., 1989; McPhee et al., 1991) and Ornstein et al. (Ornstein et al., 1995; Ornstein et al., 1991; Ornstein et al., 1989; Ornstein et al., 1993), the rate of patient refusal for screening tests, when recommended by a physician, ranged from 0 to 18%. According to the study by McDonald et al. (1984), physicians inappropriately disregarded reminders to perform screening 30-92% of the time.

Based on this finding, it is clear that the dominant reason that screening does not occur in primary practice is due to physician-based barriers. Focusing on physician interventions may enhance the physicians' role as both a recall and a recruitment provider.

2.2.2   Lay facilitator approach

A creative model that provides person-to-person intensive contact is the concept of the lay facilitator. Lay facilitators, or lay health educators, are usually members of the target group, or community of interest who share similar values, and are viewed by the group (community) to be credible, influential, and genuinely interested in the welfare of group members (Bird et al., 1998; Sung et al., 1997). The use of lay facilitators has been shown to be an effective method for promoting various lifestyle health behavior modifications, including screening for cervical cancer (Bird et al., 1998; Sung et al., 1997).

As applied to smoking cessation, Lando (1987) examined the effectiveness of professional counselor and lay facilitator programs, using a prospective experimental design. Findings indicated that the effectiveness of the intervention was not diminished in a lay-led model since similar cessation rates at one-year posttreatment were reported for smokers who attended a counselor-led clinic program, as compared to those who attended a lay-led clinic program. Lacey and others (Lacey et al., 1991) reported that lay health educators represent an effective method for mobilizing participation in health promotion programs among hard-to-reach urban smokers.

2.3   Tertiary prevention - improving follow-up

Interventions focusing on improving follow-up of an abnormal Pap smear have also focused on the patient, the provider, and the system.

In a review of controlled intervention trials to improve compliance with follow-up of abnormal Pap smears, cognitive interventions led to the greatest increase in follow-up. For instance, cognitive interventions delivered through interactive telephone counseling resulted in improvements in compliance of 24 to 31% (Lerman et al., 1992; Miller et al., 1997). Written educational material contained in letters or pamphlets also increased follow-up (5 to 30% increase in compliance), but not all improvements were statistically significant (Pardini

1996). Most behavioral interventions also led to improvements in follow-up ranging from less than 1 to 21%, although several were not statistically significant. The effectiveness of interventions that combined a variety of strategies was inconsistent, even among interventions conducted within the same study.

These results are generally consistent with those reported for patient-targeted interventions elsewhere. Educational strategies, mailed reminders and telephone prompts, transportation vouchers, and other payment incentives have been shown to improve patient compliance in other settings (Yabroff et al., 1999). Sociologic strategies, such as the use of lay health workers, have been shown to increase use of mammography screening (Yabroff et al., 1999), but the single strategy we reviewed did not lead to improved compliance with follow-up for abnormal Pap smears (Marcus et al., 1992). This intervention was delivered prior to the initial Pap smear (Marcus et al., 1992); delivery of a sociologic intervention at a time more proximal to the abnormal Pap smear result may be more effective. When effective individual interventions were combined, those using multiple approaches (e.g., behavioral and cognitive or behavioral and sociologic) were not significantly better at improving compliance with follow-up than was each intervention alone.

2.4 Vaccines for HPV

Vaccines represent an important, new approach to CIN treatment and prevention, which many have enthusiastically embraced. An Institute of Medicine report on Vaccines for the 21st Century ranked HPV vaccine administered to 12 year olds as a Level II vaccine candidate. This ranking suggested the vaccination strategy would incur small costs (less than $10,000) for each quality-adjusted life year gained (Stratton et al., 1999). HPV prophylactic vaccines have tried to induce immune response with inoculations of DNA coding for capsid proteins, viral capsid proteins themselves, papillomavirus-like particles consisting of self-assembled L1 and L1/L2 proteins, or genetically engineered DNA-free, HPV virus-like particles (Jansen 1999; Muller et al., 1997; Tindle 1999). A Phase IIb study of a HPV 16 L1 VLP vaccine among 2392 women aged 16-23 with ≤ 5 life-time sexual partners or virgins seeking oral contraceptives noted excellent tolerance of an intramuscular injection at baseline, 2 and 6 months. The subjects were followed for 36 months with 41 outcome events occurring. The outcome events were defined as HPV $16 \geq 2$ consecutive assessments at least four months apart or CIN with documented HPV 16 in the lesion. All 41 of the events occurred in the placebo vaccine arm of the study with no events in the vaccine arm (Koutsky et al., 2002). A Phase IIa study of Merck's quadrivalent HPV 6, 11, 16, 18 L1 VLP in 1155 women meeting similar criteria noted excellent tolerance with over 99% seroconversion and very high titers lasting to 24 months of observation (Villa et al., 2002). A Phase III study of the quadrivalent vaccine has been launched with outcome data anticipated in 7-10 years. HPV vaccines are discussed further in Chapters 12 and 13.

2.4.1   Acceptance of HPV vaccines by women

Vaccines for HPV are not available currently, so there is only modest information about adults' perception and acceptance. However, despite the overwhelming prevalence of HPV and potentially catastrophic consequences of an HPV infection, several studies have demonstrated an enormous lack of awareness of the disease by adults (Dell et al., 2000; Gerhardt et al., 2000; Ramirez et al., 1997; Vail-Smith et al., 1992; Yacobi et al., 1999). The available printed patient education messages about HPV are non-standard and geared to an audience with reading skills that exceed the norm of the general population (Perrin et al., 2002). There appears to be ready acceptance for prophylactic HPV vaccines with over 93% of 3,200 women age 28-38 years in Copenhagen expressing willingness to be vaccinated (Munk et al., 2002). Among this same group of women, over 89% would let their daughter or son be vaccinated. However, these reports are dependent on the vaccine being described as without serious adverse effects. It remains to be determined which educational strategies will help diffuse widespread acceptance of HPV vaccines.

CONCLUSION

Cervical cancer continues to be a significant problem throughout the world. Causes of this cancer have been well established and ways to reduce risks for developing this cancer are being tested. Smoking cessation, Pap smear utilization, and prompt follow-up of abnormal cervical findings can reduce cervical cancer incidence. Strategies tested to date are somewhat successful, but need further exploration. Less attention has been paid to testing interventions to reduce the prevalence of other types of risky behaviors such as risky sexual behaviors. Thus, further research is needed. For example, efforts targeting reduction in sexually transmitted disease risk behavior must begin before the onset of somewhat stable patterns of sexual risk behavior. Among adolescents who are sexually active, interventions should include components that increase condom use self-efficacy, build skills to communicate with sexual partners about STD prevention, and address risk behaviors. School sex education that includes specific targeted methods with direct use of medical staff and peers can produce behavioral changes that lead to health benefit.

Most interventions to improve Pap smear screening that have been tested to date have resulted in only modest increases in Pap smear screening, perhaps because they do not adequately address the complex reasons why some women do not obtain screening. Based on the health beliefs model and other theoretical models of health behavior, educational strategies must impact an individual's knowledge and attitudes to have an effect on practice. Thus, changes in screening practices are not likely to be altered by interventions that have only minimal effect on knowledge about and attitudes towards Pap smear screening.

Lastly, access to educational and preventive strategies for all women at risk throughout the world must be a priority in order to reduce the worldwide burden of cervical cancer.

REFERENCES

Ahijevych K, Gillespie J, Demirci M, et al. Menthol and nonmenthol cigarettes and smoke exposure in black and white women. Pharmacology, Biochemistry and Behavior 1996; 53: 355-60.

Altman DG. Strategies for community health intervention: promises, paradoxes, pitfalls. Psychosom Med 1995; 57: 226-33.

Altman DG, Endres J, Linzer J, et al. Obstacles to and future goals of ten comprehensive community health promotion projects. J Community Health 1991; 16: 299-314.

Bastani R, Berman BA, Belin TR, et al. Increasing cervical cancer screening among underserved women in a large urban county health system: can it be done? What does it take? Med Care 2002; 40: 891-907.

Bird JA, McPhee SJ, Ha NT, et al. Opening pathways to cancer screening for Vietnamese-American women: lay health workers hold a key. Prev Med 1998; 27: 821-9.

Blackman D, Bennett E and Miller D. Trends in self-reported use of mammograms (1989-1997) and papanicolaou test (1991-1997)--behavioral risk factor surveillance system. MMWR 1999; 48: 1-22.

Bosch FX, Cardis E Cancer incidence correlations: genital, urinary and some tobacco-related cancers. Int J Cancer 1990; 46: 178-84.

Bosch FX, Munoz N, de Sanjose S, et al. Risk factors for cervical cancer in Colombia and Spain. Int J Cancer 1992; 52: 750-8.

Boyd JT, Doll R. A study of the aetiology of carcinoma of the cervix uteri. Br J Cancer 1964; 18: 419-34.

Boyes DA. The value of a Pap smear program and suggestions for its implementation. Cancer 1981; 48: 613-21.

Boyes DA, Morrison B, Knox EG, et al. A cohort study of cervical cancer screening in British Columbia. Clin Invest Med - Medecine Clinique et Experimentale 1982; 5: 1-29.

Boyes DA, Worth AJ and Anderson GH. Experience with cervical screening in British Columbia. Gynecologic Oncology 1981; 12: S143-55.

Breen N, Figueroa JB. Stage of breast and cervical cancer diagnosis in disadvantaged neighborhoods: a prevention policy perspective. Am J Prev Med 1996; 12: 319-26.

Brinton LA, Reeves WC, Brenes MM, et al. Parity as a risk factor for cervical cancer. Am J Epidemiol 1989; 130: 486-96.

Brinton LA, Reeves WC, Brenes MM, et al. The male factor in the etiology of cervical cancer among sexually monogamous women. Int J Cancer 1989; 44: 199-203.

Caraballo RS, Giovino GA, Pechacek TF, et al. Racial and ethnic differences in serum cotinine levels of cigarette smokers: Third National Health and Nutrition Examination Survey, 1988-1991 [comment]. JAMA 1998; 280: 135-9.

Carmichael J, Clarke D, Moher D, et al. Cervical carcinoma in women aged 34 and younger. Am J Obstet Gynecol 1986; 154: 264-9.

Castellsague X, Bosch FX, Munoz N, et al. Male circumcision, penile human papillomavirus infection, and cervical cancer in female partners. New Engl J Med 2002; 346: 1105-12.

CDC. Cigarette smoking among adults- United States, 1998. MMWR 1998; 49: 891-904.

CDC. Behavioral Risk Factor Surveillance System Survey Data. Atlanta, Georgia, U.S. Department of Health and Human Services. 1998-2000.

CDC. Tobacco use among middle and high school students - United States, MMWR 1999. 2000; 49: 49-53.

CDC. State-Specific prevalence of current cigarette smoking among adults, and policies and attitudes about secondhand smoke - United States, 2000. MMWR 2001; 51: 1101-6.

Celentano DD, Klassen AC, Weisman CS, et al. Cervical cancer screening practices among older women: results from the Maryland cervical cancer case-control study. J Clin Epidemiol 1988; 41: 531-41.

Christopherson WM. Mass population screening for cervix cancer. Tumori 1976; 62: 297-301.

Clarke EA, Morgan RW, Newman AM. Smoking as a risk factor in cancer of the cervix: additional evidence from a case-control study. Am J Epidemiol 1982; 115: 59-66.

Cochran SD, Mays VM, Bowen D, et al. Cancer-related risk indicators and preventive screening behaviors among lesbians and bisexual women. Am J Public Health 2001; 91: 591-7.

Cocks PS, Peel KR, Cartwright RA, et al. Carcinoma of penis and cervix. Lancet 1980; 2: 855-6.

Cramer DW. The role of cervical cytology in the declining morbidity and mortality of cervical cancer. Cancer 1974; 34: 2018-27.

Cummings KM. Programs and policies to discourage the use of tobacco products. Oncogene 2002; 21: 7349-64.

Cummings KM, Sciandra R, Davis S, et al. Results of an antismoking media campaign utilizing the Cancer Information Service. J Natl Cancer Inst Monogr 1993: 113-8.

Daling JR, Sherman KJ, Hislop TG, et al. Cigarette smoking and the risk of anogenital cancer. Am J Epidemiol 1992; 135: 180-9.

de Sanjose S, Munoz N, Bosch FX, et al. Sexually transmitted agents and cervical neoplasia in Colombia and Spain. Int J Cancer 1994; 56: 358-63.

de Vet HC, Sturmans F and Knipschild PG. The role of cigarette smoking in the etiology of cervical dysplasia. Epidemiol 1994; 5: 631-3.

Dell DL, Chen H, Ahmad F, et al. Knowledge about human papillomavirus among adolescents. Obstet Gynecol 2000; 96: 653-6.

DiClemente RJ, Wingood GM. A randomized controlled trial of an HIV sexual risk-reduction intervention for young African-American women [comment]. JAMA 1995; 274: 1271-6.

Dignan M, Michielutte R, Sharp P, et al. The role of focus groups in health education for cervical cancer among minority women. J Community Health 1990; 15: 369-75.

Eluf-Neto J. Number of sexual partners and smoking behaviour as risk factors for cervical dysplasia: comments on the evaluation of interaction. Int J Epidemiology 1994; 23: 1101-4.

Fiore M, Bailey W, Cohen S, et al. Smoking Cessation Clinical Practice Guidelines #18. Rockville, MD, U.S. Department of Health and Human Services. 1996.

Fiore M, Bailey W, Cohen S, et al. Treating tobacco use and dependence. Rockville, MD, U.S. Department of Health and Human Services. 2000.

Fiore MC, Novotny TE, Pierce JP, et al. Methods used to quit smoking in the United States. Do cessation programs help? JAMA 1990; 263: 2760-5.

Frank-Stromborg M, Wassner LJ, Nelson M, et al. A study of rural Latino women seeking cancer-detection examinations. J Cancer Educ 1998; 13: 231-41.

Fruchter RG, Boyce J, Hunt M. Missed opportunities for early diagnosis of cancer of the cervix. Am J Public Health 1980; 70: 418-20.

Gerhardt CA, Pong K, Kollar LM, et al. Adolescents' knowledge of human papillomavirus and cervical dysplasia. J Pediatr Adolesc Gynecol 2000; 13: 15-20.

Graham S, Priore R, Graham M, et al. Genital cancer in wives of penile cancer patients. Cancer 1979; 44: 1870-4.

Green G. Rising cervical cancer mortality in young New Zealand women. NZ Med J 1979; 89: 89-91.

Gulitz E, Bustillo-Hernandez M and Kent EB. Missed cancer screening opportunities among older women: A provider survey. Cancer Pract 1998; 6: 325-32.

Hakama M. Mass screening for cervical cancer in Finland. In: Miller AB, ed. Screening in cancer: a report of the UICC workshop in Toronto. UICC Technical report series, Vol. 40. Geneva: Union Internationale Contre le Cancer, 1978, pp. 93-107.

Hakama M, Rasanen-Virtanen U. Effect of a mass screening program on the risk of cervical cancer. Am J Epidemiol 1976; 103: 512-7.

Harris RWC, Brinton LA, Cowdell RH, et al. Characteristics of women with dysplasia or carcinoma in situ of the cervix uteri. Br J Cancer 1980; 42: 359-69.

Harris R, Leininger L. Preventive care in rural primary care practice. Cancer 1993; 72:1113-1118.

Healthy people 2010. Washington D.C., U.S. Department of Health and Human Services. 2000.

Hellberg D, Valentin J and Nilsson S. Smoking and cervical intraepithelial neoplasia. Acta Obstet Gynecol Scand 1986; 65: 625-31.

Hillman AL, Ripley K, Goldfarb N, et al. Physician financial incentives and feedback: failure to increase cancer screening in Medicaid managed care. Am J Prev Med 1998; 88: 1699-701.

Hulka BS. Risk factors for cervical cancer. J Chron Dis 1982; 35: 3-11.

IARC monographs on the evaluation of the carcinogenic risk of chemicals to man. Lyon, France, International Agency for Research on Cancer, 1995, 64, pp. 1-409.

Institute of Medicine (U.S.). Committee to Study Priorities for Vaccine Development, Stratton KR, Durch J, Lawrence RS. Vaccines for the 21st century: A tool for decision making. Washington, National Academy Press. 2000, 1-97.

Jansen K. HPV Vaccines for Protection Against Infection. In: Tindle R, ed. Vaccines for Human Papillomavirus Infection and Anogenial Disease. Austin, Texas: R.G. Landes, 1999, pp. 33-8.

Jarvis M, Wardle J. Social patterning of individual health behaviors: the case of cigarette smoking. Social Determinants of Health. M Marmot and R Wilkerson. Oxford, Oxford University Press, 2001, pp. 240-55.

Jha PK, Beral V, Peto J, et al. Antibodies to human papillomavirus and to other genital infectious agents and invasive cervical cancer risk. Lancet 1993; 341: 1116-8.

Johannesson G, Geirsson G, Day N. The effect of mass screening in Iceland, 1965-74, on the incidence and mortality of cervical carcinoma. Int J Cancer 1978; 21: 418-25.

Jones E, MacDonald I, Breslow L. A study of epidemiologic factors in carcinoma of the uterine cervix. Am J Obstet Gynecol 1958; 76: 1-10.

Kaplan CP, Bastani R, Belin TR, et al. Improving follow-up after an abnormal pap smear: results from a quasi-experimental intervention study. J Womens Health Gend Based Med 2000; 9: 779-90.

Kelley MJ, McCrory DC. Prevention of lung cancer: summary of published evidence. Chest 2003; 123 (1 Suppl):50S-59S.

Kessler II. Venereal factors in human cervical cancer. Cancer 1977; 39 (Suppl): 1912-9.

Khanna N, Phillips MD. Adherence to care plan in women with abnormal Papanicolaou smears: a review of barriers and interventions. J Am Board Fam Pract 2001; 14: 123-30.

Kirby D, Short L, Collins J, et al. School-based programs to reduce sexual risk behaviors: A review of effectiveness. Public Health Rep 1994; 109: 339-60.

Koutsky L, Ault K, Wheeler C, et al. A controlled trial of a human papillomavirus type 16 vaccine. N Engl J Med 2002; 347: 1645-51.

Kreuter MW, Strecher VJ. Do tailored behavior change messages enhance the effectiveness of health risk appraisal? Results from a randomized trial. Heath Educ Res 1996; 11: 97-105.

La Vecchia C, Franceschi S, Decarli A, et al. Cigarette smoking and the risk of cervical neoplasia. Am J Epidemiol 1986; 123: 22-9.

Lacey L, Tukes S, Manfredi C, et al. Use of lay health educators for smoking cessation in a hard-to-reach urban community. J Community Health 1991; 16: 269-82.

Laedtke TW, Dignan M. Compliance with therapy for cervical dysplasia among women of low socioeconomic status. South Med J 1992; 85: 5-8.

Lando H. Lay facilitators as effective smoking cessation counselors. Addict Behav 1987; 12: 69-72.

Lantz PM, Stencil D, Lippert MT, et al. Implementation issues and costs associated with a proven strategy for increasing breast and cervical cancer screening among low-income women. J Public Health Manag Practice 1996; 2: 54-9.

Lavin C, Goodman E, Perlman S, et al. Follow-up of abnormal Papanicolaou smears in a hospital-based adolescent clinic. J Pediatr Adolesc Gynecol 1997; 10: 141-5.

Lerman C, Hanjani P, Caputo C, et al. Telephone counseling improves adherence to colposcopy among lower-income minority women. J Clin Oncol 1992; 10: 330-3.

Li JY, Li FP, Blot WJ, et al. Correlation between cancers of the uterine cervix and penis in China. J Natl Cancer Inst 1982; 69: 1063-5.

Licciardone JC, Brownson RC, Chang JC, et al. Uterine cervical cancer risk in cigarette smokers: a meta-analytic study. Am J Prev Med 1990; 6: 274-81.

Lyon JL, Gardner JW, West DW, et al. Smoking and carcinoma in situ of the uterine cervix. Am J Public Health 1983; 73: 558-62.

Macgregor JE, Innes G. Carcinoma of penis and cervix. Lancet 1980; 1: 1246-7.

Marcus AC, Crane LA, Kaplan CP, et al. Improving adherence to screening follow-up among women with abnormal Pap smears. Results from a large clinic-based trial of three intervention strategies. Med Care 1992;30:216-30.

Margolis KL, Lurie N, McGovern PG, et al. Increasing breast and cervical cancer screening in low-income women. J Gen Interri Med 1998; 13: 515-21.

Martin PL. How preventable is invasive cervical cancer? A community study of preventable factors. Am J Obstet Gynecol 1972; 113: 541-8.

Martinez I. Relationship of squamous cell carcinoma of the cervix uteri to squamous cell carcinoma of the penis among Puerto Rican women married to men with penile carcinoma. Cancer 1969; 24: 777-80.

McBride CM, Scholes D, Grothaus L, et al. Promoting smoking cessation among women who seek cervical cancer screening. Obstet Gynecol 1998; 91: 719-24.

McBride CM, Scholes D, Grothaus LC, et al. Evaluation of a minimal self-help smoking cessation intervention following cervical cancer screening. Prev Med 1999; 29: 133-8.

McDonald CJ, Hui SL, Smith DM, et al. Reminders to physicians from an introspective computer medical record. A two-year randomized trial. Ann Intern Med 1984; 100: 130-8.

McPhee SJ, Bird JA, Jenkins CN, et al. Promoting cancer screening. A randomized, controlled trial of three interventions. Arch Intern Med 1989; 149: 1866-72.

McPhee SJ, Bird JA, Davis T, et al. Barriers to breast and cervical cancer screening among Vietnamese-American women. Am J Prev Med 1997; 13: 205-13.

McPhee SJ, Bird JA, Fordham D, et al. Promoting cancer prevention activities by primary care physicians. Results of a randomized, controlled trial. JAMA 1991; 266: 538-44.

Melnikow J, Chan BK and Stewart GK. Do follow-up recommendations for abnormal Papanicolaou smears influence patient adherence? Arch Fam Med 1999; 8: 510-4.

Miller A. Evaluation of the impact of screening for cancer of the cervix. Screening for cancer of the uterine cervix. In: Hakama M, Miller AB, Day NE, eds. IARC Sci Pub 76. Lyon, International Agency for Research on Cancer, 1986, 149-160.

Miller KS, Yunger J, Single N, et al. Prevalence of abnormal Pap smears in rural family practice. J Rural Health 1996; 12: 33-8.

Miller SM, Siejak KK, Schroeder CM, et al. Enhancing adherence following abnormal pap smears among low-income minority women: a preventive telephone counseling strategy. J Natl Cancer Inst 1997; 89: 703-8.

Morell ND, Taylor JR, Snyder RN, et al. False-negative cytology rates in patients in whom invasive cervical cancer subsequently developed. Obstet Gynecol 1982; 60: 41-5.

Morrison BJ, Coldman AJ, Boyes DA, et al. Forty years of repeated screening: the significance of carcinoma in situ. Br J Cancer 1996; 74: 814-9.

Mueller KJ, Ortega ST, Parker K, et al. Health status and access to care among rural minorities. J Health Care Poor Underserved 1999; 10: 230-49.

Mueller KJ, Patil K, Boilesen E. The role of uninsurance and race in healthcare utilization by rural minorities. Health Serv Res 1998; 33: 597-610.

Muller M, Zhou J, Reed TD, et al. Chimeric papillomavirus-like particles. Virology 1997; 234: 93-111.

Munk C, Svare E, Bock J, et al. Women's attitudes towards HPV vaccination - results from the Copenhagen prospective cohort study. 20th International Papillomavirus Conference, Paris, 2002.

Munoz N, Bosch F. Epidemiology of cervical cancer. In: Munoz N, Bosch FX, Jensen OM, eds. Human papillomavirus and cervical cancer. Lyon: IARC Scientific Publications, No. 94, 1989, pp. 9-39.

Navarro AM, Senn KL, McNicholas LJ, et al. Por La Vida model intervention enhances use of cancer screening tests among Latinas. Am J Prev Med 1998; 15: 32-41.

Ngelangel C, Munoz N, Bosch FX, et al. Causes of cervical cancer in the Philippines: a case-control study. J Natl Cancer Inst 1998; 90: 43-9.

Nischan P, Ebeling K, Schindler C. Smoking and invasive cervical cancer risk. Results from a case-control study. Am J Epidemiol 1988; 128: 74-7.

Norman SA, Talbott EO, Kuller LH, et al. Demographic, psychosocial, and medical correlates of Pap testing: a literature review. Am J Prev Med 1991; 7: 219-26.

Norton CH, McManus MA. Background tables on demographic characteristics, health status, and health services utilization. Health Serv Res 1989; 23: 725-56.

Oakley A, Fullerton D, Holland J, et al. Sexual health education interventions for young people: a methodological review. Br Med J 1995; 310: 158-62.

Orleans C. Understanding promoting smokingcessation: overview and guidelines for physicain intervention. Ann Rev Med 1985; 36: 51-61.

Orleans CT, Cummings KM. Population-based tobacco control: progress and prospects. Am J Health Promot 1999; 14: 83-91.

Ornstein SM, Garr DR, Jenkins RG, et al. Implementation and evaluation of a computer-based preventive services system. Fam Med 1995; 27: 260-6.

Ornstein SM, Garr DR, Jenkins RG, et al. Computer-generated physician and patient reminders. Tools to improve population adherence to selected preventive services. J Fam Pract 1991; 32: 82-90.

Ornstein SM, Garr DR, Jenkins RG, et al. Compliance with five health promotion recommendations in a university-based family practice. J Fam Pract 1989; 29: 163-168.

Ornstein SM, Musham C, Reid A, et al. Barriers to adherence to preventive services reminder letters: the patient's perspective. J Fam Pract 1993; 36: 195-200.

Orr DP, Langefeld CD, Katz BP, et al. Behavioral intervention to increase condom use among high-risk female adolescents. J Pediatr 1996; 128: 288-95.

Pardini RS. Effect of educational brochures on Cherokee women with abnormal pap smears. Public Health Rep 1996; 111: 546-7.

Parkin D, Nguyen-dinh X, Day N. The impact of screening on the incidence of cervical cancer in England and Wales. Br J Obstet Gynaecol 1985; 92: 150-157.

Parkin DM, Pisani P, Ferlay J. Estimates of the worldwide incidence of 25 major cancers in 1990. Int J Cancer 1999; 80: 827-41.

Paskett ED, Carter WB, Chu J, et al. Compliance behavior in women with abnormal Pap smears. Developing and testing a decision model. Med Care 1990; 28: 643-56.

Paskett ED, Tatum CM, D'Agostino R, Jr., et al. Community-based interventions to improve breast and cervical cancer screening: results of the Forsyth County Cancer Screening (FoCaS) Project. Cancer Epidemiol Biomarkers Prev 1999; 8: 453-9.

Penn NE, Kar S, Kramer J, et al. Ethnic minorities, health care systems, and behavior. Health Psychol 1995; 14: 641-6.

Perez-Stable EJ, Otero-Sabogal R, Sabogal F, et al. Self-reported use of cancer screening tests among Latinos and Anglos in a prepaid health plan [comment]. Arch Intern Med 1994; 154: 1073-81.

Perrin K, Daley E, Hassle C, et al. Readability and relevant HPV content in 20 HPV patient education brocures. 20th International Papillomavirus Conference, Paris, 2002.

Peters RK, Thomas D, Hagan DG, et al. Risk factors for invasive cervical cancer among Latinas and non- Latinas in Los Angeles County. J Natl Cancer Inst 1986; 77: 1063-77.

Pierce JP, Fiore MC, Novotny TE, et al. Trends in cigarette smoking in the United States. Educational differences are increasing. JAMA 1989; 261: 56-60.

Pomerleau CS, Marks JL, Pomerleau OF. Who gets what symptom? Effects of psychiatric cofactors and nicotine dependence on patterns of smoking withdrawal symptomatology. Nicotine Tob Res 2000; 2: 275-80.

Pomerleau OF, Pomerleau CS. Neuroregulators and the reinforcement of smoking: towards a biobehavioral explanation. Neurosci Biobehav Rev 1984; 8: 503-13.

Poppe W, Drijkoningen M, Ide P, et al. Langerhans' cell and L1 anigen expression in normal and abnormal squamous epithelium of the cervical transformation zone. Gynecol Obstetric Invest 1996; 41: 207-13.

Potosky AL, Breen N, Graubard BI, et al. The association between health care coverage and the use of cancer screening tests. Results from the 1992 National Health Interview Survey. Med Care 1998; 36: 257-70.

Prokopczyk B, Cox JE, Hoffmann D, et al. Identification of tobacco-specific carcinogen in the cervical mucus of smokers and nonsmokers. J Natl Cancer Inst 1997; 89: 868-73.

Rakowski W, Clark MA, Ehrich B. Smoking and cancer screening for women ages 42-75: associations in the 1990-1994 National Health Interview Surveys. Prev Med 1999; 29:487-95.

Ramirez JE, Ramos DM, Clayton L, et al. Genital human papillomavirus infections: knowledge, perception of risk, and actual risk in a nonclinic population of young women. J Womens Health 1997; 6: 113-21.

Ries L, Eisner M, Kosary C, et al. SEER Cancer Statistics Review, 1973-1997. Bethesda, MD, National Cancer Institute, 2000.

Rimer BK, Conaway MR, Lyna PR, et al. Cancer screening practices among women in a community health center population. Am J Prev Med 1996; 12: 351-7.

Rosenfeld JA. The natural history of Pap test screening in a rural population. Tenn Med 1998; 91: 179-82.

Rotkin ID. A comparison review of key epidemiological studies in cervical cancer related to current searches for transmissible agents. Cancer Res 1973; 33: 1353-67.

Sasson IM, Coleman DT, LaVoie EJ, et al. Mutagens in human urine: effects of cigarette smoking and diet. Mutat Res 1985; 158: 149-57.

Schootman M, Fuortes LJ. Breast and cervical carcinoma: the correlation of activity limitations and rurality with screening, disease incidence, and mortality. Cancer 1999; 86: 1087-94.

Simons AM, Phillips DH, Coleman DV. Damage to DNA in cervical epithelium related to smoking tobacco.[comment]. Br Med J 1993; 306: 1444-8.

Simons AM, Phillips DH, Coleman DV. DNA adduct assay in cervical epithelium. Diagn Cytopathol 1994; 10: 284-8.

Skaer TL, Robison LM, Sclar DA, et al. Knowledge, attitudes, and patterns of cancer screening: a self-report among foreign born Hispanic women utilizing rural migrant health clinics. J Rural Health 1996; 12: 169-77.

Smith PG, Kinlen LJ, White GC, et al. Mortality of wives of men dying with cancer of the penis. Br J Cancer 1980; 41: 422-8.

Somkin CP, Hiatt RA, Hurley LB, et al. The effect of patient and provider reminders on mammography and Papanicolaou smear screening in a large health maintenance organization. Arch Intern Med 1997; 157: 1658-64.

Song F, Raftery J, Aveyard P, et al. Cost-effectiveness of pharmacological interventions for smoking cessation: a literature review and a decision analytic analysis. Med Decis Making 2002; 22: S26-37.

Stanton B, Fang X, Li X, et al. Evolution of risk behaviors over 2 years among a cohort of urban African American adolescents. Arch Pediatr Adolesc Med 1997; 151: 398-406.

Stellman SD, Austin H, Wynder EL . Cervix cancer and cigarette smoking: a case-control study. Am J Epidemiol 1980; 111: 383-8.

Sung JF, Blumenthal DS, Coates RJ, et al. Effect of a cancer screening intervention conducted by lay health workers among inner-city women. Am J Prev Med 1997; 13: 51-7.

Szarewski A, Maddox P, Royston P, et al. The effect of stopping smoking on cervical Langerhans' cells and lymphocytes. Br J Obstet Gynecol 2001; 108: 295-303.

Taylor SM, Ross NA, Cummings KM, et al. Community Intervention Trial for Smoking Cessation (COMMIT): changes in community attitudes toward cigarette smoking. Health Educ Res 1998; 13: 109-22.

Terris M, Wilson F, Smith, H et al. The relationship of coitus to carcinoma of the cervix. Am J Pub Health 1967; 57: 840-7.

The health consequences of smoking; nicotine addiction. A report of the surgeon general. Rockville, MD, U.S. Department of Health and Human Services, Office on Smoking and Health, 1988.

Tindle,R. Immunomodulation of HPV Infection and Disease: An Overview. In: Tindle R, ed. Vaccines for Human Papillomavirus Infection and Anogenital Disease. Austin, Texas: R.G. Landes, 1999, pp. 1-12.

Trevathan E, Layde P, Webster LA, et al. Cigarette smoking and dysplasia and carcinoma in situ of the uterine cervix. JAMA 1983; 250: 499-502.

Trosclair A, Husten C, Pederson L, et al. Cigarette smoking among adults - United States, 2000. MMWR 2002; 51: 642-5.

Turner BJ, Day SC, Borenstein B. A controlled trial to improve delivery of preventive care: physician or patient reminders? J Gen Intern Med 1989; 4: 403-9.

Vail-Smith K, White DM. Risk level, knowledge, and preventive behavior for human papillomaviruses among sexually active college women. J Am Coll Health 1992; 40: 227-30.

van der Graaf Y, Zielhuis GA, Peer PGM, et al. The effectiveness of cervical screening: A population-based case-control study. J Clin Epidemiol 1988; 41: 21-6.

Villa L, Costa R, Petta C, et al. A dose ranging safety and immunogenicity study of a quadrivalent HPV (types 6/11/16/18) L1 VLP vaccine in women. 20th International Papillomavirus Conference, Paris, France, 2002.

Vyslouzilova,S, Arbyn M, Van Oyen H, et al. Cervical cancer mortality in Belgium, 1955-1989, a descriptive study. Eur J Cancer 1997; 33: 1841-5.

Wewers ME, Ahijevych K, Page JA. Evaluation of a mass media community smoking cessation campaign. Addict Behav 1991; 16: 289-94.

Wilcox LS, Mosher WD. Factors associated with obtaining health screening among women of reproductive age. Public Health Rep 1993; 108: 76-86.

Winkelstein WJ. Smoking and cancer of the uterine cervix: hypothesis. Am J Epidemiol 1977; 106: 257-9.

Yabroff KR, Mandelblatt JS. Interventions targeted to patients to increase mammography use. Cancer Epidemiol Biomarkers Prev 1999;8:749-57.

Yacobi E, Tennant C, Ferrante J, et al. University students' knowledge and awareness of HPV. Prev Med 1999; 28: 535-41.

Chapter 10

Screening for Cervical Cancer

Jack Cuzick, Ph.D.
Cancer Research UK, Department of Epidemiology, Mathematics and Statistics, Wolfson Institute of Preventative Medicine

INTRODUCTION

World-wide, there are estimated to be almost half a million new cases and a quarter of a million deaths from cervical cancer each year, accounting for about 10% of all female cancers (Parkin, 2001) and making cervix cancer the second commonest cancer among women, being exceeded only by breast cancer (Table 1). The cumulative incidence rate up to age 74 ranges from over 5% in parts of Latin America to around 0.5% in parts of the Middle East and in Finland. In most European countries it is around 1% (WHO, 1997).

The incidence of cervical cancer in most countries has decreased substantially since the 1960s (WHO, 1993). In the UK, mortality from cervical cancer has been declining since 1950 except in young women (aged 20-39), in whom rates more than doubled between 1970 and the mid 1980s (Sasieni, 1991). The incidence rates of cervical cancer show strong birth cohort effects (Beral, 1974). It is estimated that, in the absence of screening, the cumulative risk of cervical cancer up to age 74 in women in the UK during the 1960s would be around 4-5% (Sasieni and Adams, 2000) which is similar to that in high risk areas. That would make cervical cancer third in importance after breast and lung in women, and underlines the need for an effective screening programme.

Table 1. Estimated worldwide cancer incidence and mortality (by site) for the year 2000 (thousands) (Parkin et al., 2001)

SITE	MALE INCIDENCE	MALE MORTALITY	FEMALE INCIDENCE	FEMALE MORTALITY
All	5300	4700	4700	2700
Lung	902	810	337	293
Breast	-	-	1050	370
Colon/Rectum	499	255	446	234
Stomach	558	405	318	241
Liver	398	384	166	165
Prostrate	543	204	-	-
Cervix Uteri	-	-	471	233
Oesophagus	279	227	133	111
Bladder	260	99	76	33
Non-Hodgkin Lymphoma	167	93	121	68
Leukaemia	144	109	113	86
Oral Cavity	170	81	97	47
Pancreas	116	112	101	101
Kidney	119	57	71	34
Ovary	-	-	192	114

After adjusting for cohort effects, the incidence rates of cervical cancer, in most countries, rise steeply between ages 25 and 39 and are then fairly constant for a further 40 years. Thus, cervical cancer has one of the earliest ages of onset of any of the major cancers and can have a devastating effect when it strikes the mothers of families with young children.

1   SCREENING PROGRAMS

The parameters of national screening programmes or policies vary widely, ranging from annual screening following sexual debut in the United States and Germany to 5-yearly screening starting at age 30 in Finland and the Netherlands (Table 2).

The effectiveness of screening is more related to the implementation of organized programmes employing quality control measures than the intensity with which screening is offered. This is well illustrated by the UK programme. This programme was introduced in the mid 1960s, but had virtually no impact on deaths from this disease. Death rates were declining at roughly 2% per year since 1950 and continued to do so at the same rate after the introduction of screening (Figure 1). This was in stark contrast to the results in Sweden, Finland and Iceland, where programmes introduced about the same time led to dramatic falls in mortality within 5-10 years. In the UK the problem was that all that was introduced was a *policy* for screening

Table 2. Screening recommendations in different countries (van Ballegooijen et al. 2002)

Country	Age to Start	Age to Stop	Frequency	Program
USA	3 years after 1st intercourse but before 21 years	69	Annual or 2 years with liquid based sample or after 3 normal tests	Opportunistic
UK	20	64	3-5 years	Organised
Finland	30	60	5	Organised
Sweden	20	59	3	Organised and Opportunistic
Netherlands	30	60	5 years	Organised
Germany	20	None	Annual	Opportunistic
Denmark	23	59	3 years	Mostly Opportunistic

without adequate infrastructure or coordination and monitoring. Overall the number of smears taken was adequate (over 3 million per year) but they were unevenly spread. Some women had very frequent smears (every 6-12 months), while other women were not screened at all. Coverage was estimated at 30-40%, but no reliable national figures were available and no attempt was made to manage the programme. In contrast, for Sweden and Finland, an organized programme was introduced from the beginning. By the mid 1980s the UK accepted the error of its ways, and in 1987 a new programme involving a computerized call and recall system and quality control measures was introduced. The results were rapid and spectacular. Coverage increased dramatically to about 85% (Figure 1) and mortality rates began to decrease within about 2-3 years reaching a 7% annual decline by 1998 (Figure 2). Mortality rates decreased by about 44% from 1985 to 1998.

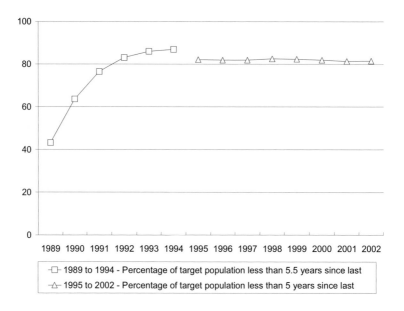

Figure 1: Cervical screening: coverage of target age group (25-64), 1988 to 2002

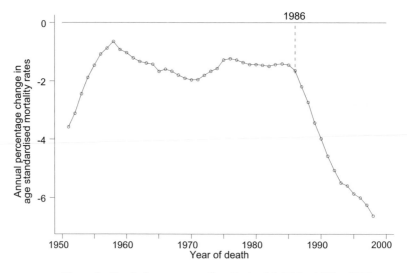

Figure 2: Cervical cancer mortality: England & Wales 1950 – 1998

In the absence of randomised trials, researchers have sought evidence from studies that looked at screening at the individual level rather than in populations. These have mostly been carried out as case-control studies, comparing the screening experience of women diagnosed with or dying from cervical cancer to that of healthy women (Table 3). This is potentially susceptible to bias, due to different lifestyle of women who are not screened, especially with regard to sexual behaviors, cigarette smoking and diet. Nevertheless, considering both case-control data and population trends, one sees a clear picture in which cancer rates are falling, and women who have been screened are much less likely to develop cancer than those who have not.

A meta-analysis of 10 case-control studies carried out in eight countries showed that cervical screening was effective in preventing the development of cervical cancer (IARC, 1986). The study found that:

- women with two or more negative smear results were less likely to develop cervical cancer than women with just one previous negative smear;
- compared to women who had never been screened, women with two or more negative smears were 15 times less likely to develop cervical cancer within a year of having a negative test, 8 times less likely 24-35 months later, 5 times 36-47 months later, 3 times 48-59 months later and 3 times 60-71 months later;

The fact that having two negative smears was associated with a substantially lower risk of developing cancer than having only one suggests that smear tests have limited sensitivity. This has been directly shown in several studies now and in the best hands cytology has about a 70% sensitivity for high grade CIN (Table 4).

Table 3. Summary of Epidemiological studies looking at the differences of cervical screening at an individual level (Sasieni et. Al., 2003)

First Author— Year	Area	Type of Study	Years of Diagnosis	No. of Invasive Cancers	Choice of Comparison Group	Notes	Summary or Results
Aristizabal 1984	Colombia	Case-control interview	1977-81	204	2 controls/ case: 1 health centre, 1 neighbourhood	Only 22% of potential cases participate. Analysis biased for screen-detected cases (in favour of screening)	4% of cases screened 12-72 months prior to diagnosis, 52% of health-centre controls, 31% of neighbourhood controls
La Vecchia 1984	Milan	Case-control interview	1981-83	191	191 hospital controls	98% participation. 61% stage I	Relative protection decreased with time since last -ve, and was greater with 2+ -ve's.
Berrino 1986	Milan	Case-control Clinical records	1978	121	3 controls/case	Hospital controls	Risk within 24 months of -ve smear 15% of that in those with no such smear.
Choi 1986	Manitoba	Cohort	1968-75	86	Historical cohort	Cases had negative smear between 1963 and 1972.	Incidence decreased with no. of -ve smears, but did not increase with time since -ve.
Clarke 1986	Toronto	Case-control interview	1973-76	156	5 Controls /case	Squamous, stage 1B+. 67% of potential cases consented.	Relative protection decreased with time since last -ve, and lasted up to 48 months.

Table 3. Summary of Epidemiological studies looking at the differences of cervical screening at an individual level (Sasieni et. Al., 2003), *continued*

First Author—Year	Area	Type of Study	Years of Diagnosis	No. of Invasive Cancers	Choice of Comparison Group	Notes	Summary or Results
Geirsson 1986	Iceland	Case-control. Clinical records	1969-84	101	5 controls/case	Cases (59% screen-detected) and controls screened at least once.	Relative protection decreased with time since last -ve, was substantial and lasted up to 119 months
Lynge 1986	Denmark	Cohort	1962-82	53	Historical cohort		Relative protection decreased with time since last -ve, and was greater with 2+ -ve's
Macgregor 1986	Aberdeen	Case-control. Clinical records	1968-83	85	5 controls/case	Cases (59% screen-detected) and controls screened at least once.	Relative protection decreased with time since last -ve, and was greater with 2+ -ve's
Magnus 1986	Norway	Cohort	1959-82	73	Neighbouring Counties		No clear effect of -ve smears
Pettersson 1986	Sweden	Cohort	1967-80	446	Historical cohort	Cases had negative smear. Only recorded organised screening	Incidence increases with time since last -ve, up to 5 yrs. Risk less after two-ve's
Raymond 1986	Geneva	Case-control	1970-76	186	1 control/case		Relative protection greatest within 12 months of -ve smear
van Oortmarssen 1986	British Columbia	Cohort	1949-69	68	Unscreened part of population	Cases had negative smear	No clear trend in incidence with time since last -ve.
Wangsu-phachart 1987	Thailand	Case-control. Interview	1979-83	189	1023 controls	Hospital controls	Relative protection ~4 for annual screening, ~2.5 for 2-5 yearly

Table 3. Summary of Epidemiological studies looking at the differences of cervical screening at an individual level (Sasieni et. Al., 2003), *continued*

First Author—Year	Area	Type of Study	Years of Diagnosis	No. of Invasive Cancers	Choice of Comparison Group	Notes	Summary or Results
Olesen 1988	Denmark	Case-control. GP questionnaire	1983	428	1 control/case. GP matched	82% of potential cases enrolled.	Relative protection ~4 with 1 previous smear, ~6 with 2+.
Sobue 1988	Japan	Case-control. Clinical records	1965-87	28	10 controls/case	Controls matched for screening in year of diagnosis. Paper also reports on deaths.	Risk greatest in those with no -ve's, and least in those -ve with 4 years. 2 smears better than 1.
vander Graaf 1988	Netherlands	Case-control. Interview	1979-85	36	6 controls/case	Stage 1B+. 30% of potential cases did not survive (or too ill) to interview. Control response rate 55%	Protection greatest 2-5 years after smear, but still 3-fold after 5 years
Klassen 1989	Maryland	Case-control. Interview	1982-84	101	396 controls	16% of potentail cases did not survive (or too ill) to interview. Telephoned controls. 73% response.	Relative protection decreased with time since last smear, and lasted 5-10 years
Herrero 1992	Latin America	Case-control. Interview	1986-87	759	2 controls/case	Hospital and community controls. Participation >96%.	Protection greatest within 4 years of smear, but last for 10 years.
Cohen 1993	Manitoba	Case-control. Clinical records	1981-1984	341	27164 controls	5% of cases could not be linked to screening databases, 18% had <5 years "follow up". Smears taken in year prior to diagnosis ignored	Relative risk for smear 2-5 years prior to diagnosis ~0.5 overall. Effect least in women aged 25-34

Table 3. Summary of Epidemiological studies looking at the differences of cervical screening at an individual level (Sasieni et. Al. 2003), *continued*

First Author— Year	Area	Type of Study	Years of Diagnosis	No. of Invasive Cancers	Choice of Comparison Group	Notes	Summary or Results
Macgregor 1994	Aberdeen	Case-control Clinical records	1982-91	282	2 controls/case	22% of cases were screen-detected	Risk greatest when last -ve smear was over 9 years ago (or never). Risk greater if within 3 years than 3-9 years
Makino 1995	Japan	Case-control Clinical records & questionnaire	1984-89	198	2 controls/case	65% of cases were screen-detected	Relative protection decreased with time since last -ve, and was greatest within 2 years
Mitchell 1996	Australia	Case-Cohort	1993	233	Cohort negatively screened 1990-93	Includes all diagnoses	Incidence greatest in those never screened and least in those screened within 3.5 years.
Herbert 1996	England	Cohort	1991-93	83	Cohort (116022)	72% of cases, stage I. Used proportion of cohort screened within 3.5 & 5.5 years.	Relative protection decreased with time since last -ve.
Sasieni 1996	UK	Case-control. Clinical records	1992	348	2 controls/case	26% micro-invasive analysed separately	Risk least in those screened at least every 4 years and least in those never screened.
Hernandez-Avila 1998	Mexico	Case-control. Interview	1990-92	397	1005 controls	Participation 95% (cases) 85% (controls). Recorded gynaecological symptoms.	

Table 3. Summary of Epidemiological studies looking at the differences of cervical screening at an individual level (Sasieni et. Al., 2003), *continued*

First Author—Year	Area	Type of Study	Years of Diagnosis	No. of Invasive Cancers	Choice of Comparison Group	Notes	Summary or Results
Jimenez-Perez 1999	Mexico	Case-control. Interview	1991-94	143	311 controls	Health centre controls. Response 94%	Risk greatest in those never screened and least in those screened within 5 years. Proportion screened less in advanced cancers
Nieminen 1999	Helsinki	Case-control. Questionnaire	1987-94	179	1507 controls	Cases had to survive until 1994. Response 87% (cases), 76% (controls)	No data on screening interval. Organised screening more protective than spontaneous screening.
Viikki 1999	Finland	Cohort	1971-1994	48	Cohort (n=45572) with normal smear in 1971-76		Relative protection of screening 2.3
Andersson-Ellstrom 2000	Sweden	Case-control. Clinical records	1990-97	112	112 controls	61% stage I.	50% cases and 55% of controls screened within 3 years. But 69% of stage I and 9% of stage III-IV
Kinney 2001	California	Case-control. Clinical records	1983-95	482	2 controls/case	Abstract only	Risk within 18 months of -ve half that within 19-42 months

The lower risk of cervical cancer following a negative smear is due to the test being able to identify those who are at risk of developing cancer. It is only through effective treatment of precursor lesions that cancer is prevented. This does not always occur. A substantial minority of cervical cancers in the UK are now being diagnosed in women who have a past history of positive cytology (Sasieni et al., 1996). This is due to mismanagement of women with abnormal smears and/or unsuccessful treatment. Thus, the IARC estimates that three- or five-yearly screening could reduce cervical cancer incidence by 91% and 84% respectively are likely to be overly optimistic.

Table 4. Summary statistics for studies of the conventional Papanicolaou test. Studies with complete or random colposcopy evaluation of seven negatives are listed separately (Nanda et al., 2000)

Threshold (cystology histology)	Studies, n	Sensitivity (median)	Specificity (median)	Median prevalence of histologic disease
ASCUS/CIN-I				
Overall	37	0.74	0.68	0.51
Verification				
All or random	21	0.68	0.75	0.36
Some or unclear	16	0.78	0.60	0.73
LSIL/CIN-I				
Overall	71	0.69	0.81	0.64
Verification				
All or random	38	0.62	0.90	0.43
Some or unclear	33	0.75	0.71	0.72
LSIL/CIN-II-III				
Overall	54	0.83	0.66	0.32
Verification				
All or random	31	0.81	0.77	0.24
Some or unclear	23	0.87	0.46	0.47
LSIL/CIN-II-III				
Overall	43	0.58	0.92	0.41
Verification				
All or random	25	0.53	0.96	0.28
Some or unclear	18	0.62	0.78	0.54

The extent to which these findings are likely to over-estimate the benefits of screening can be judged by a more recent UK study in which 8% of cancers in women under 70 had been preceded by a smear history requiring referral to colposcopy at least 6 months prior to diagnosis (Sasieni et al., 1996). That paper also estimated the protective effect of participating in screening by studying the risk of cancer within three years of any screening test regardless of the outcome. When these criteria were used, the benefit of screening was less and the reduction of incidence was found to be about 70%.

2   SCREENING PARAMETERS

A number of issues are still open concerning the use of the conventional pap smear. In particular there is controversy about the ages at which screening should start, when it can be stopped, and how frequent the screening interval should be.

2.1   When should screening start?

Most cervical screening programmes start between the ages of 20 and 30 years. The rationale for starting at a younger age is based on the fact that high-grade abnormality rates (and HPV infection rates) are very high even a few years after coitarche and are greatest after about 10 years. Those that start later are more influenced by the low rates of cervical cancer under the age of 30 and extremely low rates under the age of 25. There is currently no evidence that screening under age 30 has any impact on cancer incidence rates, but it is associated with a large number of referrals for low-grade disease. It has been suggested that one value of early screening is to overcome the low sensitivity of cytology by ensuring that 2-3 negative screens are obtained before the age of 30. With newer, more sensitive screening methods becoming available (see section 5), it may be more appropriate to begin screening at age 25 or 30.

2.2   When should screening stop?

In some countries there is no upper age-limit for cervical screening, but in many countries screening ceases after the age of 60 or 65 years. The reasons for not continuing to screen older women are: (i) the rate of high-grade lesions detected on screening in women over the age of 50 is low compared to the rates in younger women; (ii) cervical screening is more uncomfortable in older women and the gain in terms of added years of cancer-free life decreases with increasing age; (iii) it is believed that almost all cervical cancer in older women results from HPV infection under the age of 35, so that older women who have had two or three recent negative screens are at extremely low risk of developing cancer in the future. Indeed it has been argued that screening could cease at age 50 in women who have been previously well screened (van Wijngaarden and Duncan, 1993) based on the extremely rare finding of incident high-grade disease in such women. Those who argue for continued screening of older women would point to the increasing mortality rates over the age of 65 observed in many countries.

2.3   Screening interval

There have been no randomised studies comparing the efficacy of cytological screening at different intervals and so decisions need to be made based on observational studies and available resources. Cytological screening has variously been carried out at intervals of 1, 3 and 5 years. Annual screening is the norm in the United States and Germany, whereas 5 yearly screening is recommended in countries such as the Netherlands and Finland with a public health based screening programme. Most European countries aim at 3 yearly screening starting at age 20-30 and continuing until age 59-65. Although there are certain overheads associated with running a screening programme that are independent of the amount of screening undertaken, these are small. The major determinant of cost is the number of smears taken each year. The latter is determined by the number of smears offered per woman in her lifetime and the compliance with the programme policy. Although there is some evidence that the rate of high-grade abnormalities increases with the screening interval, the rate of low-grade abnormalities appears to be independent of the screening interval (Sigurdsson and Adalsteinsson, 2001). Thus, roughly speaking, annual screening is three times as expensive as three-yearly screening which in turn is 66% more expensive than five-yearly screening.

For many years, the meta-analysis conducted by IARC (1986), provided the best estimates of the relative effectiveness of cytological screening at different intervals and provided the "input parameters" for many of the models looking at the effectiveness of different screening policies. That paper suggested that whereas annual screening could prevent 93.5% of cervical cancer, three-yearly screening was almost as good (90.8%), whilst five-yearly screening was slightly less effective (83.6%). Based on these figures, it was generally believed that annual screening was excessive, but the choice between 3 and 5 yearly screening was more difficult.

Two more recent studies from the UK also provide estimates of the relative benefit of different screening intervals. A UK-based audit (Sasieni et al., 1996) included the screening histories of 348 women with invasive cervical cancer in a case-control study, and Herbert et al.(1996) studied the screening histories of 83 women with invasive cancer and compared them to known performance indicators of the local screening programme. Both studies found a substantial difference in the risk of cancer associated with three- and five-yearly screening. Sasieni et al. (1996) considered both time since last negative smear and time since last smear (regardless of result, but excluding all smears taken within 6 months of diagnosis). In both analyses, the relative risk 5 years after screening compared to no screening is around 65%, whereas the relative risk after 3 years is around 30-35%. Thus, it would appear that even the marginal cost of 3-yearly screening compared to 5-yearly screening is justified by the marginal benefit. Herbert et al. (1996) also found that the benefit of 5-yearly screening (compared to no screening) was less than in the IARC (1986) overview and that the relative benefit of 3 compared to 5 yearly screening was greater. Whether or not they excluded screen-detected cancers, they found the relative benefit of three- compared to five-yearly screening to be similar to the relative benefit of five-yearly screening compared to no screening.

In Table 5, we compare the "effectiveness" of screening at different intervals as estimated from the IARC study and from the UK audit. The table includes the effect of imperfect sensitivity on the results from the IARC study. Assuming the relative rates obtained from the IARC study apply to a test with 100% sensitivity, we also look at what the results would be for a test with either 75% or 60% sensitivity. Such sensitivities are typical when cytology is compared to other screening tests such as HPV testing. The effect of taking into account imperfect sensitivity is to reduce the effectiveness of screening (at any interval) and to increase the relative benefit of more frequent screening (assuming the results of cytology taken at different times in a given woman are conditionally independent, given her true disease status).

Table 5. IARC vs UK audit

Months since last negative smear	Relative protection	
	IARC	**UK Audit**
0-11	15	8
12-35	10	5
36-47	5	1.7
48-65	3	1.6
65+/Never	1	1

3   NEW METHODS FOR CERVICAL SCREENING

The achievement of cervical screening by Pap smears in reducing mortality is unprecedented in cancer control. This is particularly clear in the UK and in parts of Scandinavia where well-organized national programmes have produced striking benefits with drops in mortality of 50-70%.

However, it is not clear how much further UK rates will decrease, and evidence from an audit suggests that they may be nearing the limit of what is achievable by this technology. In particular, in this audit 47% of 205 invasive cancers in women age 70 are now occurring in women who appear to have an adequate and negative screening history (Sasieni et al.,1996). The reasons for this are now becoming clear. Despite the demonstrated ability of cervical cytological screening in reducing cervical cancer mortality, the conventional smear test is less sensitive than it was previously believed to be. Also, cytological screening is not very effective for adenocarcinoma, which is rapidly accounting for a larger fraction of cancers (Sasieni and Adams, 2001). The tediousness of the job of the cyto-screener must also be acknowledged, and the regularity with which scandals appear in the popular press highlights all of these weaknesses.

An ideal screening test should be performed infrequently and be capable of detecting high-grade precursor lesions or early micro-invasive cancers with great accuracy; that is, it should have very high sensitivity.

We define sensitivity as the proportion of truly diseased persons in the screened population who are identified by the screening test. In other words, sensitivity assesses the propensity of a test to avoid false-negative results (i.e., giving a negative result when disease is actually present in the women). Cervical screening aims to detect and treat disease before it becomes invasive cancer, and it is conventional to expect a perfect test to detect all high grade CIN (CIN2/3 or HSIL). False-negative results can arise in a variety of ways:

- when there are no abnormal cells on the specimen because of failure in collecting cells from lesions or transferring such cells to the slide

- when there are abnormal cells present in the sample that have not been detected or have been misinterpreted in the laboratory

- when the disease is rapidly progressing and the lesion itself was not present at the time of sampling. This situation is considered to be quite uncommon, except possibly in very young women.

Conversely, specificity refers to the ability of a test to correctly identify women without disease and is defined as the proportion of women without disease who are found to have a negative test. This is very closely approximated by 100% minus the false positive rate, which is the proportion of women with a positive test who turn out not to have disease after faulty investigations.

Screening studies unaffected by work-up bias have provided estimates of the sensitivity of conventional smear screening ranging from 30% to 87% (mean 47%) and specificity ranging from 86% to 100% (mean 95%) (Nanda et al., 2000). The smear test is more sensitive when a higher threshold of disease is used. In studies where other tests have also been employed to refer women with negative smears for colposcopy, sensitivities for cytology of 50-80% for high grade (CIN) have been reported (see Table 11).

A range of different approaches are currently under investigation for improving the sensitivity of the basic screening test.

3.1   Liquid-based cytology

Liquid-based cytology for cervical screening aims to improve the quality of the conventional cervical smear through an improved sample collection and slide preparation technique. This is designed to produce a more representative sample of the specimen, with reduced obscuring background material.

The liquid-based cytology technique involves transferring material collected on a plastic 'broom' device into a liquid preservative medium by agitation. A cell suspension is formed that is used to deposit a monolayer of cells on the slide. Almost all of the cells collected from the cervix are transferred to the fluid. The subsequent stage of the procedure results in a sample of cells being deposited on the glass slide, which is smaller, but more representative than is obtained in a conventional smear. Cellular preservation is also enhanced, the preparation is more of a monolayer, and contamination (blood cells, pus and mucus) is reduced. Moreover, improved fixation allows more consistent staining. Most evaluations have been conducted on one of two commercially available products (Thin Prep, Cytyc Corp or Autocyte Prep, Tripath Corp), but several other approaches are also now available and more are being developed. As a result, these preparation techniques reduce the proportion of specimens classified as technically unsatisfactory for evaluation. A further advantage is that the unused portion of the cell suspension in preservative can be retained and used for additional testing for HPV, chlamydia, and other molecular markers, as required.

3.2   Comparisons of liquid-based and conventional cytology

Two main types of study have been used to evaluate liquid-based cytology. Both are based on the cytological detection rate of abnormalities. There is little information regarding the histological abnormality rate and none on the impact on invasive cancer rates or mortality. Any attempt to determine the effect of liquid-based cervical cytology on these outcome measures can currently only be arrived at by modelling studies with all their attendant assumptions and subsequent uncertainties about the conclusions.

3.2.1 Split-sample studies

The most frequent study design employed a split-sample method. For these studies a conventional smear is first produced. Then the remaining cells on the spatula are deposited in the liquid collection medium. In some cases a further sample is also obtained and agitated into the liquid. Thus two specimens are produced for each patient screened – a conventional smear and a liquid-based preparation. These can be directly compared at each screening exam. The main outcome comparison in most of these studies is a diagnosis of LSIL or higher. This outcome threshold avoids the lack of reproducibility and time-dependent positivity rate of ASCUS smears, but still has enough positive results to provide a powerful comparison. Use of HSIL is more informative, especially as histology is usually not studied, but this was not always available.

Table 6 summarizes these results. Overall, the liquid-based method seems to result in more slides being classified as LSIL+ which were classified as a lower diagnosis (e.g., negative or ASCUS) by conventional smears than the reverse situation. These studies are of variable size and of variable quality (e.g., in the blinding of cytologists to the results from the other specimen obtained) and cannot all be given equal weight in evaluation. It is important also to note that there is a considerable variation between studies in respect of the prevalence of significant abnormality and hence the type of population that was studied. This is apparent from the last column of Table 6 where positivity of rates by both methods varied from 1% to over 50%.

Table 6. ThinPrep split-sample studies using either ThinPrep or Autocyte Prep (Payne et al., 2000)

Study/country	No. of samples/women	Conv>Liq LSIL+	Liq>Conv LSIL+	Both LSIL+
Hutchison et al., 1991 USA	443	0.45%	1.13%	18.7%
Hutchison et al., 1991 USA	2655	0.68%	2.64%	12.3%
Awen et al., 1995 USA	1000	0.0%	0.5%	1.3%
Laverty et al., 1995 Australia	1872	2.4%	3.3%	7.5%
Wilbur et al., 1994 USA	3218	0.8%	3.1%	17.0%
Aponte-Cipriani et al., 1995 USA	665	0.5%	0.8%	3.0%
Sheets, 1995 USA	782	1.5%	3.3%	29.4%
Tezuka et al., 1996 Japan	215	2.3%	0.0%	54.4%
Ferenczy et al., 1996 Canada/USA	364	7.7%	8.8%	33.5%
Wilbur et al., 1996 USA	259	3.1%	1.9%	13.5%
Lee et al., 1997 USA	6747	1.9%	3.3%	6.1%
Roberts et al., 1997 Australia	35,560	0.3%	0.5%	1.7%
Corkill et al., 1998 USA	1583	0.8%	3.7%	1.9%
Hutchison et al., 1999 Costa Rica	8636	2.5%	2.8%	2.4%
Bur et al., 1995 USA	128	1.6%	1.6%	19.5%
Vassilakos et al., 1996 Switzerland	560	0.5%	1.3%	3.2%
Takahashi & Naito, 1997 Japan	2000	0.4%	0.3%	3.2%

Table 6. ThinPrep split-sample studies using either ThinPrep or Autocyte Prep., *continued*

Study/country	No.of samples/women	Conv>Liq LSIL+	Liq>Conv LSIL+	Both LSIL+
Howell et al., 1998 USA	852	0.8%	1.1%	2.5%
Geyer et al., 1993 USA	551	0.0%	0.7%	12.5%
Sprenger et al., 1996 Germany	2863	2.0%	5.1%	36.2%
Bishop, 1997 USA	2032	1.1%	6.1%	2.9%
Laverty et al., 1997 Australia	2064	3.9%	1.6%	5.0%
Wilbur et al., 1997 USA	277	1.1%	6.1%	2.9%
Data on file, CellPath, 1997	8983	1.6%	2.15	5.7%
Stevens et al., 1998 Australia	1325	1.3%	0.2%	3.9%
McGoogan & Reith, 1996 Scotland	3091	1.0%	0.3%	3.6%

A review of split-sample studies has been carried out by Austin and Ramzy (1998). These authors used the LSIL+ detection as a summary measure and concluded that the liquid-based methods showed overall increased detection of epithelial cell abnormalities. Results varied considerably from study to study and appeared to be influenced by the type of collection device used. Newer liquid-based preparatory methodologies using plastic 'broom' brushes appear to be associated with enhanced detection.

3.2.2   Two-cohort studies

The next type of study commonly used is a two-cohort analysis. This examines two groups of women, usually from two different time periods, whose cervical cytology specimens have been examined by one or the other (but not both) of the slide preparation techniques. Again, the outcome measure most often used is the proportion of specimens classified as LSIL or higher. A basic assumption is that the women in the two cohorts come from the same underlying population, with similar levels of cervical cancer and pre-cancerous changes. Once again, of the studies identified, an increase in classification of specimens as LSIL+ was found with liquid-based methods. Studies in this category are shown in Table 7. Not all the studies in this table provide full details of the proportions of specimens graded as HSIL+, but the two largest studies do. Vassilakos et al. (1997) found that this increased from 0.38% to 0.68% with the use of the AutoCyte liquid-based cytology method, and Diaz-Rosario and Kabawat (1999) found a similar increase from 0.27% to 0.53% using ThinPrep. Both of these two large studies also found a decrease in specimens graded as ASCUS.

Table 7. Two-cohort studies (Payne et al., 2000)

Study Year Country	Method	Number conventional smear	Number liquid-based	Conventional smears LSIL+	Liquid-based LSIL+
Vassilakos et al., 1999 Switzerland & France	AutoCyte	88,569	111,358	1.58%	2.52%
Vassilakos et al., 1998 Switzerland	CytoRich	15,402	32,655	1.10%	3.60%
Weintraub, 1997 Switzerland	ThinPrep	35,000	18,000	0.70%	2.27%
Bolick & Hellman, 1998 USA	ThinPrep	39,408	10,694	1.12%	2.92%
Dupree et al., 1998 USA	ThinPrep	22,323	19,351	1.19%	1.67%
Papillo et al., 1998 USA	ThinPrep	18,569	8,541	1.63%	2.48%
Carpenter & Davey, 1999 USA	ThinPrep	5000	2,727	7.70%	10.50%
Diaz-Rosario & Kabawat, 1999 USA	ThinPrep	74,573	56,095	1.85%	3.24%
Guidos & Selvaggi, 1999 USA	ThinPrep	5423	9,583	1.11%	3.70%

3.2.3   Other studies

A few studies have provided histologically confirmed CIN on all patients. None of these were screening studies (which is not feasible or ethical), but usually considered women with a known previous cytological abnormality who had been referred for colposcopy. The results are shown in Table 8. Sensitivities and especially specificities must be considered as relative, because of the type of population, but the results support an increase in sensitivity without an apparent loss of specificity.

Table 8. Summary of results of studies with histologic verification of disease
(Payne et al. 2000)

Study Year Population	Method	Smear sensitivity	Smear specificity	Liquid-based sensitivity	Liquid-based specificity	Definition of Positives and of Reference standard
Sheets et al., 1995 Colposcopy clinic Ref's, USA	Thin Prep	67.3% (107/159)	76.9% (220/286)	73.6% (117/159)	76.2% (218/286)	Colposcopic biopsy
Ferenczy et al.,1996 Colposcopy clinic Referrals, USA	Thin Prep	70.1% (n not stated)	74.7% (n not stated)	78.0% (n not stated)	73.6% (n not stated)	LSIL= based on histology in women referred for colposcopy.
Bishop et al., 1998 Mixed hospital and HMO-served populations, USA	Auto Cyte Prep	78.5% (73/93)	--	89.2% (83/93)	--	LSIL= based on positive Biopsy patients
Bollick & Hellman, 1998. Routine clinical Practice, USA	Thin Prep	85.1% (57/67)	36.4% (8/22)	95.2% (40/42)	58.3% (7/12)	LSIL= based on biopsy Results (part of a larger study)
Inhorn et al., 1998 Known cases of cervical cancer	Thin Prep	93.6% (44/47)	--	95.7% (45/47)	--	Invasive cervical cancer based on biopsy confirmation
Asfaq et al., 1999 Population with high glandular abnormality rates, USA	Thin Prep	68.7% (222/323)	--	87.9% (284/323)	--	Glandular lesions based on biopsy confirmation.
Hutchison et al., 1999 Population with high incidence of cervical cancer, Costa Rica.	Thin Prep	68.7% (222/323)	--	87.9% (284/323)	--	LSIL= based on a final diagnosis, which was made by a combination of cytology, histology and cervicography
Vassilakos et al., 2000 Random sample from large Swiss population	Auto Cyte Prep	88.6% (124/140)	--	91.0% (690/758)	--	HSIL + confirmed by histology after colposcopy, but includes only ASCUS+ smears so may overestimate sensitivity

4   HPV TESTING

The human papillomavirus (HPV) has now been clearly established as the primary cause of cervical cancer in nearly all cases (Walboomers et al., 1999). Thus, it should not be surprising that testing for HPV should have a role in measures aimed at control of this disease. The ultimate goal must be eradication of HPV by vaccination (Koutsky et al., 2002), but a more immediate prospect is to utilize the detection and monitoring of the virus as part of the screening and diagnostic process. Testing for HPV has 3 potential roles: triage of patients with atypical squamous cells of undetermined significance (ASCUS) and low-grade cervical smears; surveillance of high-grade cervical intraepithelial neoplasia and localised (micro) invasive disease after treatment; and as a primary screening test – either alone or in combination with cytology.

4.1   Triage of borderline smears

The most clearly established role for HPV testing is in the triage of women with borderline or low-grade cytological abnormalities (Table 9). Early studies established that HPV testing had discriminatory power in women with abnormal smears that was typically better than that obtained from a repeat smear (Cuzick et al., 1992; Cox et al., 1995; Schneider et al., 1996). Subsequent studies have focussed on this particular group and found a very high sensitivity and reasonable specificity for borderline (ASCUS) smears (Kjellberg et al., 1998; Manos et al., 1999; Nobbenhuis et al., 1999; Solomon et al., 2001). However, the ALTS study suggested that for LSIL (mild/moderate) smears the HPV positivity rate was too high and the specificity was too low to justify additional testing. In particular, 83% of such women were found to be positive for high-risk HPV types, so that few women could be spared immediate colposcopy on the basis of HPV negativity. These data have led the UK Health Technology Assessment panel to recommend a careful, controlled introduction of HPV testing for borderline or mildly dyskaryotic smears (Cuzick et al., 1999) and pilot studies are currently underway in 3 districts. A number of logistical issues are important here for determining a cost-effective implementation of this approach. If liquid-based cytology is used, then HPV testing can be done as required on the remaining material. However, liquid-based sampling is currently an expensive addition to cytology which itself has yet to prove its cost-effectiveness. The other options of routinely taking a second sample for HPV testing or recalling the 5-10% of women with low grade cytological abnormalities for a second test are not optimal either, and one would hope a cheap liquid-based approach will be developed which will cater both for the needs of HPV testing and cytology.

Table 9. HPV testing in women with abnormal cytology (selected studies)

Study	Population	n	CIN2/CIN3 on histology (%)	HPV test	Sensitivity	Positivity rate	PPV	NPV	Comments
Cuzick, 1992	Mild/ Moderate	55	23(41.8)	TS-HPV 16	65	29	94	79	HPV 16 alone gives good PPV, but poor sensitivity, viral load important
Nobbenhuis, 1999	Any dyskaroysis	353	133(37.7)	GP5+/6+	80% (+14% transient or acquired)	35 (persistent)	88	88	Study confirms importance of persistence for disease progression.
Cox, 1995	ASCUS	217	15(6.9)	HC-II	93	37	17	99.3	HPV better than repeat cytology, viral load important
Manos, 1999	ASCUS	973	65(6.7)	HC-II	89	39	15	98.8	
Solomon, 2001	ASCUS	2324	267(11.5)	HC-II	95	55	20	99.4	HPV effective for ASCUS but not LSIL.

4.2   Follow up after treatment of HSIL

HPV testing also offers scope for better follow-up of women who have been treated for CIN. Currently, these women receive annual smears for at least 5 years and often for the rest of their life. Several reports suggest that the persistence of HPV positivity after treatment is an accurate method of assessing treatment failures and could be used to safely return negative women to routine screening after one or two follow-ups at 6-24 months (Bollen et al., 1996; Elfgren et al., 1996) (Table 10). At the same time the persistence of HPV positivity after 12 months indicates treatment failure and the need for additional treatment.

4.3   Primary screening

Use as a primary screening test is where HPV testing offers the greatest promise, but also where the greatest uncertainties lie. Several studies have shown sensitivities of approximately 90% or greater for the second-generation Hybrid Capture test or consensus primer PCR tests, and comparative studies indicate a higher sensitivity than that achieved by cytology (Womack et al., 2000; Clavel et al., 1999; Schiffman et al., 2000; Ratnam et al., 2000) (Table 11). Specificity is now the major concern and false-positive rates of 5% to 20% have been reported. Sensitivity appears to be high regardless of age, but false-positive rates are higher in younger women suggesting that HPV is likely to be more cost-effective in older women. Persistence is a key attribute of infections related to high-grade disease. This can currently only be directly verified by repeated testing. Transient infections are much more common in younger women, and restricting HPV testing to women over age 30 (at least for primary screening) substantially reduces the false positive rate from about 15-20% to about 5% or less.

Table 10. Post treatment

Study	Population	Follow up	Residual/ Recurrent Disease (%)	HPV Test	HPV Pos (%) (recurrent)	HPV Pos (%) (non-recurrent)
Nuovo, 1992	85 CIN2+	4-60 mo	10 (12)	TS-PCR 16,18,31,33,35	7/10 (70%)	N/A
Elfgren, 1996	22 CIN2+	16-27 mo	4 (18)	GP 5/6	4/4	0/18
Bollen, 1996	40 CIN2+ 18 Abn. FU cyto	43 mo mean	6 (15)	CPI/II G	6/6	10/34 (30) 3/22 normal cyto
Chua, 1997	48 CIN3 (case-control)	3 mo FU smear	26 (54)	MY09/11 then GP5/6	24/26 (92)	0/22
Bollen, 1999	43 CIN2+ & Abn FU cyto	13-206 mo 48 mo mean	16 (37)	CPI/II G	16/16	15/27 (56)
Nagai, 2000	58 CIN3	12-72 mo 32 mo mean	5 (9)	Yoshikawa L1-consensus	5/5	6/53 (11)
Kjellberg, 2000	112 CIN	22-46 mo 36 mo mean	0	MY09/11 then GP5/6	-	3/112 (3)
Nobbenhuis, 2001	184 CIN 2+	24 mo	29 (16)	GP5+/6+	26/29(90) 6 mo 27/29(93) 24 mo	13/155 (8) 6 mo 2/155 (1) 24 mo
Lin, 2001	75 CIN3 with involved margins	6 wks	27 (36)	HC-II	27/27	25/48 (52)

Table 11. Screening studies using Hybrid Capture II (High Risk) with histologic CIN 2/3 outcome

Study	N	HPV Sensitivity	HPV Specificity	Cytology ≥ ASCUS Sensitivity	Cytology ≥ ASCUS Specificity
Schneider, 1996*	967	50.0	95.7	29.0	95.6
Cuzick, 1999	1703	95.2	95.1	85.7	95.7
Clavel, 1999	1518	100	85.2	85.3	94.9
Ratnam, 2000	2098	85.3	90.6	55.9	91.6
Wright, 2000	1415	83.9	82.6	67.9	85.6
Womack, 2000	2140	80.9	62.0	44.3	90.6
Schiffman, 2000	8554	88.4	89.0	77.7	94.2
Schneider, 1996*	967	50.0	95.7	29.0	95.6
Denny, 2000	2944	73.3	87.8	86.7	89.9
Clavel, 2001 (LBC)	7932	100	87.3	68.1 87.8	95.3 93.1
Petry, 2002	8466	97.8	95.3	43.5	98.0
Cuzick, 2002	10358	96.9	93.4	79.3	95.9
Kulasingam, 2002	4075	90.8	72.6	57.2	89.9

*First generation Hybrid Capture Tube test used.

One way to use HPV testing is as an adjunct to cytology to improve sensitivity. This is only viable in older women (above the age of 30 or 35), and even if done infrequently (every 5-10 years), could make an important contribution in dealing with the increasingly large proportion of women who develop cancer after apparently normal cytology smears (Sasieni et al., 1996). By detecting more abnormalities at each screen, it also could allow the screening interval to be safely extended to 5 years or longer in women who are both cytologically and HPV-negative. Studies of archival smears show that HPV is detectable many years before cancer (Walboomers et al., 1995; Wallin et al., 1999). Thus, screening failures are more often due to the failure to collect or identify the abnormal cells on the smears than to rapidly developing disease that develops *de novo* in less than 5 years.

A more radical approach is to employ HPV as the sole primary test, and then do cytology only on HPV-positive women to determine appropriate management. The very high sensitivity of HPV testing makes this a logical option, even for younger women. As the HPV test is automatable, the more tedious cytological review of smears could be focussed on the few women who are HPV-positive (typically 5% over the age of 35 and 15-20% in younger women). A key issue here is cost – high volume HPV testing needs to be no more expensive than cytology for this to be viable. A second issue is the appropriate management of HPV-positive but cytology negative women. A substantial fraction of the younger women (15%) will fall into this group, and at least for them, re-testing at one year, at which time most of the HPV infections will have disappeared, seems the most sensible option. Women with HPV DNA persisting for at least one year are likely to have a significant lesion and probably should be referred for colposcopy regardless of the cytological result. A possible algorithm for this approach is shown in Figure 3. Similar issues arise in women with borderline or mild lesions, which in many cases reflect HPV infections that are transient and will resolve spontaneously within one year.

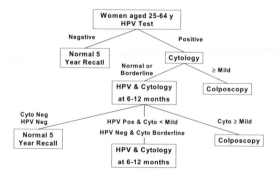

Figure 3: Proposed new screening algorithm.

When considering the most appropriate role for HPV testing, it must be recognised that this will be highly dependent on the existing screening infrastructure. For clinical settings in which an effective, well-organised, cytology-based program is in place, the issue is whether HPV testing adds to the existing program and questions of cost-effectiveness, quality control, and added value to current practice come to the fore. In contrast, for settings such as those commonly found in the developing world, where screening is non-existent or is ineffective because of poor-quality cytology or inherent limitations due to a high rate of inflammatory smears, the more basic questions of sensitivity, specificity, cost, and simplicity of testing procedures become paramount. Here it may make more sense to consider periodic HPV testing, possibly coupled with visual inspection, rather than to try to make cytology work.

4.4 Self sampling

HPV testing also has the potential for being performed on a self-collected sample taken at home. To date, most studies have shown that these samples are not as good as physician or nurse taken samples, but they are still at least as sensitive as routine cytological smears (Wright et al., 2000.) However, better collection devices may provide samples on which the sensitivity of HPV testing is as good as that on samples obtained by medical personnel (Sellors et al., 2000). An accurate self-sampled HPV test could have enormous implications. For developing countries, it is not clear if this would offer an advantage over the use of a trained nurse who performs visual inspection and HPV testing in the community. In areas where organised screening is in place, self-sampling offers an additional approach for reaching women who refuse to have conventional screening. It may also have a role in surveillance or the monitoring after the treatment of HPV-positive cytology-negative women, in which follow-up testing at short intervals is needed. A clear priority is to determine the reasons for lower sensitivity (such as use of a vaginal swab) and to find ways to make a self-sampled test as good as a test performed by a clinician.

4.5 Conclusion

The discovery of the central role of HPV in cervical carcinogenesis is just beginning to lead to its use in controlling the disease. Initial results show great promise, but more studies are urgently needed to fully define its role in primary screening. A full evaluation of HPV testing should provide information on the length of protection of a negative result and ideally demonstrate a reduction in cancer incidence. This is likely to require a study (or studies) involving several hundred thousand women and a cluster randomised pilot programme would seem to be the most appropriate way of achieving this.

5   VISUAL INSPECTION

5.1   Background

Unfortunately, screening programmes using cytology are only viable in the developed world where a substantial medical infrastructure exists. Most cancers are now occurring in the developing world, and attempts to introduce cytology screening there have mostly failed. There are a number of reasons for this. It is clear that cervical screening only saves lives where a good infrastructure exists with the ability to take good smears, read them accurately, get patients back for treatment, and provide high quality treatment and follow-up. In addition, there are more intrinsic issues related to the amount of genital infections in this population. This is illustrated by some data from Recife, Brazil (Table 12) in which the majority of smears are found to be 'inflammatory' and CIN rates are not dissimilar from those in Europe or North America, despite the fact that this region has one of the highest cervix cancer incidence rates in the world. The problem is that most of the disease is masked by the inflammation and when viewed colposcopically many of these women have cancer or high-grade lesions. One simpler approach that does not require as much infrastructure or expertise is direct visual inspection of the cervix. The naked-eye visualisation of the cervix after application of 3-5% acetic acid is termed visual inspection with acetic acid (VIA), direct visual inspection (DVI), acetic acid test (AAT), visual inspection of the cervix (VIA) or sometimes cervicoscopy. VIA has been investigated as a low-cost alternative to cytological screening programmes. VIA with or without magnification has shown similar or better sensitivity than cytology in detecting pre-cancerous lesions. VIA may become part of screening programmes in countries where cytology has not been successfully implemented yet.

5.2   Studies

The first report indicating that a cervix at risk can be identified by recognising acetowhite areas with the naked eye was that of Ottaviano and La Torre (1982) in Florence, Italy. It was not a screening study but one to evaluate the need of using a colposcope when examining the cervix. The cervices of 2,400 patients with normal or abnormal cervical cytology were examined by VIA and colposcopy. An atypical transformation zone (ATZ)

Table 12. Cervical screening results Recife, Brazil 1991

Diagnosis	Negative	Inflammatory	CIN I	CIN II	CIN III	CIS	Cancer	Inadequate	Total
Total	12347	44961	1978	760	497	281	233	2318	63315
%	19.5	71	3.1	1.2	0.8	0.4	0.4	3	100

was found in 312 women with colposcopy, and 307 (98.4%) women with VIA. VIA and colposcopy detected all confirmed cervical lesions (143) and misclassified 169 benign lesions. Based on the high percentage of agreement between both visual exams, the authors concluded that colposcopic magnification was not essential in clinical practice to identify a cervix at risk, but only to decide what treatment is required.

Many studies to evaluate the performance of VIA as a cervical screening method have followed (Table 13). They differed greatly in population (number, age-group and reason to attend, screening history) and methodology: VIA characteristics (performers and their training, classification and report of results), other screening tests used (cytology, cervicography, HPV DNA), positivity definition of tests and choice of gold standard.

In most studies, VIA showed a higher sensitivity but a lower specificity than cytology for detecting confirmed high-grade lesions (HSIL) (Cecchini et al., 1993; Frisch et al., 1994; Sankaranarayanan et al., 1998; Anonymous, 1999; Denny et al., 2000). Slawson et al. (1992) reported that VIA improved the detection of cervical disease by 30%. But, this was the case when histological abnormalities included condylomas as well as squamous intraepithelial lesions (SIL). Instead, when only HSIL or worse lesions were considered positive VIA sensitivity was 29%, the lowest of all studies.

In the second phase of the JHPIEGO/University of Zimbabwe study (Anonymous, 1999), where 98% of 2,203 women underwent colposcopy, VIA sensitivity and specificity were 77% (95% CI:70-82) and 64% (95% CI: 62-66) to detect HSIL, as compared with 44% (95% CI: 37-51) and 91% (95% CI:89-92) for cytology (considered positive if LSIL or worse lesions). In 2001, Belinson et al. (2001) carried out a study in the Shanxi Province of rural China, where all 1,997 women aged 35 to 45 underwent colposcopy with biopsy/curettage. VIA was performed by gynaecologic oncologists as compared with nurses, midwifes, or health workers being the providers in other studies. They estimated a sensitivity of 71% (95% CI: 60-80) and a specificity of 74% (95% CI:72-76) of VIA to detect HSIL lesions, as compared to Thin Prep cytology, sensitivity of 87% (95% CI:78-93) and specificity of 94% (95% CI:92-95). VIA failed to identify one of three cancers in the group. One possible explanation for the low performance of VIA is a high prevalence of acute cervicitis making VIA difficult to perform.

5.3   Conclusion

The universal disadvantage of VIA is its low specificity, which increases the number of women called for further evaluation, and hence the cost of a screening programme especially in low-income countries. Different approaches have been suggested to overcome the low specificity of VIA. One of them is to use two-stage screening in which only those women positive in a high sensitivity-low specificity test are screened by a more specific second test such as cytology or even HPV. This approach will

Table 13. Results of visual inspection after acetic acid (VIA) studies

Authors	Number screened	% with HSIL	% VIA pos in HSIL pos	% VIA pos in LSIL pos	% VIA pos in <LSIL	% VIA pos in <HSIL	Women with colposcopy No.(%)	Screening tests/exams used for referral
Ottaviano & La Torre Italy,1982	2,400	2.6	100.0			10.5	2,400 (100)	All women underwent colposcopy
Cecchini et al., Italy,1993	2,105	0.4	87.5			16.5	486 (23)	VIA, cytology>=ASCUS or cervicography
Slawson et al., USA,1992	2,753	1.1	29.0	37.7	2.2	2.9	221 (8)	VIA or cytology>=ASCUS
Frisch et al., USA,1994	95	4.2	100.0	92.3	70.5	73.6	52 (55)	VIA, cytology>=ASCUS or Cervicography
Megevand et al., South Africa,1996	2,426	1.3	64.5	13.8	1.0	2.3	330 (14)	VIA or cytology>=LSIL
Chirenje et al., Zimbabwe,1999	1,000	3.8	68.4			23.3	213 (21)	VIA or cytology>=HSIL
JHPIEGO Zimbabwe,1999	**Phase I** 8,731	4.7	65.5			17.9	1,584 (18)	VIA or cytology>=LSIL and a 10% of those with VIA negative or atypical
	Phase II 2,203	9.5	76.7	54.1	32.7	35.9	2,147 (98)	All women referred to colposcopy
Denny et al., South Africa,2000	2,944	2.9	67.4	49.5	18.3	16.7	760 (26)	VIA, cytology>=LSIL, HPV DNA (viral load>10 pg/mL) or cervigrams "warranting colposcopy" or >=LSIL
Belinson et al., China,2001	1,997	4.3	70.9	44.1	24.4	25.7	1997 (100)	All women referred to colposcopy
Cronje et al., South Africa,2001	6,301	2.6		49.4	16.0		1,747 (28)	VIA, cytology>=LSIL, cervigrams "warranting colposcopy" or >=LSIL
Denny et al., South Africa,2002	VIA ² 2,754	4.2	72.6	57.8	20.7	22.2	1,156 (42)	VIA, cytology>=LSIL, HPV DNA (viral load>1pg/mL) or cervigrams "warranting colposcopy" or >=LSIL
	VIA ³ 2,754	4.2	76.1	59.8	23.4	24.8		
Rodriguez-Reyes et al., Mexico, 2002	376	13.6	92.2	100	40.3	41.2	376 (100)	All women underwent colposcopy

1: HSIL not including CIN II or moderate dysplasia.
2: VIA without magnification. 3: VIA with magnification (Aviscope™).

increase specificity at the cost of some sensitivity reduction. Another approach is the "screen and treat", in which those women with positive VIA will be treated immediately using simple, cheap, low-complication treatment methods such as cryotherapy. There are several studies ongoing in order to evaluate the efficacy of combined cervical screening tests, and screen and treat approaches in Asia, Africa and Latin America. The results of these studies should be available in the next few years.

6   OTHER METHODS

Several other approaches to screening have been developed over the years. One long-standing area is automated or computer-assisted cytology. Early promise has not led to widespread adoption (Banda-Gamboa et al., 1992; Koss et al., 1992), but the use of liquid-based thin-layer cytology has encouraged a re-evaluation, as the near mono-layer produced for the slides may be more amenable to computerised evaluation. Several systems are currently available or under test (Lee et al., 1998).

A more recent development is the use of antibodies against cell-cycle markers as a screening test. One group is developing tests based on the cell proliferation markers Cdc 5 and Mcm2 and has reported encouraging early results (Williams et al., 1998), while another group is developing a test based on p16^{INK4A} (Klaes et al., 2001). Results for biopsy specimens look promising, but further development is needed for an assay useable on cytologic preparations. These tests appear to be highly specific and may be useful second stage tests following, for example, HPV testing.

Further methods involve electrical and light scattering probes (Coppleson et al., 1994) and infrared spectroscopy (Wong et al., 1991). All other methods are at an early stage of development and further work is planned to see if any can be of value as screening tests.

CONCLUSION

Screening for precursors to cervix cancer has been one of the great success stories in cancer prevention. Well-organized programmes have cut mortality by 50-80% in several countries. However the requirements for a successful programme are not really achievable in much of the developing world, where the cervical cancer problem remains acute. The Pap smear was first described in 1928 (Papanicolaou, 1928) and much has been learned about the natural history of cervix cancer since then. Foremost is the discovery of the causal link with high risk types of the human papillomavirus. This may eventually lead to the eradication of cervix cancer by universal vaccination. This is some decades away, however, and the imperative now is to use this knowledge to integrate HPV testing with improved cytology, new molecular markers, and, for the developing countries, simple visual inspection-based regimes, to reduce the cancer burden worldwide in a feasible and cost-effective manner.

REFERENCES

Andersson-Ellstrom A, Seidal T, Grannas M, et al. The pap-smear history of women with invasive cervical squamous carcinoma. A case-control study from Sweden. Acta Obstet Gynecol Scand 2000;79:221-6.

Anonymous. Visual inspection with acetic acid for cervical-cancer screening: test qualities in a primary-care setting. University of Zimbabwe/JHPIEGO Cervical Cancer Project. Lancet 1999;353:869-73.

Aponte-Cipriani S, Teplitz C, Rorat E, et al. Cervical smears prepared by an automated device versus the conventional method. A comparative analysis. Acta Cytol 1995;39:623-30.

Aristizabal N, Cuello C, Correa P, et al. The impact of vaginal cytology on cervical cancer risks in Cali, Colombia. Int J Cancer 1984;34:5-9.

Ashfaq R, Gibbons D, Vela C, et al. ThinPrep Pap test. Accuracy for glandular disease. Acta Cytol 1999;43:81-5.

Austin R, Ramzy I. Increased detection of epithelial cell abnormalities by liquid-based gynecologic cytology preparations. A review of accumulated data. Acta Cytol 1998; 42:178-84.

Awen C, Hathway S, Eddy W, et al. Efficacy of ThinPrep preparartion of cervical smears: a 1,000-case, investigator-sponsored study. Diagn Cytopathol 1994;11:33-6.

Banda-Gamboa H, Ricketts I, Cairns A, et al. Automation in cervical cytology: an overview. Anal Cell Pathol 1992; 4:25-48.

Belinson J, Qiao YL, Pretorius R, et al. Shanxi province cervical cancer screening study: a cross-sectional comparative trial of multiple techniques to detect cervical neoplasia. Gynecol Oncol 2001;83:439-44.

Beral V. Cancer of the Cervix: a sexually transmitted infection? Lancet 1974; 1:1037-40.

Berrino F, Gatta G, d'Alto M, et al. Efficacy of screening in preventing invasive cervical cancer: a case-control study in Milan, Italy. IARC Sci Publ 1986:111-23.

Bishop J. Comparison of the CytoRich system with conventional cervical cytology. Preliminary data on 2,032 cases from a clinical trial site. Acta Cytol 1997;41:15-23.

Bishop J, Bigner S, Colgan TJ, et al. Multicenter masked evaluation of AutoCyte PREP thin layers with matched conventional smears. Including intitial biopsy results. Acta Cytol 1998;42:189-97.

Bolick D, Hellman DJ. Laboratory implementation and efficacy assessment of the ThinPrep cervical cancer screening system. Acta Cytol 1998;42:209-13.

Bollen LJM, Tjong-A-Hung SP, van der Velden J, et al. Human papillomavirus DNA after treatment of cervical dysplasia: Low prevalence in normal cytologic smears. Cancer 1996; 77: 2538-43.

Bollen LJM, Tjong-A-Hung SP, van der Velden J, et al. Prediction of recurrent and residual cervical dysplasia by human papillomavirus detection among patients with abnormal cytology. Gynecol Oncol 1999;72:199-201.

Bur M, Knowles K, Pekow P, et al. Comparison of ThinPrep preparations with conventional cervicovaginal smears. Practical considerations. Acta Cytol 1995;39:631-42.

Carpenter A, Davey DD. ThinPrep Pap test: performance and biopsy follow-up in a university hospital. Cancer 1999;87:105-12.

Cecchini S, Bonardi R, Mazzotta A, et al. Testing cervicography and cervioscopy as screening tests for cervical cancer. Tumori 1993;79:22-5.

Chirenje ZM, Chipato T, Kasule J, et al. Visual inspection of the cervix as a primary means of cervical cancer screening: results of a pilot study [published erratum appears in Cent Afr J Med 1999 Mar;45(3):79]. Cent Afr J Med 1999;45:30-3.

Choi NW, Nelson NA. Results from a cervical cancer screening programme in Manitoba, Canada. IARC Sci Publ 1986:61-7.

Chua K.-L, Hjerpe A. Human papillomavirus analysis as a prognostic marker following conization of the cervix uteri. Gynecol Oncol 1997;66:108-113.

Clarke EA, Hilditch S, Anderson TW. Optimal frequency of screening for cervical cancer: a Toronto case-control study. IARC Sci Publ 1986:125-31.

Clavel C, Masure M, Bory J-P, et al. Hybrid Capture II-based human papillomavirus detection, a sensitive test to detect in routine high-grade cervical lesions: a preliminary study on 1518 women. Br J Cancer 1999; 80: 1306-11.

Clavel C, Masure M, Bory J-P, et al. Human papillomavirus testing in primary screening for the detection of high-grade cervical lesions: a study of 7932 women. Br J Cancer 2001;89:1616-23.

Cohen MM. Using administrative data for case-control studies: the case of the Papanicolaou smear. Ann Epidemiol 1993;3:93-8.

Coppleson M, Reid B, Sklanev V, et al. An electronic approach to the detection of pre-cancer and cancer of the uterine cervix: a preliminary evaluation of Polarprobe. Int J Gynecol Cancer 1994. 4;79-83.

Corkill M, Knapp D, Hutchison ML. Improved accuracy for the cervical cytology with the ThinPrep method and the endocervical brush-spatula collection procedure. J Lower Genital Tract Dis 1998;2:12-16.

Cox JT, Lorincz AT, Schiffman MH, et al. Human papillomavirus testing by hybrid capture appears to be useful in triaging women with a cytologic diagnosis of atypical squamous cells of undetermined significance. Am J Obstet Gynecol 1995; 172: 946-54.

Cox JT. Clinical role of HPV DNA testing. In: Lorincz AT, Reid R, (eds.) Obstetrics and Gynecology Clinics of North America: Human Papillomavirus II. 2nd ed. Philadelphia; WB Saunders, 1996.

Cronje HS, Cooreman BF, Beyer E, et al. Screening for cervical neoplasia in a developing country utilizing cytology, cervicography and the acetic acid test. Int J Gynaecol Obstet 2001; 72:151-7.

Cuzick J, Terry G, Ho L, et al. Human papillomavirus type 16 DNA in cervical smears as predictor of high-grade cervical intraepithelial neoplasia. Lancet 1992; 339: 959-60.

Cuzick J, Szarewski A, Terry G, et al. Human papillomavirus testing in primary cervical screening. Lancet 1995; 345:1533-7.

Cuzick J, Sasieni P, Davies P, et al. A systematic review of the role of human papillomavirus testing within a cervical screening programme. Health Technology Assessment 1999; 3: No. 14.

Cuzick J. Time to consider HPV testing in cervical screening. Ann Oncol 2001;12:1511-4.

Cuzick J. Role of HPV testing in clinical practice. Virus Research 2002;89:263-9.

Cuzick J. Management of HPV positive, cytology negative/borderline women – Results from the HART study. To be published, 2003.

Denny L, Kuhn L, Pollack A, et al. Evaluation of alternative methods of cervical screening for resource-poor settings. Cancer 2000;89:826-33.

Denny L, Kuhn L, Pollack A, et al. Direct visual inspection for cervical cancer screening: an analysis of factors influencing test performance. Cancer 2002;94:1699-707.

Diaz-Rosario LA, Kabawat SE. Performance of a fluid-based, thin layer Papanicolaou smear method in the clinical setting of an independent laboratory and an outpatient screening population in New England. Arch Pathol Lab Med 1999;123:817-21.

Dupree WB, Suprun HZ, Beckwith D, et al. The promise of a new technology. The Leigh Valley Hospital's experience with liquid-based cytology. Cancer 1998;84:202-7.

Elfgren K, Bistoletti P, Dillner L, et al. Conization for cervical intraepithelial neoplsia is followed by disappearance of human papillomavirus deoxyribonucleic acid and a decline in serum and cervical mucus antibodies against human papillomavirus antigens. Am J Obstet Gynecol 1996; 174: 937-42.

Ferenczy A, Franco E, Arseneau J, et al. Diagnostic performance of Hybrid Capture human papillomavirus deoxyribonucleic acid assay combined with liquid-based cytologic study. Am J Obstet Gynecol 1996;175:651-6.

Ferenczy A, Robitaille J, Franco E, et al. Conventional cervical cytologic smears vs. ThinPrep smears. A paired comparison study on cervical cytology. Acta Cytol 1996;40:1136-42.

Frisch LE, Milner FH, Ferris DG. Naked-eye inspection of the cervix after acetic acid application may improve the predictive value of negative cytologic screening. J Fam Prac 1994;39:457-60.

Geirsson G, Kristiansdottir R, Sigurdsson K, et al. Cervical cancer screening in Iceland: a case-control study. IARC Sci Publ 1986:37-41.

Geyer JW, Hancock F, Carrico C, et al. Preliminary evaluation of Cyto-Rich: an improved automated cytology preparation. Diagn Cytopathol 1993;9:417-22.

Guidos BJ, Selvaggi SM. Use of the ThinPrep Pap Test in clinical practice. Diagn Cytopathol 1999; 20:70-3.

Herbert A, Stein K, Bryant TN, et al. Relation between the incidence of invasive cervical cancer and the screening interval: is a five year interval too long? J Med Screen 1996;3:140-5.

Hernandez-Avila M, Lazcano-Ponce EC, de Ruiz PA, Romieu I. Evaluation of the cervical cancer screening programme in Mexico: a population-based case-control study. Int J Epidemiol 1998; 27:370-6.

Herrero R, Brinton LA, Reeves WC, et al. Screening for cervical cancer in Latin America: a case-control study. Int J Epidemiol 1992;21:1050-6.

Howell LP, Davis RL, Belk T, et al. The AutoCyte preparation system for gynecologic cytology. Acta Cytol 1998;42:171-7.

Hutchison ML, Cassin C, Ball H. The efficacy of an automated preparation device for cervical cytology. Am J Clin. Pathol 1991;96:300-5.

Hutchison ML, Agarwal P, Denault T, et al. A new look at cervical cytology. ThinPrep multicenter trial results. Acta Cytol 1992;36:499-504.

Hutchison ML, Zahniser DJ, Sherman ME, et al. Utility of liquid-based cytology for cervical carcinoma screening: results of a population-based study conducted in a region of Costa Rica with a high incidence of cervical carcinoma. Cancer 1999;87:48-55

IARC Working Group on evaluation of cervical cancer screening programmes. Screening for squamous cervical cancer: duration of low risk after negative results of cervical cytology and its implications for screening policies. Br Med J 1986; 293:659-64.

Inhorn SL, Wilbur D, Zahniser D, et al. Validation of the ThinPrep Papanicolaou test for cervical cancer diagnosis. J Lower Genital Tract Dis 1998;2:208-12.

Jiminez-Perez M, Thomas DB. Has the use of pap smears reduced the risk of invasive cervical cancer in Guadalajara, Mexico? Int J Cancer 1999;82:804-9.

Kinney WK, Miller M, Sung H, et al. Risk of invasive squamous carcinoma of the cervix associated with screening intervals of 1,2, and 3 years: a case-control study. Obstet Gynecol 2001;97:S3.

Kjellberg L, Wiklund F, Sjoberg I, et al. A population-based study of human papillomavirus deoxybribonucleic acid testing for predicting cervical intraepithelial neoplasia. Am J Obstet Gynecol 1998; 179: 497-502.

Kjellberg L, Wadell G, Bergman F, et al. Regular disappearance of the human papillomavirus genome after conization of cervical dysplasia by carbon dioxide laser. Am J Obstet Gynecol 2000;183:1238-42.

Klaes R, Friedrich T, Spitkovsky D, et al. Over expression of p16^{INK4A} as a specific marker for Dysplastic and Neoplastic Epithelial cells of the cervix uteri. Int J Cancer 2001; 92:276-84.

Klassen AC, Celentano DD, Brookmeyer R. Variation in the duration of protection given by screening using the Pap test for cervical cancer. J Clin Epidemiol 1989;42:1003-11.

Koss LG, ed. Diagnostic Cytology and Its Histopathologic Bases. 4th ed. Philadelphia, Pa: JB Lippincott Co. 1992.

Koutsky LA, Ault KA, Wheeler CM, Brown DR, Barr E, Alvarez FB, Chiacchierini LM, Jansen KU. A controlled trial of a human papillomavirus type 16 vaccine. N Engl J Med. 2002; 347:1703-5.

Kulasingam SL, Hughes JP, Kiviat NB, Mao C, Weiss NS, Kuypers JM, Koutsky LA. Evaluation of Human Papillomavirus Testing in Primary Screening for Cervical Abnormalities. Comparison of Sensitivity, Specificity, and Frequency of Referral. JAMA 2002; 288:1749-57.

La Vecchia C, Franceschi S, Decarli A, Fasoli M, Gentile A, Tognoni G. "Pap" smear and the risk of cervical neoplasia: quantitative estimates from a case-control study. Lancet 1984;2:779-82.

Laverty CR, Thurloe JK, Redman NL, et al. An Australian trial of ThinPrep: a new cytopreparatory technique. Cytopathol 1995;6:140-8.

Laverty CR, Farnsworth A, Thurloe JK, et al. Evaluation of the CytoRich slide preparation process. Anal Quant Cytol Histol 1997;19:239-45.

Lee KR, Ashfaq R, Birdsong G, et al. Comparison of conventional Papanicolaou smears and a fluid-based, thin-layer system for cervical cancer screening. Obstet Gynecol 1997;90:278-84.

Lee JSJ, Kuan L, Oh S, et al. A Feasibility Study of the AutoPap System Location-Guided Screening. Acta Cytologica 1998;42:221-5.

Lin C-T, Tseng C-J, Lai C-H, et al. Value of human papillomavirus deoxyribonucleic acid testing after conization in the prediction of residual disease in the subsequent hysterectomy specimen. Am J Obstet Gynecol 2001;184:940-5.

Londhe M, George SS, Seshadri L. Detection of CIN by naked eye visualization after application of acetic acid. Indian J Cancer 1997;34:88-91.

Lynge E, Poll P. Risk of cervical cancer following negative smears in Maribo County, Denmark, 1996-1982. IARC Sci Publ 1986,69-86.

Macgregor JE, Moss S, Parkin DM, Day NE. Cervical cancer screening in north-east Scotland. IARC Sci Publ 1986:25-36.

Macgregor JE, Campbell MK, Mann EM, et al. Screening for cervical intraepithelial neoplasia in north east Scotland shows fall in incidence and mortality from invasive cancer with concomitant rise in preinvasive disease. Brit Med J 1994;308:1407-11.

Magnus K, Langmark F. Cytological mass screening in Ostfold County, Norway. IARC Sci Publ 1986:87-90.

Makino H, Sato S,Yajima A, et al. Evaluation of the effectiveness of cervical cancer screening: a case-control study in Miyagi, Japan. Tohoku J Exp Med 1995;175:171-8.

Manos MM, Kinney WK, Hurley LB, et al. Identifying women with cervical neoplasia: using human papillomavirus DNA testing for equivocal Papanicolaou results. JAMA 1999; 281:1605-10.

Martin-Hirsch P, Lilford R, Jarvis G, et al. Efficacy of cervical-smear collection devices: a systematic review and meta-analysis. Lancet 1999; 354:1763-70.

McGoogan E, Reith A. Would monolayers provide more representative samples and improved preparations for cervical screening? Overview and evaluation of systems available. Acta Cytol 1996;40:107-19.

Megevand E, Denny L, Dehaeck K, et al. Acetic acid visualization of the cervix: an alternative to cytologic screening. Obstet Gynecol 1996;88:383-6.

Mitchell HS, Giles GG. Cancer diagnosis after a report of negative cervical cytology. Med J Aust 1996;164:270-3.

Nagai Y, Maehama T, Asato T, et al. Persistence of human papillomavirus infection after therapeutic conization for CIN 3: is it alarm for disease recurrence? Gynecol Oncol 2000; 79: 294-9.

Nanda K, McCrory DC, Myers ER, et al. Accuracy of the Papanicolaou test in screening for and follow-up of cervical cytologic abnormalities: a systematic review. Ann Intern Med 2000; 132:810-9.

National Audit Office. Report of the Comptroller and Auditor General: The Performance of the NHS Cervical Screening Programme in England. The Stationery Office: London, 1998.

Nieminen P, Kallio M, Anttila A, et al. Organised vs. spontaneous Pap-smear screening for cervical cancer: A case-control study. Int J Cancer 1999;83:55-8.

Nobbenhuis MAE, Walboomers JMM, Helmerhorst TJM, et al. Relation of human papillomavirus status to cervical lesions and consequences for cervical cancer screening: a prospective study. Lancet 1999; 354:20-25.

Nobbenhuis M, Meijer CJLM, van den Brule AJC, et al. Addition of high-risk HPV testing improves the current guidelines on follow-up after treatment for cervical intraepithelial neoplasia. Br J Cancer 2001;84:796-801.

Nuovo G, Moritz J, Kowalik A, et al. Human papillomavirus types and cervical squamous intraepithelial lesions that recur after cold-knife conization. Gynecol Oncol 1992;46:304-8.

Olesen F. A case-control study of cervical cytology before diagnosis of cervical cancer in Denmark. Int J Epidemiol 1988;17:501-8.

Ottaviano M, La Torre P. Examination of the cervix with the naked eye using acetic acid test. American J Obstet Gynecol 1982; 143: 139-42.

Papanicolaou GN. New Cancer Diagnosis. In: Proceedings of the Third Race Betterment Conference. Battle Creek, Michi: Race Betterment Foundation; 1928:528-34.

Papillo JL, Zarka MA, St John TL. Evaluation of the ThinPrep Pap test in clinical practice. A seven-month, 16,314-case experience in northern Vermont. Acta Cytol 1998;42:203-8.

Parkin DM. Global cancer statistics in the year 2000. Lancet Oncol 2001;2:533-43.

Payne N, Chilcott J, McGoogan E. Liquid-based cytology in cervical screening: a rapid and systematic review. Health Technology Assessment 2000;4.

Petry K-U, Menton S, Menton M, et al. Inclusion of HPV testing in routine cervical cancer screening in Germany: results for 8466 patients. Bri J Cancer 2003;88:1570-7.

Pettersson F, Naslund I, Malker B. Evaluation of the effect of Papanicolaou screening in Sweden: record linkage between a central screening registry and the National Cancer Registry. IARC Sci Publ 1986:91-105.

Quinn M, Babb P, Jones J, et al. Effect of screening on incidence of and mortality from cancer of cervix in England: evaluation based on routinely collected statistics. BMJ 1999; 318: 904-8.

Ratnam S, Franco EL, Ferenczy A. Human papillomavirus testing for primary screening of cervical cancer precursors. Cancer Epidemiol Biomarkers Prev 2000; 9: 945-51.

Raymond L, Obradovic M, Riotton G. Additional results on relative protection of cervical cancer screening according to stage of tumour from the Geneva case-control study. IARC Sci Publ 1986:107-10.

Roberts JM, Gurley AM, Thurloe JK, et al. Evaluation of the ThinPrep Pap test as an adjunct to the conventional Pap smear. Med J Aust 1997;167:466-500.

Rodriguez-Reyes ER, Cerda-Flores RM, Quinonez-Perez JM, et al. Acetic acid test: a promising screening test for early detection of cervical cancer. Anal Quant Cytol Histol 2002;24:134-6.

Sankaranarayanan R, Wesley R, Somanathan T, et al. Visual inspection of the uterine cervix after the application of acetic acid in the detection of cervical carcinoma and its precursors. Cancer 1998;83:2150-6.

Sasieni P. Trends in cervical cancer mortality. Lancet 1991;338:818-9.

Sasieni P, Cuzick J, Farmery E. Accelerated decline in cervical cancer mortality in England & Wales. Lancet 1995; 346: 1566-7.

Sasieni PD, Cuzick J, Lynch-Farmery E and the NCN Working Group. Estimating the efficacy of screening by auditing smear histories of women with and without cervical cancer. Br J Cancer 1996; 73: 1001-5.

Sasieni P, Adams J. Effect of screening on cervical cancer mortality in England and Wales: analysis of trends with age period cohort model. BMJ 1999; 318: 1244-5.

Sasieni PD, Adams J. Analysis of Cervical Cancer mortality and incidence data from England and Wales: evidence of a beneficial effect of screening. JR Stat Soc [A] 2000; 163:191-209.

Sasieni P, Adams J. Changing rates of adenocarcinoma and adenosquamous carcinoma of the cervix in England. Lancet 2001; 357: 1490-3.

Sasieni P et al. Cervical Screening in Evidence Based Oncology. To appear 2003.

Schiffman M, Herrero R, Hildesheim A, et al. HPV DNA testing in cervical cancer screening. Results from women in a high-risk province of Costa Rica. JAMA 2000; 283: 87-93.

Schneider A, Zahm DM, Kirchmayr R, et al. Screening for cervical intraepithelial neoplasia grade 2/3. Am J Obstet Gynecol 1996; 174: 1534-41.

Sellors JW, Lorincz AT, Mahony JB, et al. Comparison of self-collected vaginal, vulvar and urine samples with physician-collected cervical samples for human papillomavirus testing to detect high-grade squamous intraepithelial lesions. Can Med Assoc J 2000; 163: 513-8.

Sheets E, Constantine N, Dinisco S, et al. Colposcopically directed biopsies provide a basis for comparing the accuracy of ThinPrep and Papanicolaou smears. J Gynecol Tech 1995;1:27-33.

Sigurdsson K, Adalsteinsson S. Risk variables affecting high grade Pap smears at second visit. Effects of screening interval, year, age and low-grade smears. Int J Cancer 2001; 94:884-8.

Singh V, Sehgal A, Parashari A, et al. Early detection of cervical cancer through acetic acid application - an aided visual inspection. Singapore Med J 2001;42:351-4.

Slawson DC, Bennett JH, Herman JM. Are Papanicolaou smears enough? Acetic acid washes of the cervix as adjunctive therapy: a HARNET study. Harrisburg Area Research Network. J Fam Prac 1992;35:271-7.

Sobue T, Suzuki T, Hashimoto S, et al. A case-control study of the effectiveness of cervical cancer screening in Osaka, Japan. JPN J Cancer Res 1988;79:1269-75.

Solomon D, Schiffman M, Tarone R for the ALTS Group. Comparison of three management strategies for patients with atypical squamous cells of undetermined significance: Baseline results from a randomized trial. J Natl Cancer Inst 2001; 93: 293-9.

Sprenger E, Schwarzmann P, Kirkpatrick M, et al. The false negative rate in cervical cytology. Comparison of monolayers to conventional smears. Acta Cytol 1996;40:81-9.

Stevens MW, Nespolon WW, Milne AJ, et al. Evaluation of the CytoRich technique for cervical smears. Diagn Cytopathol 1998;18:236-42.

Takahashi M, Naito M. Application of the CytoRich monolayer preparation system for cervical cytology. A prelude to automated primary screening. Acta Cytol 1997;41:1785-9.

Tezuka F, Oikawa H, Shuki H, et al. Diagnostic efficacy and validity of the ThinPrep method in cervical cytology. Acta Cytol 1996;40:513-8.

van Ballegooijen M, et al. EJC 2002. CA: A Cancer Journal for Clinics. NOV/DEC 2002.

van der Graaf Y, Zielhuis GA, Peer PG, et al. The effectiveness of cervical screenings: a population-based case-control study. J Clin Epidemiol 1988;41:21-6.

van Oortmarssen GJ, Habbema JD. Cervical cancer screening data from two cohorts in British Columbia. IARC Sci Publ 1986:47-60.

van Wijngaarden WJ, Duncan ID. Rationale for stopping cervical screening in women over 50. BMJ 1993; 306:967-71.

van Wijngaarden WJ, Duncan ID, Hussain KA. Screening for cervical neoplasia in Dundee and Angus – 10 years on. B J Obstet & Gynecol 1995; 102: 137-42.

Vassilakos P, Griffin S, Megevand E, et al. CytoRich liquid-based cervical cytologic test. Screening results in a routine cytopathology service. Acta Cytol 1998;42:198-202.

Vassilakos P, Saurel J, Rondez R. Direct-to-vial use of the AutoCyte PREP liquid-based preparation for cervical-vaginal specimens in three European laboratories. Acta Cytol 1999; 43:65-8.

Vassilakos P, Schwartz D, de Marual F, et al. Biopsy-based comparison of liquid-based, thin-layer preparations to conventional Pap smears. J Reprod Med 2000;45:11-16.

Viikki M, Pukkala E, Hakama M. Risk of cervical cancer after a negative Pap smear. J Med Screen 1999;6:103-7.

Walboomers JMM, De Roda Husman A-M, Snijders PJF, et al. Human papillomavirus testing in false negative archival cervical smears: implications for screening for cervical cancer. J Clin Pathol 1995; 48: 728-32.

Walboomers JMM, Jacobs MV, Manos MM, et al. Human papillomavirus is a necessary cause of invasive cervical cancer worldwide. J Pathol 1999; 189: 12-19.

Wallin KL, Wiklund F, Angstrom T, et al. Type-specific persistence of human papillomavirus DNA before the development of invasive cervical cancer. N Engl J Med 1999; 341: 1633-8.

Wangsuphachart V, Thomas DB, Koetsawang A, et al. Risk factors for invasive cervical cancer and reduction of risk by 'Pap' smears in Thai women. Int J Epidemiol 1987;16:362-6.

Weintraub J. The coming revolution in cervical cytology: a pathologist's guide for the clinician. References en gynecologie obstetrique 1997;5:1-6.

WHO. Trends in Cancer Incidence and Mortality. In: Coleman MP, Esteve J, Daniecki P, et al. eds. (IARC Scientific Publications No. 121). Lyon: International Agency for Research on Cancer, 1993.

WHO. Age-specific and standardized incidence rates. In: Parkin DM, Muir CS, Whelan SL, et al, eds. Cancer Incidence in Five Continents, Vol VII (IARC Scientific Publications No. 143). Lyon: International Agency for Research on Cancer, 1997.

Wilbur DC, Cibas ES, Merritt S, et al. ThinPrep Processor. Clinical trials demonstrate an increased detection rate of abnormal cervical cytologic specimens. Am J Clin Pathol 1994; 101:209-14.

Wilbur DC, Dubeshter B, Angel C, et al. Use of thin-layer preparations for gynecologic smears with emphasis on the cytomorphology of high-grade intraepithelial lesions and carcinomas. Diagn Cytopathol 1996;14:201-11.

Wilbur DC, Facik MS, Rutkowski MA, et al. Clinical trials of the CytoRich specimen-preparation device for cervical cytology. Preliminary results. Acta Cytol 1997;41:24-9.

Williams GH, Romanowski P, Morris L, et al. Improved cervical smear assessment using antibodies against proteins that regulate DNA replication. Proc Natl Acad Sci USA 1998; 95: 14932-7.

Womack SD, Chirenje ZM, Blumenthal PD, et al. Evaluation of a human papillomavirus assay in cervical screening in Zimbabwe. Br J Obstet Gynecol 2000; 107: 33-8.

Wong P, Wong R, Caputo T, et al. Infrared spectroscopy of exfoliated human cervical cells: Evidence of extensive structural changes during carcinogenesis. Proc Nat Acad Sci USA 1991; 88:10988-92.

Wright TC Jr, Denny L, Kuhn L, et al. HPV DNA testing of self-collected vaginal samples compared with cytologic screening to detect cervical cancer. JAMA 2000; 283: 81-6.

Chapter 11

Chemoprevention of Cervical Cancer

Michele Follen, M.D., Ph.D.[1], Frank L. Meyskens, Jr., M.D.[2], E. Neely
Atkinson, Ph.D.[3], David Schottenfeld, M.D.[4]
[1]Center for Biomedical Engineering, The University of Texas M.D. Anderson Cancer Center;
[2]Chao Family Comprehensive Cancer Center, University of California-Irvine; [3]Department of
Biomathematics, The University of Texas M.D. Anderson Cancer Center; [4]Department of
Epidemiology, The University of Michigan, School of Public Health.

INTRODUCTION

Cervical cancer is the third leading cause of cancer deaths in women
worldwide (Parkin et al., 1999). It represents an important and costly
problem in the developed world, and a devastating problem in the
developing world, where resources and infrastructure are inadequate.
Nevertheless, cervical cancer has long been thought to be one of the most
preventable of cancers because it has a predictable preclinical phase, the
affected organ is accessible to examination and biopsy, there is a reasonably
good screening test, and vaccines are being developed against infection with
human papillomavirus (HPV), which plays a central role in the etiology of
the disease (see Chapters 7, 12 and 13). Furthermore, there is emerging
evidence that risk of development of cervical cancer might be reduced
through the use of chemopreventive agents.

Chemoprevention has been defined as the use of drugs or other agents to
inhibit, delay, or reverse the progressive genetic damage and the associated
tissue damage that accrue during carcinogenesis (O'Shaughnessy et al.,

2002). Chemoprevention has some advantages over the surgical removal of cancer precursors, because surgery can cause substantial morbidity, and unlike chemoprevention, it does not treat the entire epithelial field at risk. The cervix is an ideal organ for the study both of progression from benign neoplasia to invasive cancer and of factors that interfere with progression. The course of the disease can be studied using cytology, histopathology, and colposcopy, and these are the tools used to follow patients during chemoprevention trials.

Littenberg suggested a paradigm for the evaluation of new technologies and new therapies (Littenberg, 1992). He proposed that these technologies and therapies be evaluated for their biologic plausibility, technical feasibility, clinical effectiveness, patient satisfaction, and societal benefit. These concepts apply to many areas relevant to cervical cancer detection and prevention. Table 1 outlines the paradigm and shows how it applies to trials of cervical chemopreventive agents. In this chapter, the current state of knowledge concerning the chemoprevention of cervical cancer is reviewed within the framework proposed by Littenberg (1992).

1   BIOLOGIC PLAUSIBILITY

1.1   Chemoprevention agents and HPV expression

Four classes of agents have been used in chemoprevention trials in the cervix: retinoids, micronutrients, polyamine synthesis inhibitors, and adduct reducers (Table 2) (Current Clinical Trials Oncology, 1994a, 1994b; Bell et al., 2000; Butterworth et al., 1992a; Butterworth et al., 1992b; Childers et al., 1995; de Vet et al., 1991; Fairley et al., 1996; Follen et al., 2001a; Graham et al., 1986; Keefe 1998; Mackerras et al., 1999; Manetta et al., 1996; Meyskens et al., 1983; Meyskens et al., 1994; Mitchell et al., 1998; Romney et al., 1987; Romney et al., 1985; Romney et al., 1997; Ruffin et al., 1999; Surwit et al., 1982; Weiner et al., 1986)

Retinoids have inhibitory effects on the growth of HPV; specifically, there are several mechanisms by which retinoic acid is thought to affect the HPV E6 and E7 transforming proteins. Bartsch et al. (1992) have demonstrated that in the presence of retinoic acid there is decreased expression of HPV messenger RNA. Additionally, retinoic acid has also been shown to increase the secretion of TGF-β1 and TGF-β2 in cells immortalized by HPV (Batova et al., 1992). TGF-β can suppress the expression of the E6 and E7 proteins in cervical epithelial cells (Batova et al., 1992; Pietrantoni et al., 1995; Woodworth et al., 1990).

Table 1. Development of a logical rationale for cervical chemoprevention trials
following the paradigm of technology assessment

BIOLOGIC PLAUSIBILITY

- Choosing an agent that decreases HPV expression or decreases growth of HPV-positive cell lines or tissue cultures
- Identifying and validating relevant surrogate end point biomarkers

TECHNICAL FEASIBILITY; NATURAL HISTORY OF THE DISEASE

- Taking natural history of the disease into account when calculating the sample size
- Accounting for regression rates in the placebo arm
- Designing the trial to accommodate the desired difference in response rates between placebo and treated groups

TECHNICAL FEASIBILITY: TRIAL DESIGN AND EXECUTION

- Performing a phase I trial to determine dose or range of doses prior to the phase II study
- Performing a phase I trial to determine duration of treatment
- Defining response—partial and complete—and doing so explicitly, quantitatively, and reproducibly.
- Using colposcopically directed biopsy as an entry and exit test

PATIENT SATISFACTION

- Determining what factors encourage participation in chemoprevention trials
- Determining what incentives are meaningful to encourage fulfilling study requirements and participating to trial end
- Determining benefits of participation

SOCIETAL BENEFIT

- Obtaining results from the intervention that improve patient care and represent an advance over the standard of care
- Obtaining results that can be extrapolated to benefit the underserved: the medication must be cost-effective, of low toxicity, and easy to administer

Table 2. Agents used in chemoprevention trials in the cervix

Class	Agent	Trial
Retinoids	Retiny-acetate gel	Romney et al. (1985)
	All-*trans*-retinoic acid (topical)	Surwit et al. (1982), Meyskens et al. (1983, 1994), Weiner et al. (1986), Graham et al. (1986), Meyskens et al. (1994), Ruffin et al. (1999)
	4-Hydroxyphenylretinamide	Follen et al. (2001a)
Micronutrients	Vitamin C	Romney et al. (1987)
	β-carotene	Romney et al. (1997 and protocol 09315), Manetta et al. (1996), Berman et al. (protocol 09088), Keefe et al. (1998), de Vet et al. (1991), Fairley et al. (1996), Mackerras et al. (1999)
	Folate	Butterworth et al. (1992a, 1992b), Childers et al. (1995)
Polyamine synthesis inhibitors	Difluoromethlyornithine	Mitchell et al. (1998), Follen et al. (unreported)
Adduct reducers	Indole-3-carbinol	Bell et al. (2000)

Source: Adapted, with permission, from Follen and Schottenfeld (2001).

These studies show that retinoid compounds affect the expression levels of these E6 and E7 proteins, which therefore may serve as markers of responsiveness.

With respect to micronutrients, the biologic mechanisms underlying the chemopreventive effects of beta-carotene and folate have been investigated. Specifically, it has been reported that tissue levels of TGF-β1 were higher after beta-carotene treatment than before treatment (Comerci et al., 1997). Statistically significant increases in TGF-β1 were seen across parabasal, midepithelial, and superficial epithelia. With respect to folate, red blood cell folate levels below 660 nmol/l have been shown to enhance the susceptibility of patients to HPV infection. A possible explanation for this is that folic acid acts as a coenzyme in DNA synthesis for normal cellular growth, proliferation, and differentiation. In a study that supports these biologic concepts, Pietrantoni et al. (1995) examined the regulation of HPV oncogene expression in cell lines treated with folic acid, specifically focusing on c-*fos*, c-*jun*, and HPV E6 expression in CaSki (HPV-positive) cell lines. They found diminished c-*fos* and c-*jun* expression using Western blot analysis when concentrations of folate greater than 100 nM were used. E6 protein expression was also diminished at folate concentrations of greater than 100 nM, suggesting that the mechanism by which the transcription regulators c-*fos* and c-*jun* were controlled involved diminished viral E6 expression.

The adduct reducer indole-3-carbinol has been validated as a chemopreventive agent in an animal model. Indole-3-carbinol has been shown to prevent cervical cancer in HPV type 16 transgenic mice during 6 months of treatment (Jin et al., 1999). Nineteen of 25 control mice developed cancer with estradiol administration, whereas only 2 of 24 mice fed indole-3-carbinol and given estradiol developed cancer (Jin et al., 1999).

1.2 Identifying and validating relevant surrogate end point biomarkers

The study of surrogate end point biomarkers (SEBs) allows understanding of the biologic progression and regression of disease. In chemopreventive studies, surrogate end point biomarkers are defined as intermediate indicators of cancer incidence reduction. According to Kelloff et al. (1994), biomarkers must meet certain criteria before they are deemed useful as chemopreventives. These include: *(a)* the SEB must be expressed differentially in normal and high-risk tissues; *(b)* it should appear at a well-defined stage of carcinogenesis; *(c)* the assay for the biomarker should have acceptable sensitivity, specificity, and accuracy; *(d)* easy measurement should be a hallmark; *(e)* it should be clear that chemopreventive agents modulate the marker; and *(f)* the SEB's modulation should correlate with a decrease in the rate of cancer incidence (Kelloff et al., 1994).

Table 3 lists the classes of biomarkers that have been studied in the cervix. Pilot and phase I studies provide an ideal opportunity for the study and validation of SEBs (Boone et al., 1990; Kelloff et al., 1995; Mitchell et al., 1995a). Several authors have critically reviewed the studies of SEBs in the cervix following the paradigm outlined by Kelloff (Daly 1993; Kelloff et al., 1994; Kelloff et al., 1992; Sporn, 1993). The best-validated marker is ploidy, or DNA content, because it has been validated in chemoprevention and chemotherapy trials and has been shown to correlate with survival. Interested readers are encouraged to examine reviews by Follen and others (Boone et al., 1990; Boone et al., 1992; Follen and Schottenfeld, 2001; Mitchell et al., 1995a) addressing the value of these markers.

Table 3. Classes of biomarkers in the cervical epithelium

QUANTITATIVE HISTOPATHOLOGIC AND CYTOLOGIC MARKERS

- Nuclei (abnormal size, shape, texture, pleomorphism)
- Nucleoli (abnormal number, size, shape, position, pleomorphism)
- Nuclear matrix (tissue architecture)

PROLIFERATION MARKERS

- Proliferating cell nuclear antigen
- Ki-67, MIB-1
- Labeling indices (thymidine, bromodeoxyurdidine)
- Mitotic frequency (MPM-2)

REGULATION MARKERS

- Tumor suppressors (p53, Rb)
- Human papillomavirus viral load and oncoprotein expression
- Oncogenes (ras, myc, c-erb B-2)
- Altered growth factors and receptors (epidermal growth factor receptor, transforming growth factor-β, cyclin-dependent kinases, retinoic acid receptors)
- Polyamines (ornithine decarboxylase, arginine, ornithine, putrescine, spermine, spermidine)
- Arachidonic acid

DIFFERENTIATION MARKERS

- Fibrillar proteins (cytokeratins, involucrin, cornifin, filaggrin, actin, microfilaments, microtubules)
- Adhesion molecules (cell-cell: gap junctions, desmosomes) (cell-substrate: integrins, cadherins, laminins, fibronectin, proteoglycans, collagen)
- Glycoconjugates (lectins, lactoferrin, mucins, blood group substances, glycolipids, CD44)

Table 3. Classes of biomarkers in the cervical epithelium–*Continued*

GENERAL GENOMIC INSTABILITY MARKERS

- Chromosome aberrations (silver-stained nucleolar organizer region proteins, micronuclei, three-group metaphases, double minutes, deletions, insertions, translocations, inversions, isochromosomes, fragile histidine triad)
- DNA abnormalities (DNA hypomethylation, loss of heterozygosity, point mutations, gene amplification
- Aneuploidy (measured by flow cytometry)

TISSUE MAINTENANCE MARKERS

- Metalloproteinases
- Telomerases
- Apoptosis and antiapoptotic markers

Source: Reprinted, with permission, from Follen and Schottenfeld (2001) and based on Mitchell et al. (1995a)

2 TECHNICAL FEASIBILITY OF CLINICAL TRIALS: NATURAL HISTORY OF THE DISEASE

2.1 Natural history of the disease and sample size

Cervical intraepithelial neoplasia (CIN) or cervical squamous intraepithelial lesions (SILs) have been the subject of two reviews that have focused on transition probabilities using crude statistical methodology (Table 4) (Follen et al., 2002; Mitchell et al., 1994; Oster, 1993). These reviews suggest that low-grade lesions or HPV and CIN 1 lesions have a high probability for regression (see chapter 2 also); thus, sample sizes for studies that include these precursors must be sufficiently powered to allow for these high regression rates. Indeed, for a simple randomized trial involving a treatment and placebo group, taking natural history into account in planning would produce sample sizes that range from 8 to 392 depending on the anticipated difference between placebo and treated arms (Follen et al., 2002; Mitchell et al., 1994; Oster, 1993).

Several trials of cervical cancer chemoprevention agents have been conducted (Table 5) (Follen et al., 2002). While several phase I trials have shown promising results, only two phase II trials, one of all-*trans*-retinoic acid (Meyskens et al., 1994), and the other of indole-3-carbinol (Bell et al., 2000) have shown statistically significant differences in outcomes, both in favor of the agent being tested compared to placebo.

Table 4. Natural history of CIN in cohorts of untreated patients from two reviews

Case Classification	Behavior of lesion				
	Regression (%)	Persistence (%)	Progression (%)		
	To lower grade of CIN	At same grade of CIN	To higher grade of CIN	To carcinoma in situ	To invasive cervical cancer
	Studies clustered by CIN grade (Oster 1993)				
CIN 1	57.0	32.0	—	11.0	—
CIN 2	43.0	35.0	—	22.0	—
CIN 3	32.0	56.0	—	12.0	—
Overall all grades of CIN					1.7
	Studies clustered by study design (Mitchell et al. 1994)				
CIN 1–3 (no carcinoma in situ) followed by Papanicolaou smear only	34.0	41.0	25.0	10.0	1.0
CIN 1–3 (no carcinoma in situ) followed by Papanicolaou smear and biopsy	45.0	31.0	23.0	14.0	1.4

Source: Reprinted, with permission, from Follen et al. (2002). Data from Oster (1993) and Mitchell et al. (1994).

Table 5. Cervical cancer chemoprevention trials by type of medication

Chemopreventive and study	Results[a]		
	Pilot/Phase I	Phase II/III	
		CR	CR + PR
Retinoids			
Retinyl acetate gel (topical) Romney et al. (1985)	Toxicity: 50% at 3 mg, 21% at 6 mg; 75% at 9 mg; 100% at 18 mg Response: None reported Results: Selected 9-mg dose		
All-TRA (topical) Surwit et al. (1982)	Toxicity: 55% (10/18) overall Response: 11% (2/18) CR Results: Designed next phase I study		
All-TRA (topical) Meyskens et al. (1983)	Toxicity: Moderate—24% (5/21) at 0.21%–0.372%; 100% (3/3) at 0.484% Response: 33% (7/21) CR + PR at 6 months Results: Selected 0.372% dose as least toxic and probably most active		
All-TRA (topical) Weiner et al. (1996)	Response:14% (2/14) at 0.05%–0.12%; 45% (10/22) at 0.15%–0.48%		
All-TRA (topical) Graham et al. (1986)		50% (10/20)	
All-TRA (topical) Meyskens et al. (1994)		TRA: 43% (32/75) Placebo: 27% (18/66)	

Table 5. Cervical cancer chemoprevention trials by type of medication, *continued*

Chemopreventive and study	Results[a]		
	Pilot/Phase I	Phase II/III	
		CR	CR + PR
Micronutrients			
Vitamin C Romney et al. (1987)	Toxicity: None Response: Vitamin C slightly favored over placebo (not quantified) Results: Recommendation to proceed to phase I study		
β–Carotene Romney et al. (1994, 1997)			β–Carotene: 46% (18/39) Placebo: 50% (15/30)
β–Carotene Manetta et al. (1996)	*β–Carotene: 70% (21/30)*		
β-Carotene Berman (1994) and Keefe et al. (1998)		β-Carotene: 32% Placebo: 32%	
β-Carotene De Vet et al. [24]		β-Carotene: 16% (22/137) Placebo: 11% (15/141)	β-Carotene: 32% (44/137) Placebo: 32% (45/141)
β-Carotene Fairley et al. (1996)			Results[a]
β-Carotene, vitamin C Mackerras et al. (1999)		β-Carotene: 44% (16/36) Vitamin C: 26% (9/35) Both: 23% (8/35) Placebo: 29% (10/35)	

Table 5. Cervical cancer chemoprevention trials by type of medication, *continued*

Chemopreventive and study	Results[a]		
	Pilot/Phase I	Phase II/III	
		CR	CR + PR
Folate, vitamin C Butterworth et al. (1992a)		Folate: 14% (3/22) Placebo (vitamin C): 4% (1/25)	β-Carotene: 63% (37/59) Placebo: 60% (31/52)
Folate, vitamin C Butterworth et al. (1992b)		Folate: 64% (58/91) Placebo (vitamin C): 52% (45/86)	
Folate Childers et al. (1995)		Folate: 7% (9/129) Placebo: 6% (7/117)	Folate: 36% (8/22) Placebo (vitamin C): 16% (4/25)
Polyamine synthesis inhibitors			
DFMO (oral) Mitchell et al. (1998)	Response: 50% (15/30) CR + PR Result: Selected doses of 0.125 and 0.5 g/m^2/day		
Adduct reducers			
Indole-3-carbinol (oral) Bell et al. (2000)		200 mg: 50% (4/8) CR 400 mg: 44% (4/9) CR Placebo: 0% (0/10)	

Note: CR, complete response; PR, partial response; CIS, carcinoma in situ; all-TRA, all-*trans*-retinoic acid; 4-HPR, N-(4-hydroxyphenyl)retinamide; DFMO, α-difluoromethylornithine
[a] Published reports do not consistently include toxicity results; response, including CR + PR data; and decision regarding next phase

2.2   Accounting for placebo arm regression rates

Clearly these trials give us valuable information for the design and conduct of future trials of chemopreventive agents (and of vaccines). The regression rates in the placebo arms vary from 0 to 66%, depending on the precursor lesions in the patient population. Regression rates are highest when the precursor lesion is a low-grade lesion and lowest when the precursor lesion is a high-grade lesion. Regression rates also vary with duration of follow-up. Even a high-grade lesion followed over a long period of time will have a higher regression rate than a high-grade lesion followed over a shorter period of time. Surprisingly, Follen et al. (2001a) reported a partial and complete response rate of 44% in the placebo arm of their high-grade trial in which patients were randomized between treatment with 4-HPR and placebo and followed for one year. With regression rates of this magnitude, one would need to have 100 patients per arm to observe a 20% difference between treated groups, 40 patients per arm to observe a 30% difference between treated groups, and 20 patients per arm to observe a 40% difference between treated groups.

2.3   Allowing for response rate differences in trial design

Data from previous studies (Table 5) can be used to generate suggested sample sizes for future trials. The sample sizes, which take into account the anticipated differences between the placebo and treated groups, range from fewer than 10 per group when the difference is 70%, to 70 or more when the difference is 10% (Follen et al., 2002). The minimum detectable statistically significant difference between the intervention and control groups can also be calculated for the phase II studies reported to date (Follen et al., 2002). This reveals that, with the exception of the studies by Meyskens et al. (1994) and Bell et al. (2000), none of the studies has been sufficiently powered to detect the desired difference.

3   TECHNICAL FEASIBILITY: TRIAL DESIGN AND EXECUTION

Four steps are fundamental to constructing a chemoprevention study: *(a)* identifying high-risk cohorts; *(b)* selecting appropriate medications whose choice is governed by a biologic rationale and whose toxicity is low; *(c)* ensuring the investigation follows the logical progression of phases in order (phase I, IIa, IIb, and III); and *(d)* incorporating SEBs. Following these steps rigorously is critical to success (Boone et al., 1992; Mitchell et al., 1995b).

From pilot to phase III, Table 6 defines each phase and describes the objectives of each, including identifying when such elements as side effect evaluation, toxicity evaluation, and efficacy evaluation are appropriately included (Follen et al., 2002; Goodman, 1992). Increasingly, researchers weave measurement of biomarkers into chemoprevention trials.

3.1 Phase I trial preceding phase II trial

In phase I chemotherapy trials, researchers evaluate drug toxicity as they test escalating doses. De-escalating doses, on the other hand, are used in phase I and IIa chemoprevention trials, when researchers try to find the lowest dose at which SEBs may be biologically modulated and toxicity is at a minimum. It is important to remember here that the definition of the "correct" dose will vary between organ systems. As part of the phase I, I–II, IIa trial designs, researchers should integrate into the study design a test of the drug in various tissues of interest. If SEBs modulated by the agent under study have not already been identified, they may be selected during phase I, IIa trials (see Goodman, 1992).

In phase II trials, the focus is on the effectiveness of an agent in a specific organ. Phase II chemoprevention trials incorporate a placebo group because researchers must have a measure of any spontaneous regression that may occur. Though both phase IIa and phase IIb include a placebo group, these two phases may vary in duration and inclusion of SEBs. Both may be either long- or short-term, but SEB inclusion is optional in I, IIa studies but required in phase IIb studies.

Phase III chemoprevention studies are large, doubly blinded trials conducted at multiple clinical sites. They focus on patients at high risk for cancer and examine SEB modulation. Using SEB modulation rather than cancer incidence as an end point permits shorter trials, lowers costs, and allows smaller sample sizes (Boone et al., 1992; Mitchell et al., 1995b).

The logical paradigm described by Goodman demonstrates the rationale for progressing from one study to the next. Secure foundations lead to a reliable base from which sample sizes, drug dose, drug durations, and response validity can be determined. Table 6 outlines the Goodman (Goodman, 1992) paradigm as modified in Follen et al. (2002). In Table 7, the studies outlined in Table 5 are arranged so that one can see how the paradigm of Goodman has or has not been followed in the cervical cancer chemoprevention trials performed to date for each agent tested. For example, phase I trials of retinyl acetate gel (Romney et al., 1985), all-TRA (Surwit et al., 1982; Meyskens et al., 1983; Weiner et al., 1986), and DFMO (Mitchell et al., 1998) for chemoprevention of cervical neoplasia were conducted before phase II studies were conducted. In contrast, there have never been phase I trials of folate, indole-3-carbinol, or 4-HPR (Follen et al., 2002).

Table 6. Achievable objectives in study designs for chemoprevention trials

Design and objective	Type of trial					
	Pilot[a]	Phase I	Phase I–II[a]	Phase IIa	Phase IIb	Phase III
Definition	Exploratory study	Dose escalation study or dose–de-escalation study involving a single arm, used to evaluate toxicity and tolerance	Single-arm study used to explore response in the disease of interest, not dose finding	Randomized, double-blinded, placebo-controlled trial, used to evaluate response, may evaluate multiple dose levels	Randomized, double-blinded, placebo-controlled trial used to evaluate biomarkers and response, may evaluate multiple dose levels	Randomized, double-blinded, placebo-controlled trial used to evaluate response in a multicenter setting
Objectives						
Side effect evaluation	Maybe	Short-term: yes Long-term: no	Short-term: yes Long-term: No	Short-term: yes Long-term: yes	Short-term: yes Long-term: yes	Short-term: yes Long-term: yes
Dose/toxicity evaluation	No	Yes	Maybe	Yes	Yes	Yes
Recruitment evaluation	No	No	No	Yes	Yes	Yes
Pharmacokinetics evaluation	Maybe	Yes	No	Yes	Yes	Yes
Efficacy evaluation	No	No	Yes	Yes	Yes	Yes
Duration	< 1 year	< 1 year	< 1 year	1–5 years	1–5 years	At least 1–5 years
Target population	Appropriate target population	Appropriate target population	Appropriate target population	Appropriate target population	Appropriate target population	Appropriate target population
Accrual goal	20	25–100	25–100	100–1000	100–1000	>1000

Source: Adapted from Goodman (1992) and reprinted, with permission, from Follen et al. (2002).
[a] Not defined in Goodman (1992) but used by many investigators.

3.2   Defining treatment duration and measuring response

Each of the phase II/III trials listed in Table 5 was of different duration. Additionally, each study used different response criteria, and none of the responses was measured quantitatively. All of these differences render direct comparison of the trials difficult.

3.3   Colposcopically directed biopsy as entry and exit test

Eligibility for cervical chemoprevention trials should be ascertained on the basis of colposcopically directed biopsy, for which the sensitivity and specificity are estimated to be 96% and 48%, respectively (Fahey et al., 1995), compared with ~60% and ~60%, respectively, for the Papanicolaou smear (Mitchell et al., 1999). Using the Papanicolaou smear or colposcopy without biopsy could lead to the misclassification of 15% to 40% of patients at study entry (Butterworth et al., 1982; Butterworth et al., 1992a; Fairley et al., 1996). While biopsy may induce a slightly higher rate of regression than is observed with Papanicolaou smears, the increased accuracy in study entry and response ascertainment probably outweigh the negative effects of the biopsy approach. Similarly, response needs to be ascertained with the same test at study entry as at study end. Using a different test at study entry and study end, a common practice in phase II studies reported to date (Butterworth et al., 1982; Butterworth et al., 1992a; Childers et al., 1995; de Vet et al., 1991; Mackerras et al., 1999), introduces the error of the test differences. The difficulty in comparing these studies is evident from the differences between entry and exit tests both within and between studies (Follen et al., 2002).

Table 7. Study designs used in cervical cancer chemoprevention trials by agent

Medication	Study design					
	Pilot	Phase I	Phase I–II	Phase IIa	Phase IIb	Phase III
Retinoids						
Topical retinyl acetate gel			Romney et al. (1985)			
Topical all-TRA		Meyskens et al. (1983) Weiner et al. (1986)	Surwit et al. (1982)	Graham et al. (1986)	Meyskens et al. (1994)[a] Ruffin et al. (2000)	
4-Hydoxyphenyl-retinamide					Follen et al. (2001)	
Micronutrients						
Vitamin C	Romney et al. (1987)				Mackerras et al. (1999)	
Folate					Butterworth et al. (1992a) Butterworth et al. (1992b)	
α-Difluoromethyl-ornithine		Mitchell et al. (1998)		Follen et al . [ongoing/unreported]		
Adduct Reducers						
Indole-3-carbinol				Bell et al. (2000)[a]		

Source: Reprinted, with permission, from Follen et al. (2002).
[a] Statistically significant response rate.

4 PATIENT SATISFACTION – ENCOURAGING PARTICIPATION IN CHEMOPREVENTION TRIALS

Patient satisfaction is an important consideration in recruiting patients for chemoprevention trials. Ensuring patient satisfaction is probably even more difficult than enlisting patients for clinical trials. Unlike patients who have already experienced disease and who are likely to believe they will benefit, patients in chemoprevention trials are asymptomatic; thus, the benefits of participating in the trial are much less obvious. Factors such as the duration of study, medication schedule, cost, time, follow-up visits, and drug side effects become important considerations to patients who are otherwise asymptomatic. Participation rates of women and minority women in prevention and screening trials remain low; most participants in cancer prevention trials are white, middle class, and highly educated (Swanson and Ward, 1995; Yeomans-Kinney et al., 1998). Among socially disadvantaged women there are barriers such as transportation, length of participation, and time away from work. Attitudes, lack of knowledge, and cultural characteristics can be additional barriers. The fact that cervical cancer incidence and mortality are higher among minorities increases the importance of their participation in cervical cancer chemoprevention trials.

Qualitative interviews with women in two colposcopy clinics in Houston by Karen Basen-Enquist and colleagues were designed to explore how African-American, Hispanic, and non-Hispanic white women with abnormal Pap smear findings perceived cervical cancer chemoprevention trials (Basen-Enquist K, Tortolero-Luna G, Pounds K, Torres I, Follen M. Participation in cervical cancer chemoprevention trials as perceived by Hispanic, African-American, and white women. Unpublished manuscript, 2003). Motivating factors included the opportunity to help others, the hope of helping to prevent cancer, and the desire by participants to have their own health monitored. Major barriers identified by participants included transportation problems, difficulties in meeting family responsibilites during participation, and taking medications. Possibilities for improving recruitment include hiring bilingual and bicultural staff, providing transportation subsidies, and extending clinic hours, but finding funding to meet these needs and overcome these obstacles will be difficult.

5 SOCIETAL BENEFIT – ADVANCING BEYOND THE STANDARD OF CARE

Once a clinical chemoprevention trial has been conducted it can be subjected to a cost-effectiveness analysis and a cost-benefit analysis. In a cost-effectiveness analysis, we compare management strategies in terms of their cost per unit of output, where output is additional years of life, utility, or additional cases of newly detected disease. A cost-benefit analysis is a comparison of management strategies in which the costs and benefits are both expressed in the same terms (Sox et al., 1988).

Data from chemoprevention trials can be modeled to see if the chemopreventive agent would be useful, for example, in the developing world to prevent or delay cancers. Data from actual trials can be subjected to cost-effectiveness analysis or cost-benefit analysis and compared against analyses of the standard of care to identify the better course. Such comparisons advance decision-making and allocation of limited resources. In the developed world, for example, it is important that the medication be of low toxicity and easy to administer. In the developing world, where resources are scarce, it is important that the medication be inexpensive, of extremely low toxicity, easy to administer, easy to store and transport, capable of being stored without refrigeration, and able to be administered by untrained health care workers. In both worlds, these interventions should have been shown to be cost-effective, ethical, and of societal benefit.

6 ISSUES IN TRIAL DESIGN

Rules designed to improve the reporting of randomized clinical trials have been published as the Consolidated Standards of Reporting Trials (CONSORT) criteria. The criteria hold that the protocol must prospectively clearly express the hypothesis under study, identify the study population using inclusion and exclusion criteria, lay out the planned interventions and the schedule on which they will be implemented, describe primary and secondary outcome measures, identify the projected sample size and the theoretical foundation of the statistical analysis, define conditions under which the trial could be stopped, and profile blinding and randomization. Reports of the results of the trial are to include a description of the participant flow and detailed analyses (Begg et al., 1996).

For cervical chemoprevention trials, the null hypothesis is that the agent being studied will produce no difference in regression rates between placebo and treatment arms. The alternative hypothesis is that the agent will produce a higher regression rate in the treatment arm than in the placebo arm by a given delta error. A primary hypothesis may be paired with a secondary hypothesis based on SEB modulation, asserting no change against the alternative hypothesis of an increasing or decreasing measure, depending on the marker.

CONCLUSION

What the results of extant studies teach us is the fundamental necessity of following the principles of good study design. Advances in cervical cancer prevention depend on researchers understanding factors that have limited the validity and generalizability of previous interventions (Follen et al., 2001b). As discussed above, advances require meeting rigorous standards during the design of randomized clinical trials: identifying suitable cohorts and carefully selecting a treatment modality in relation to both primary and secondary outcome measures, the biologic rationale, and the anticipated response.

Because untreated SIL/CIN is known to have regression rates of 32% to 57%, researchers must calculate sample size based on projected spontaneous regression rates and the predetermined therapeutic objectives. Cohorts may have any grade of CIN, but researchers must include in their calculations the rate of regression associated with that grade as determined by the method of follow-up.

Undergirding such initial steps as choosing the medication must be a biologic rationale, and on that choice, the decision of which SEBs it would be appropriate to incorporate in the trial will be based. Of interest in all studies are viral load and HPV oncoprotein expression. Preclinical laboratory work, including showing suppression of HPV oncoprotein expression in cell lines or prevention of HPV-induced tumors in mice, contribute to the biologic rationale.

Incorporating biomarkers is integral to good chemoprevention trial design. Essential in carefully designed pilot, phase I, IIa, IIb, and III studies in patients with CIN are SEB validation and variability determination, which are critical to study success; measures of toxicity; and tests at study entry and termination that are identical. These studies create a foundation for phase IIb placebo-controlled studies and multicenter phase III studies.

All measures, including baseline values, primary and secondary outcome measures, and response criteria, need to be well defined. Because it has the highest sensitivity, colposcopically-directed biopsy should be the test patients undergo at study entry and at study exit, and on it all diagnoses should be based. To ensure reliability, consensus panels of pathologists who are blinded to study outcome should perform evaluations. In this way, the large variation in reading of cervical biopsy specimens can be overcome.

Adding value in the future will be quantitative and reproducible measures of pathology that are now beginning to emerge, which add value by quantitatively rather than qualitatively assessing response. In addition, researchers could serve their colleagues and their aim by reporting as much raw data as possible, including at least the entry diagnosis and, after treatment, partial and complete response rates.

Overall, cervical cancer chemoprevention studies require that investigators have deep knowledge, be familiar with biologic and epidemiologic principles, and be persistent. What is now known about the natural history and pathobiology of cervical cancer—and it is much— must be employed to construct rigorous trial designs that ensure progress in the future.

ACKNOWLEDGMENTS

This work was supported by National Cancer Institute Grant CN-25483-02.

REFERENCES

Bartsch D, Boye B, Baust C, et al. Retinoic acid-mediated repression of human papillomavirus 18 transcription and different ligand regulation of the retinoic acid receptor beta gene in non-tumorigenic and tumorigenic HeLa hybrid cells. EMBO J 1992;11:2283–91.

Batova A, Danielpour D, Pirisi L, et al. Retinoic acid induces secretion of latent transforming growth factor ß1 and ß2 in normal and human papillomavirus type 16-immortalized human keratinocytes. Cell Growth Differ 1992;3:763–72.

Begg C, Cho M, Eastwood S, et al. Improving the quality of reporting of randomized controlled trials. The CONSORT statement. JAMA 1996;276:637–9.

Bell MC, Crowley-Nowick P, Bradlow HL, et al. Placebo-controlled trial of indole-3-carbinol in the treatment of CIN. Gynecol Oncol 2000;78:123–9.

Boone C, Kelloff G, Malone W. Identification of candidate cancer chemopreventive agents and their evaluation in animal models and human clinical trials: a review. Cancer Res 1990; 50:2–9.

Boone C, Kelloff G, Steele V. Natural history of intraepithelial neoplasia in humans with implications for cancer chemopreventive strategy. Cancer Res 1992;52:1651–69.

Butterworth C, Hatch K, Gore H, et al. Improvement in cervical dysplasia associated with folic acid therapy in users of oral contraceptives. Am J Clin Nutr 1982;35:73–82.

Butterworth C, Hatch K, Soong S, et al. Oral folic acid supplementation for cervical dysplasia: A clinical intervention trial. Am J Obstet Gynecol 1992a;166:803–9.

Butterworth CJ, Hatch K, Macaluso M, et al. Folate deficiency and cervical dysplasia. JAMA 1992b;267:528–33.

Childers J, Chu J, Voigt L, et al. Chemoprevention of cervical cancer with folic acid: A Phase II Southwest Oncology Group Intergroup Study. Cancer Epidemiol Biomarkers Prev 1995; 4:155–9.

Comerci J, Runowicz C, Fields A, et al. Induction of transforming growth factor β-1 in cervical intraepithelial neoplasia in vivo after treatment with β-carotene. Clin Cancer Res 1997; 3:157–60.

Current Clinical Trials Oncology. National Cancer Institute PDQ. Volume 1, Number 2 (March–April 1994) (protocol 09088), 1994a.

Current Clinical Trials Oncology. National Cancer Institute PDQ. Volume 1, Number 2 (March–April 1994) (protocol 09315), 1994b.

Daly M. The chemoprevention of cancer: Directions for the future. Cancer Epidemiol Biomarkers Prev 1993;2:509–12.

de Vet HC, Knipschild PG, Willebrand D, et al. The effect of beta-carotene on the regression and progression of cervical dysplasia: a clinical experiment. J Clin Epidemiol 1991; 44:273–83.

Fahey M, Irwig L, Macaskill P. Meta-analysis of Pap test accuracy. Am J Epidemiol 1995; 141:680–9.

Fairley C, Tabrizi S, Chen S, et al. A randomized clinical trial of beta carotene vs. placebo for the treatment of cervical HPV infection. Int J Gynecol Cancer 1996;6:225–30.

Follen M, Atkinson E, Schottenfeld D, et al. A randomized clinical trial of 4-hydroxyphenylretinamide for high-grade squamous intraepithelial lesions of the cervix. Clin Cancer Res 2001a;7:3356–65.

Follen M, Meyskens F Jr, Atkinson E, et al. Why most randomized phase II cervical cancer chemoprevention trials are uninformative: lessons for the future. J Natl Cancer Inst 2001b; 95:1293–6.

Follen M, Schottenfeld D. Surrogate endpoint biomarkers and their modulation in cervical chemoprevention trials. Cancer 2001;91:1758–76.

Follen M, Vlastos A, Meyskens Jr F, et al. Why phase II trials in cervical chemoprevention are negative: what have we learned? Cancer Causes and Control 2002;13:855–73.

Goodman G. The clinical evaluation of cancer chemoprevention agents: Defining and contrasting phase I, II, and III objectives. Cancer Res 1992;92(Suppl):2752s–7s.

Graham V, Surwit E, Weiner S, Meyskens F. Phase II trial of β-ALL-*trans*-retinoic acid for cervical intraepithelial neoplasia via collagen sponge and cervical cap. West J Med 1986; 145:192–5.

Jin L, Oi M, Chen D. Indole-3-carbonol prevents cervical cancer in human papilloma virus type 16 (HPV 16) transgenic mice. Cancer Res 1999;59:3991–7.

Keefe K. Abstract 144. Paper presented at: Twenty-ninth Annual Meeting of the Society of Gynecologic Oncologists, Walt Disney World Dolphin Resort, February 7–11, 1998.

Kelloff G, Boone C, Crowell J, et al. Surrogate endpoint biomarkers for phase II cancer chemoprevention trials. J Cell Biochem Suppl 1994;19:1–9.

Kelloff G, Johnson J, Crowell J, et al. Approaches to the development and marketing approval of drugs that prevent cancer. Cancer Epidemiol Biomarkers Prev 1995;4:1–10.

Kelloff G, Malone W, Boone C, et al. Intermediate biomarkers of precancer and their application in chemoprevention. J Cell Biochem Suppl 1992;16G:15–21.

Littenberg B. Technology assessment in medicine. Acad Med 1992;67:424–8.

Mackerras D, Irwig L, Simpson JM, et al. Randomized double-blind trial of beta-carotene and vitamin C in women with minor cervical abnormalities. Br J Cancer 1999;79:1448–53.

Manetta A, Schubbert T, Chapman J, et al. b-Carotene treatment of cervical intraepithelial neoplasia: A Phase II study. Cancer Epidemiol Biomarkers Prev 1996;5:929–32.

Meyskens F, Jr, Graham V, Chvapil M, et al. A phase I trial of β-all-trans-retinoic acid delivered via a collagen sponge and a cervical cap for mild or moderate intraepithelial cervical neoplasia. J Natl Cancer Inst 1983;71:921–5.

Meyskens F, Jr, Surwit E, Moon T, et al. Enhancement of regression of cervical intraepithelial neoplasia II (moderate dysplasia) with topically applied all-trans-retinoic acid: A randomized trial. J Natl Cancer Inst 1994;86:539–43.

Mitchell M, Cantor S, Brookner C, et al. Screening for squamous intraepithelial lesions with fluorescence spectroscopy. Obstet Gynecol 1999;94:889–96.

Mitchell M, Hittelman W, Hong W, et al. The natural history of cervical intraepithelial neoplasia: An argument for intermediate endpoint biomarkers. Cancer Epidemiol Biomarkers Prev 1994;3:619–26.

Mitchell M, Hittelman W, Lotan R, et al. Chemoprevention trials and surrogate end point biomarkers in the cervix. Cancer 1995a;76 (Suppl 10):1956–77.

Mitchell M, Hittelman W, Lotan R, et al. Chemoprevention trials in the cervix: Design, feasibility, and recruitment. J Cell Biochem Suppl 1995b;23:104–12.

Mitchell M, Tortolero-Luna G, Lee J, et al. Phase I dose de-escalation trial of α-difluoromethylornithine in patients with grade 3 cervical intraepithelial neoplasia. Clin Cancer Res 1998;4:303–10.

O'Shaughnessy JA, Kelloff GJ, Gordon GB, et al. Treatment and prevention of intraepithelial neoplasia: an important target for accelerated new drug development. Recommendations of the American Association for Cancer Research Task Force on the Treatment and Prevention of Intraepithelial Neoplasia. Clin Cancer Res 2002;8:314-46.

Oster G. Natural history of cervical intraepithelial neoplasia: a critical review. Int J Gynecol Cancer 1993;12:186–92.

Parkin DM, Pisani P, Ferlay J. Estimates of the worldwide incidence of 25 major cancers in 1990. Int J Cancer 1999;80:827-41.

Pietrantoni M, Taylor D, Gercel-Taylor C, et al. The regulation of HPV oncogene expression by folic acid in cultured human cervical cells. J Soc Gynecol Invest 1995;2:228.

Romney S, Basu J, Vermund S, et al. Plasma reduced and total ascorbic acid in human uterine cervix dysplasias and cancer. Ann N Y Acad Sci 1987;498:132–43.

Romney S, Dwyer A, Slagle S, et al. Chemoprevention of cervix cancer: Phase I-II. A feasibility study involving the topical vaginal administration of retinyl acetate gel. Gynecol Oncol 1985;20:109–19.

Romney S, Ho G, Palan P, et al. Effects of beta-carotene and other factors on outcome of cervical dysplasia and human papillomavirus infection. Gynecol Oncol 1997;65:483–92.

Ruffin M, Bailey J, Underwood D, et al. The potential use of HPV copy number and E6/E7 expression as biomarkers in cervical dysplasia [abstract 2850]. Proc Amer Assoc Cancer Res 1999;40.

Sox HC, Blatt MA, Higgins MC, et al. Medical decision making. Boston: Butterworth-Heinemann, 1988

Sporn M. Chemoprevention of cancer. Lancet 1993;342:1211–13.

Surwit E, Graham V, Droegemueller W, et al. Evaluation of topically applied trans-retinoic acid in the treatment of cervical intraepithelial lesions. Am J Obstet Gynecol 1982;143:821–3.

Swanson GM, Ward AJ. Recruiting minorities into clinical trials: Toward a participant-friendly system. JNCI 1995;87:1747-59.

Weiner S, Surwit E, Graham V, Jr MF. A phase I trial of topically applied trans-retinoic acid in cervical dysplasia-clinical efficacy. Invest New Drugs 1986;4:241–4.

Woodworth C, Notario V, DiPaolo J. Transforming growth factors ß1 and 2 transcriptionally regulate human papillomavirus (HPV) type 16 early gene expression in HPV-immortalized human genital epithelial cells. J Virol 1990;64:4767–75.

Yeomans-Kinney A, Richards C, Vernon S, et al. The effect of physician recommendation on enrollment in the breast cancer chemoprevention trial. Prev Med 1998;27:713-9.

Chapter 12

Preventive Human Papillomavirus Vaccines

John T. Schiller, Ph.D. and Douglas R. Lowy, Ph.D.

Laboratory of Cellular Oncology, National Cancer Institute, NIH

INTRODUCTION

Prophylactic vaccines against infectious diseases are among the most successful and cost effective public health interventions ever devised. They have led to the eradication of small pox and will likely soon lead to the eradication of polio. Prophylactic vaccination has also effectively controlled other infectious diseases, including rubella, mumps, tetanus, and diphtheria (Ulmer and Liu, 2002). Perhaps the most important implication of the establishment of sexually transmitted HPV infection as the central cause of cervical cancer (Bosch et al., 2002) is the potential for cervical cancer prevention through prophylactic vaccination against the oncogenic HPVs. This chapter will focus on the development of vaccines to prevent infection and neoplastic disease by oncogenic HPV types that infect the genital tract. However, similar vaccines are being developed to prevent infection by the non-oncogenic types that are largely responsible for genital warts.

The development of prophylactic HPV vaccines has paralleled in many ways the earlier development of the successful recombinant hepatitis B (HBV) vaccine. A substantial fraction of hepatocellular carcinomas is caused by persistent HBV infection. Since HBV cannot be efficiently grown in culture, the developers of the hepatitis B vaccine used recombinant DNA technologies to produce empty shells of the virus composed of the HBV surface protein in a lipid bilayer. These particles induce high titers of HBV neutralizing antibodies in vaccinees that prevent acute hepatitis and chronic HBV infection (Hilleman, 2001). Recent studies indicate that childhood vaccination in Taiwan has led to a dramatic reduction in hepatocellular carcinoma in children in that country. Large reductions in adult liver cancer rates are expected in the future (Kao and Chen, 2002).

The current HPV prophylactic vaccine candidates are also based on virus-like particles (VLPs) produced using recombinant DNA technology (Schiller, 1999). As with the HBV and other prophylactic vaccines, they are based on the principle of inducing virion-neutralizing antibodies to prevent or control virus infection (Robbins et al., 1995). Will a VLP-based HPV prophylactic vaccine be as effective as the hepatitis B subunit vaccine? Although the results outlined below are certainly encouraging, it is difficult to predict the long-term outcome of HPV prophylactic vaccination based on the HBV model. This is because of the unique life cycle of the papilloma-viruses, as detailed in Chapters 3 and 4. In contrast to HBV, HPV infections are normally confined to stratified squamous epithelial surfaces, with no systemic viremia (Stubenrauch and Laimins, 1999). Therefore, to prevent or control the sexually transmitted HPV infections that cause cervical cancer, sufficient virion neutralizing antibodies presumably have to reach the mucosal surface of the female genital tract. There is no successful vaccine against a sexually transmitted infection on which to base prophylactic HPV vaccine development.

1 PRECLINICAL STUDIES

Live attenuated viruses have been successfully developed as prophylactic vaccines for several viral diseases, including polio, measles, mumps and rubella, and vaccines from inactivated wild type virus was successfully developed for polio. However, these approaches were not viable options for an HPV vaccine. First, the viruses cannot be efficiently propagated in cultured cells (Hagensee and Galloway, 1993). Second, the viral genome contains oncogenes (zur Hausen, 1999). The possibility of vaccine-induced carcinogenesis would preclude the use of a vaccine based either on a live attenuated virus or inactivated virions intended for use in healthy young women, the vast majority of whom are not destined to develop cervical cancer in their lifetime. Therefore, HPV vaccine developers turned to a subunit approach. Initial attempts to develop vaccines in animal models based on denatured forms of the major capsid protein L1, or fragments thereof, were unsuccessful, because the antibodies they induced were unable, or weakly able, to prevent virus infection (Pilacinski et al., 1986). However, in the early 1990s it was discovered that L1, in the absence of all other papillomavirus proteins, would spontaneously assemble into VLPs that were morphologically and antigenically similar to authentic virions (Kirnbauer et al., 1992; Hagensee et al., 1993; Kirnbauer et al., 1993; Zhou et al., 1993) (Figure 1). Most importantly, injection of the L1 VLPs in experimental animals induced high titers of antibodies that prevented infection of cultured cells by the corresponding viral type. Denaturation of the VLPs abrogated their ability to induce virus-neutralizing antibodies, confirming that the virion surface epitopes recognized by neutralizing antibodies are conformation dependent. The L2 minor capsid protein was shown to co-assemble with L1 into VLPs with the same 1:30 ratio seen in authentic viruses, but the titers of neutralizing antibodies induced by L1/L2 VLPs were no greater than the titers induced by L1 only VLPs (Lowy et al., 1994). Therefore, most subsequent prophylactic vaccine development has centered on L1 VLPs.

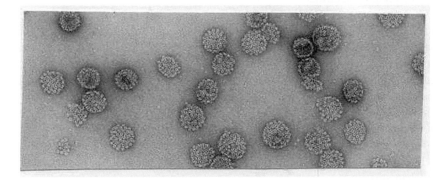

Figure 1. HPV16 L1 VLPs purified form recombinant baculovirus infected insect cells.

Since more than a dozen genital HPV types are believed to be causative agents of cervical cancer (Bosch et al., 1995), it was important to evaluate whether neutralizing antibodies raised after VLP vaccination were type-specific or able to cross-neutralize infection by other types. The results of in vitro infection assays using authentic virions or pseudovirions, in which the virion shell carries a plasmid with a marker gene, predict that protection will be largely type-specific (Roden et al., 1996; Unckell et al., 1997; White et al., 1998; Giroglou et al., 2001). A degree of cross-neutralization was detected in some assays for certain closely related types, e.g., HPV 16 with HPV 31 or 33, and HPV 18 with HPV 45. However, homologous neutralizing titers were generally at least 50-fold higher than cross-neutralizing titers. It is unclear whether these cross-neutralizing titers are high enough to produce significant cross-protection in people. Fortunately, the existence of serologic subtypes within a specific genotype does not appear to be a concern for VLP vaccination, at least with regard to HPV 16, the most prevalent oncogenic HPV type (Pastrana et al., 2001).

Prophylactic vaccination with L1 VLPs produced excellent protection from experimental challenge in three animal PV models: cottontail rabbit papillomavirus (CRPV) infection of domestic rabbits, canine oral papillomavirus (COPV) infection of dogs, and bovine papillomavirus type 4 (BPV 4) infection of cattle (Breitburd et al., 1995; Suzich et al., 1995; Christensen et al., 1996; Kirnbauer et al., 1996). In each model, the virus was applied to scarified skin or oral mucosa, in order to expose the basal epithelial cells to the virus. Type-specific protection from high dose challenge was seen after low dose vaccination (low microgram amounts) even in the absence of adjuvant or even when vaccine-specific antibody titers were low. Protection from experimental viral challenge could be passively transferred to naïve animals via VLP immune sera, indicating that neutralizing antibodies alone can mediate protection.

No cross-type protection has been observed after VLP vaccination. In addition, VLP vaccination did not induce regression of preestablished viral papillomas. So, although the animal studies indicated that the L1 VLPs were promising prophylactic vaccines, there was no indication that they could act therapeutically. This was the expected result, since intact L1 is not found on the surface of infected cells, and therefore is not subject to antibody-mediated mechanisms of immune regression. Also, L1 is not expressed in the basal cells of the stratified squamous epithelium in which the viral infection is maintained (Stubenrauch and Laimins, 1999). Therefore, these cells would not be directly targeted by L1-specific cell-mediated immune mechanisms.

L2 proteins or peptides are a potentially interesting alternative to L1 VLPs for a prophylactic vaccine. In contrast to L1 VLPs, HPV L2s induce the production of broadly cross-neutralizing antibodies in animal models (Kawana et al., 1999; Roden et al., 2000; Kawana et al., 2001). Antibodies to the L2s of HPV 16, HPV 18, and HPV 6 are each able to cross-neutralize the other two heterologous types, and short peptides containing cross-neutralizing epitopes have been identified. It is interesting that cross-neutralizing antibodies are not induced when L2 is presented in its normal context of an L1/L2 VLP. Either the relevant L2 epitopes are not exposed on the surface of the VLPs or they are subdominant to the L1 epitopes, perhaps because they are more widely dispersed and/or at lower copy number than L1 in the VLPs. The titers of neutralizing antibodies induced by the current L2 vaccines are much lower than the neutralizing titers induced by L1 VLPs, approximately 50-fold lower for homologous type neutralization and 500-fold lower for heterologous type neutralization. These titers may not be sufficient to induce long-term protection from genital tract HPV infection. A challenge for the future will be to devise vaccines that induce higher titer cross-neutralizing antibodies to L2.

2   CLINICAL STUDIES

Three groups have produced clinical grade L1 VLPs for oncogenic types and have tested them in early phase trials. VLPs generated in recombinant baculovirus infected insect cells have been tested by Medimmune, in collaboration with GlaxoSmithKline (GSK), and by the U.S. National Cancer Institute (NCI), while *Sacchromyces cerevisiae* (bread yeast) derived VLPs have been tested by Merck. Published phase I/II trials and meeting reports of unpublished trials indicate that the VLP vaccines consistently induce high titers of virion antibodies after intramuscular injection in young women (and in the few young men examined) (Brown et al., 2001; Evans et al., 2001; Harro et al., 2001; Koutsky et al., 2002). Three injections of 10-50 micrograms of VLPs, usually on the 0, 1 or 2, and 6 month schedule developed for the HBV vaccine, produced geometric mean VLP-specific serum IgG titers that were approximately 50-fold higher in vaccinated naïve individuals than the mean VLP IgG serum titers induced after natural HPV infection. There has been almost 100% seroconversion after vaccination, with relatively little variance from the mean titer. One phase I study evaluating adjuvants reported that antibody titers were at least as high without adjuvant as with alum or MF59 (a squalene emulsion adjuvant) (Harro et al., 2001). The long-term durability of the serum IgG response to vaccination has not been reported. However, the three-fold drop in titer observed six months after the third VLP injection without adjuvant in an NCI phase II trial is on par with the results seen with other subunit vaccines (our unpublished results). The vaccines were well tolerated. No serious vaccine-related adverse events have been reported in the trials. Local pain at the injection site was the most common side effect, most notably when an alum-based adjuvant was used, but the reactogenicity was not higher than that reported for vaccinees receiving adjuvant alone.

Since the objective of the HPV prophylactic vaccines under development is to prevent or reduce HPV infection at the cervix, it is important to evaluate the VLP-specific antibody levels at the cervix. The female genital tract is somewhat unusual for a mucosal tissue in that secretory IgA does not dominate the antibody response. A considerable proportion of the antibody in genital tract secretions is IgG, much of which is believed to be transudated from the serum (Mestecky and Russell, 2000). Therefore, the induction of serum IgG after parenteral VLP immunization should result in VLP-specific IgG in cervical secretions, although the vaccine would not be expected to generate specific secretory IgA (Bouvet et al., 2002). Consistent with this prediction, an early study demonstrated readily detectable VLP-specific IgG in cervico-vaginal lavage samples after intramuscular VLP vaccination of macaques (Lowe et al., 1997). A recently published study in young women detected specific IgG in Weck-cell samples of cervical secretions after intramuscular vaccination with HPV 16 VLPs without adjuvant (Nardelli-Haefliger et al., 2003). In women taking oral contraceptives, the VLP antibody titers were relatively constant and approximately 10-fold lower than the serum titers. In women with normal menstrual cycles, there was a consistent 10-fold drop in mucosal titers around the time of ovulation. The drop in VLP-specific IgG titers paralleled the drop in total cervical IgG at the time of ovulation. This raises the possibility that the vaccine might be more effective in women taking oral contraceptives.

An important proof-of-concept efficacy trial was recently reported (Koutsky et al., 2002). The investigators evaluated approximately 1500 young women who had been randomized to be vaccinated three times (0, 2, and 6 months) with 40 micrograms of HPV16 VLPs in alum or with placebo. The vaccinated women, who were HPV16 DNA negative and HPV16 VLP seronegative at enrollment and after a complete vaccination series, were periodically evaluated for acquisition of persistent genital tract HPV16 infection as the primary end point. Persistent infection was operationally defined as genital tract HPV16 DNA positivity at two consecutive visits four or more months apart. All cases of persistent HPV16 infection and all cases of HPV16-associated cervical dysplasia occurred in the placebo group (Table 1). These are certainly excellent efficacy results, but there are two caveats. The first is that relatively short-term protection was measured; the mean length of follow-up was 17 months. Second, it is unclear whether the study adequately evaluated protection in ovulating women. The percentage of the study women taking oral contraceptives was not reported, although it is likely to be high in a sexually active group of U.S. women with the reported low pregnancy rate.

Table 1. HPV16 VLP Vaccine Proof of Concept Efficacy Trial*

	Placebo	HPV16 VLP
Number	765	768
HPV16 DNA Pos.		
Persistent:	41	0
Transient:	27	6
CINs		
HPV16 DNA Pos.:	9	0
Other Types:	22	22

*Data from Koutsky et al., 2002

HPV16 DNA was detected at a single time in 6 vaccine recipients, compared with 27 placebo recipients, but none of these women had cervical intraepithelial neoplasia. It is unclear whether the single time HPV detections represent transient new infections, transient detection of previously acquired latent infection, sporadic detection of lower genital tract infections, contamination from an infected partner, or a combination of these possibilities. Equal numbers of HPV16-independent cervical neoplasia (CIN) were found in the HPV16 VLP and placebo control groups. The results suggest that VLP vaccines can produce excellent type-specific protection, but probably will not afford appreciable cross-protection against other types, consistent with the type-restricted neutralizing activity of VLP antisera in in vitro assays.

Given the encouraging clinical trial results to date, it is likely that Merck, GSK and the NCI will proceed with plans for larger scale efficacy trials. GSK has indicated that it plans to test a bivalent vaccine consisting of insect cell-derived HPV16 L1 and HPV18 L1 VLPs. Merck has indicated that it will test a yeast-derived tetravalent vaccine including L1 VLPs of types 6, 11, 16 and 18. It will therefore target genital warts as well as cervical cancer. It is important to note that no immunogenicity interference among the VLP types was observed in early phase trials of the tetravalent vaccine. For instance, the titers induced against HPV16 in the tetravalent vaccine were at least as high as the titers induced by the monovalent HPV16 VLP vaccine (see http://www.IPVSoc.org for 19th International Papillomavirus Conference abstract #O51). Each trial will enroll more than 10,000 women, and the women will be followed for several years for acquisition of type-specific HPV infection and cervical neoplasia. The Merck and GSK studies will be multi-centric, involving sites in North America, South America, Europe, and perhaps South East Asia. The NCI trial will be conducted in Guanacaste province, Costa Rica, the site of a large natural history study of HPV and cervical cancer.

The end point that should be required for licensure of the prophylactic HPV VLP vaccines is currently a hotly debated subject. Although the ultimate goal of the vaccines is to prevent cervical cancer, it is unethical to allow women to develop cancer in clinical trials with active follow-up. In addition, it would take more than a decade to accrue a sufficient number of cancer cases, even if the trial size was very large. High-grade cervical dysplasia (CIN 3) is an attractive surrogate endpoint since it is universally recognized as the immediate precursor lesion to cervical cancer. However, CIN 3 is a relatively infrequent outcome of oncogenic HPV infection and typically develops many years after initial HPV infection (Schiffman and Burk, 1997). Using CIN 3 as the primary end point for vaccine efficacy would necessitate a large and relatively long-term efficacy trial. It is also possible that standards of routine care will evolve during the course of the trials to the point where it will no longer be ethically permissible to follow persistent low-grade lesions to CIN 3, if they are positive for an oncogenic HPV. CIN 1 is the most frequent and earliest neoplastic manifestation of oncogenic HPV infection. A CIN 1 clinical end point could be reached with a rather modest size trial of short duration. However, most CIN 1 resolves spontaneously, and there is some question of whether it is on the causal pathway to cervical cancer (Kiviat and Koutsky, 1996). CIN 2 is an intermediate category that contains a mixture of CIN 3/cancer precursors and lesions that are more similar to CIN 1, in that they are destined to resolve spontaneously. Because of its intermediate nature, this is also a histologic classification for which it is difficult to reach consensus among pathologists (Stoler and Schiffman, 2001). A consensus panel assembled by the U.S. Food and Drug Administration has recommended that CIN 2-3 be used as the clinical endpoint for licensure, in part because these clinical entities are normally treated by ablative surgery (http://www.fda.gov/ohrms/dockets/ac/ 01/minutes/3805ml.pdf). Study sizes for the efficacy trials outlined above appear to be calculated with demonstration of protection of HPV16 induced CIN 2-3 in mind.

There has also been considerable discussion of using persistent type-specific HPV DNA as a virologic endpoint for licensure. Persistent infection by an oncogenic HPV, especially HPV16, is the most important risk factor for progression to high grade cervical dysplasia and cancer (Ho et al., 1998; Nobbenhuis et al., 1999). Measurements of HPV DNA are also more reliable and reproducible across investigators than are cytologic or histologic measures of HPV-induced disease. However, oncogenic HPV infections, even persistent ones, are usually asymptomatic and are not a treatable disease per se. Also, the length of time that an infection must persist to place it at high risk for progression is not well established (Einstein and Burk, 2001). For practical reasons, the planned trials will likely use six to twelve months as the operational definition of persistence. If interim analyses in the upcoming large-scale efficacy trials point to a vaccine efficacy against persistent infection of close to one hundred percent, then it is possible that accelerated approval of the vaccines based on this end point will be sought. It is difficult to predict how this request would be viewed by national regulatory agencies.

3   IMPLEMENTATION ISSUES

The increasing likelihood that the VLP-based vaccines will prove to be safe and effective at preventing cervical HPV infection, and thereby cervical cancer, should prompt increasing attention to issues of HPV vaccine implementation. Several concerns apply to implementation in all settings, while others are more relevant to developed countries or developing countries, respectively. As described below, adequately addressing some of these issues will likely require further advances in vaccine technology, while addressing others may require public health information campaigns.

3.1 General Issues

Three issues will be important for HPV prophylactic vaccine implementation in all settings. The first is the acceptance of the vaccine by the general public. It is difficult to predict whether parents will be willing to have their adolescent or preadolescent girls, and perhaps boys (see below), vaccinated against a sexually transmitted infection (STI) (Zimet et al., 2000). None of the current vaccines are aimed at preventing an STI. Acceptance might be increased if the stigma generally associated with STIs were removed for genital HPV infections. However, the high prevalence of genital HPV infection in young people with relatively low-risk sexual behaviors is not widely appreciated (Mays et al., 2000). This is an area in which public awareness needs to be increased. It might be advantageous to emphasize cancer prevention, rather than STI prevention, especially since the infections are asymptomatic. However, the sexually transmitted nature of the disease cannot be ignored. There must be a rationale for vaccinating prior to the onset of sexual activity. Also, a rationale for vaccinating boys against cervical cancer must be provided, assuming that they will also be vaccinated. Acceptance might also be reduced by the fact that the primary benefits of the vaccine, prevention of cervical cancer, will be restricted to a small percentage of vaccinees and usually not realized until decades after receiving the vaccine. This is in contrast to the HBV vaccine, which prevents both an acute disease, viral hepatitis, in the short term and a cancer, hepatocellular carcinoma, in the long term.

The second general implementation issue is the development of vaccination programs for adolescents or preadolescents. No widely implemented public heath program involves multiple clinic visits by this age group. Even in the most developed countries, it will be a formidable task to establish vaccination programs that, according to current protocols, would require three clinic visits for intramuscular injections over a six-month period. It might be possible to partially overcome this problem by administering the priming dose(s) as part of the infant immunization program, followed by adolescent boosting. A particularly attractive variation of this approach would be to boost adolescents with an oral, nasal or aerosol vaccine that could be administered easily in a school setting (see below for a discussion of possible strategies). However, it would take at least 15 years to demonstrate the effectiveness of such a strategy, and it is unclear whether vaccine manufacturers will be interested in conducting such long-term studies. Incorporating the entire series of injections in infant vaccination programs is even more problematic, as the vaccine would have to generate long-term protection (for decades) without boosting. This seems unlikely if vaccine efficacy is based solely on maintenance of antibody levels sufficient to prevent initial infection of the cervix.

The third general issue is whether to vaccinate only girls or both sexes. One would assume that the greatest impact would be achieved by vaccinating both sexes if the goal is to decrease the prevalence of an STI. However, the transmission dynamics of genital HPV infections are poorly understood, so the impact of vaccinating one versus both sexes is difficult to estimate (Garnett and Waddell, 2000; Hughes et al., 2002). The decision of who to vaccinate may depend upon the setting. It is easy to justify concentrating vaccination efforts on girls in settings with limited resources, since women bear most of the HPV-associated cancer burden, especially in developing countries without effective Pap screening programs. Vaccination of both sexes might be justified in developed countries with sufficient resources. However, it is important to note that there is currently no evidence that the vaccine is effective in men. After intramuscular injection of an HPV VLP vaccine, one would expect similar immunogenicity in men and women, but it is possible that the resulting serum antibodies may be less effective at preventing infection in men. This is because there is not extensive transudation of serum IgG in the male genitalia, as there is at the cervix (Mestecky and Russell, 2000). Serum antibodies could reach the site of infection in men through direct exudation at sites of trauma that disrupt the basement membrane. However, it is not known what percentage of transmission to men involves this type of trauma. The recent demonstration of efficacy in women, but not men, for a prophylactic herpes simplex gD vaccine supports the possibility of differential efficacy in the two sexes (Stanberry et al., 2002).

Vaccination of women might also be more effective at preventing transmission than vaccinating men. The female genital tract is bathed in mucus, which in vaccinated women should contain virion-neutralizing antibodies. Therefore, most of the virus shed by vaccinated women with pre-existing or breakthrough infections might be rendered non-infectious. Note however that this possibility may be difficult to demonstrate experimentally, due to the lack of an assay that can detect relatively small numbers of infectious virions. It is uncertain where the majority of infectious virus originates in men. To the extent that it is shed from cornified skin of the external genitalia, the virions would not be expected to come in contact with neutralizing antibodies in vaccinated men with breakthrough infections. Consequently, vaccination of men might have less impact on transmission rates than vaccination of women. This might be especially true during the initial years after introduction of the vaccine, where many individuals with pre-existing infection would presumably be vaccinated.

3.2 Developed Country Issues

Certain vaccine implementation issues will be unique to developed countries, because they have Pap screening programs that function to effectively reduce cervical cancer risk. An effective vaccine would decrease the cost effectiveness of current Pap screening programs, since fewer malignant and premalignant cervical lesions would be identified. However, caution will be needed when considering possible changes in the screening policies in response to an effective vaccine (Hughes et al., 2002). It is difficult to imagine that the current vaccine candidates would be as effective as a good Pap screening program. Cervical cancer rates have decreased by more than 80% in U.S. since the implementation of routine Pap screening, despite an increase in STIs during this period (http://cancer.gov/cancerinfo/pdq/screening/cervical/healthprofessional). The current vaccines alone will almost certainly not be 80% effective at reducing cervical cancer rates. As noted above, they are likely to be type-specific and so will only target cervical cancers caused by HPV16 and 18, approximately 70-80% of cases. But they are unlikely to be 100% effective against these targeted types and vaccine coverage will not be 100%. They are also not expected to reduce the cancer risk of women with pre-existing infections (Breitburd et al., 1995; Suzich et al., 1995; Christensen et al., 1996; Kirnbauer et al., 1996).

It is therefore important to consider the potential negative impact of a licensed HPV vaccine on compliance with existing Pap screening programs. Vaccinated women could have reduced compliance because of misconceptions of the overall effectiveness of the vaccine at preventing cervical cancer and/or its effectiveness against established infections. For example, a substantial number of sexually active women, many of whom have already encountered HPV16 and/or 18, may choose to be vaccinated, despite the fact that there is little chance that vaccination will decrease their cervical cancer risk. Will they understand the need to continue their regular pelvic examinations now that they have been "vaccinated against cervical cancer"? It will be important to inform all vaccinated women that they are still at risk for developing cervical cancer and therefore should continue to participate in Pap screening programs. It may be difficult to implement a balanced public awareness campaign that effectively promotes both vaccination and continued compliance with Pap screening. It may be necessary to mount public sector efforts to emphasize the continued need for pelvic exams, since vaccine manufacturers will have a keen interest in promoting the virtues of vaccination, but not the virtues of continued screening.

The most important benefit of the current vaccines in developed countries would be the prevention of HPV16- and 18-associated cancers that are missed in screening programs. In addition, an effective vaccine could substantially reduce the cost of Pap screening programs, even if there are no changes in the screening policies or compliance rates (Hughes et al., 2002). This is because a substantial proportion of the cost of these programs is devoted to follow-up of abnormal smears, which can include repeat testing, referral to colposcopy, cervical biopsy, and ablative therapy. A large fraction of these abnormalities is caused by HPV16 and 18, and the current vaccines would be expected to greatly diminish this subset of lesions. The physical and psychological burdens associated with follow-up of cervical abnormalities would also be correspondingly reduced.

3.3   Developing Country Issues

The potential for decreasing cervical cancer deaths through HPV vaccination is greatest in developing countries, because most lack an effective Pap screening program and consequently many have high cervical cancer rates. However, the anticipated high cost of vaccination programs based on the current vaccine candidates is likely to be a major deterrent to widespread use in many low resource settings. The vaccines will be expensive to manufacture since they are multivalent subunit vaccines, based on highly purified antigens that are produced in cultured cells. The monovalent HBV vaccine produced in yeast is now available in developing countries for as low as $0.30 per dose. However, this is still too expensive for wide-spread distribution in many poor countries that could benefit from its use (Kao and Chen, 2002). Even with multi-tiered pricing, it seems unlikely that the polyvalent HPV vaccines under current development will be available at this price in the near future. The vaccines will also be expensive to administer, since they require three intramuscular injections and will likely require a cold chain for distribution. Establishing a public health program specifically designed to reach adolescents will also be expensive.

Access to an HPV prophylactic vaccine by the poor women of the world most in need of it could be facilitated in two ways. The first is to convince charitable organizations, such as the Gates Foundation or Rockefeller Foundation, to purchase large lots of the current vaccines, once they are licensed, for testing and eventual general distribution in low resource settings. The second is to develop second-generation vaccines that could be produced and delivered at lower costs. The latter approach is attractive because it could potentially lead to self-sustaining vaccination programs in countries of intermediate development, such as India, Mexico, Brazil, and China, where a large percentage of world's cervical cancer deaths occur

(Parkin et al., 2001). However, this approach has two liabilities. One is a potential lack of corporate sponsorship if the current vaccines become widely used in developed countries. The second-generation vaccines would therefore probably have to be developed as public sector initiatives. The second is that, while there are several potentially attractive strategies, none has been developed to the point of clinical trials. It is probably worthwhile to pursue both approaches.

Production costs of the vaccines could in theory be reduced using several strategies, for instance by VLP production in plants (Mason et al., 2002), use of live L1 recombinant bacterial vectors (Nardelli-Haefliger et al., 1997) or production of an L1 naked DNA vaccine (Donnelly et al., 1996; Leder et al., 2001; Liu et al., 2001). The costs of distribution could be substantially reduced by administration by oral ingestion or via a nasal or aerosol spray. Two attractive strategies that might have both low production and distribution costs would be oral delivery of crude extracts of VLP-producing bread yeast or transgenic plant, perhaps also expressing a mucosal adjuvant, or oral delivery of live enteric bacteria that express VLPs. The manufacturing processes needed to generate these vaccines would be modest, raising the possibility for local or regional production in developing countries. There have been some encouraging preclinical developments of at least some aspects of these strategies (Nardelli-Haefliger et al., 1997; Cook et al., 1999; Gerber et al., 2001). However, additional technical development and clinical assessment will be required before these approaches can be considered promising vaccine candidates for human use.

A second major concern for developing country implementation is the long lag between the time of vaccination and realization of a public health benefit from the vaccination. The current vaccine will target teenagers or preteens, but since cervical cancer death rates do not peak until after age 35 (Kiviat et al., 1998), it would take at least two decades to produce a substantial reduction in cervical cancer deaths. In competition for severely limited health care resources, it might prove difficult for public heath administrators in many developing countries to support an expensive intervention program with such a delayed benefit. A combined prophylactic/ therapeutic vaccine could address this issue, if it would induce regression of established premalignant lesions in older women. Such a vaccine could provide the best combination of short-term benefit and long-term impact. It could be used for mass immunization of sexually active as well as virgin women. Compared to a strictly prophylactic vaccine, a combined vaccine would therefore have a greater potential of having an immediate impact on HPV 16 and 18 transmission rates and overall prevalence in the population.

There are a number of candidates for a combined therapeutic/prophylactic vaccine. Chimeric VLPs are one of the most advanced candidates. They consist of polypeptides of early viral genes incorporated into VLPs as fusions with L1 or L2 (Muller et al., 1997; Greenstone et al., 1998; Liu et al., 2002). Chimeric VLPs can retain the ability to induce neutralizing antibodies and can also efficiently induce cell-mediated immune responses to the additional polypeptides. Therapeutic trials targeting high-grade cervical dysplasias with an HPV16 L1-E7 chimeric VLP are currently being conducted by Medigene (http://www.medigene.de/englisch/projekte.php). HPV pseudovirions, in which the target early viral gene is incorporated in the VLPs as a DNA plasmid, is another potential combined vaccine (Roden et al., 1996; Unckell et al., 1997; Touze and Coursaget, 1998; Shi et al., 2001). However, this approach is currently limited by the inability to produce the pseudovirions by a process that could lend itself to large-scale GMP manufacturing. A third alternative is to simply combine the current VLP vaccines with early viral protein or peptide-based vaccines being developed as strictly therapeutic HPV vaccines. One example is the Mycobacterium heat shock protein-E7 fusion protein under clinical development by Stressgen to treat cervical and anal dysplasia (Hunt, 2001). These combination vaccines could be tested without further technical development, but this approach has the disadvantage of requiring the manufacture of two distinct vaccine components.

Discussion of the rather extensive body of work on therapeutic HPV vaccines is presented in Chapter 13, and has also been addressed in a number of recent reviews (Da Silva et al., 2001; Gissmann et al., 2001; Davidson et al., 2002; Stanley, 2002). However, it is important to note that there is generally less optimism that an effective therapeutic HPV vaccine is on the horizon than that there will soon be a licensed prophylactic HPV vaccine. This is in line with the great success of prophylactic vaccines against other viruses, but very limited success of therapeutic vaccines against other chronic viral infections or tumors (Vandepapeliere, 2002). Nevertheless, HPV-induced premalignant neoplasias of the cervix, and of other genital sites, are very attractive diseases to target for therapeutic vaccine intervention. They selectively retain and express viral protein targets (E6 and E7), their natural history is reasonably well understood, their progress can be followed non-invasively, and the lesions are routinely identified in cervical cytology screening programs. Suffice it to say that the insights gained in therapeutic vaccine studies will inform the further development of combined prophylactic/therapeutic vaccines.

CONCLUSION

Exceptional progress has been made in HPV prophylactic vaccine development in the ten years since the discovery that papillomavirus L1 capsid proteins can self-assemble into VLPs that induce high titers of neutralizing antibodies. The uniformly encouraging results of recent clinical trials support the optimistic view that HPV VLPs will prove to be generally safe and effective at preventing oncogenic HPV infection and may be approved for general distribution within five years. If so, HPV VLP vaccines could follow the HBV particle vaccines as the second vaccine to successfully prevent a major virus-induced cancer. However, the record of hepatitis B immunization programs in the 20 years since it became available should be viewed as a cautionary tale with regard to the prospective implementation of prophylactic HPV vaccines. Despite the WHO recommendation that hepatitis B vaccination be incorporated into routine infant and childhood immunization programs, it has been introduced into only 130 of 216 countries, and is underutilized in many of these (Kao and Chen, 2002). As detailed above, the current HPV vaccine candidates will almost certainly have greater implementation hurdles to overcome than do the hepatitis B vaccines. It is reasonable to increase efforts to devise solutions to the expected distribution problems of a prophylactic HPV vaccine.

REFERENCES

Bosch FX, Lorincz A, Munoz N, et al. The causal relation between human papillomavirus and cervical cancer. J Clin Pathol 2002; 55: 244-65.

Bosch FX, Manos MM, Munoz N, et al. Prevalence of human papillomavirus in cervical cancer: a worldwide prospective. J Nat Cancer Inst 1995; 87: 796-802.

Bouvet JP, Decroix N, Pamonsinlapatham P. Stimulation of local antibody production: parenteral or mucosal vaccination? Trends Immunol 2002; 23: 209-13.

Breitburd F, Kirnbauer R, Hubbert NL, et al. Immunization with virus-like particles from cottontail rabbit papillomavirus (CRPV) can protect against experimental CRPV infection. J Virol 1995; 69: 3959-63.

Brown DR, Bryan JT, Schroeder JM, et al. Neutralization of human papillomavirus type 11 (HPV-11) by serum from women vaccinated with yeast-derived HPV-11 L1 virus-like particles: correlation with competitive radioimmunoassay titer. J Infect Dis 2001; 184:1183-6.

Christensen ND, Reed CA, Cladel NM, et al. Immunization with virus-like particles induces long-term protection of rabbits against challenge with cottontail rabbit papillomaviruses. J Virol 1996; 70: 960-5.

Cook JC, Joyce JG, George HA, et al. Purification of virus-like particles of recombinant human papillomavirus type 11 major capsid protein L1 from Saccharomyces cerevisiae. Protein Expr Purif 1999; 17: 477-84.

Da Silva DM, Eiben GL, Fausch SC, et al. Cervical cancer vaccines: emerging concepts and developments. J Cell Physiol 2001; 186: 169-82.

Davidson EJ, Kitchener HC, Stern PL. The use of vaccines in the prevention and treatment of cervical cancer. Clin Oncol (R Coll Radiol) 2002; 14: 193-200.

Donnelly JJ, Martinez D, Jansen KU, et al. Protection against papillomavirus with a polynucleotide vaccine. J Infect Dis 1996; 173: 314-20.

Einstein MH, Burk RD. Persistent human papillomavirus infection: definitions and clincial implications. Papillomavirus Reports 2001; 12: 119-23.

Evans TG, Bonnez W, Rose RC, et al. A Phase 1 study of a recombinant virus-like particle vaccine against human papillomavirus type 11 in healthy adult volunteers. J Infect Dis 2001; 183: 1485-93.

Garnett GP, Waddell HC. Public health paradoxes and the epidemiological impact of an HPV vaccine. J Clin Virol 2000; 19: 101-11.

Gerber S, Lane C, Brown DM, et al. Human papillomavirus virus-like particles are efficient oral immunogens when coadministered with Escherichia coli heat-labile enterotoxin mutant R192G or CpG DNA. J Virol 2001; 75: 4752-60.

Giroglou T, Sapp M, Lane C, et al. Immunological analyses of human papillomavirus capsids. Vaccine 2001; 19: 1783-93.

Gissmann L, Osen W, Muller M, et al. Therapeutic vaccines for human papillomaviruses. Intervirology 2001; 44: 167-75.

Greenstone HL, Nieland JD, de Visser KE, et al. Chimeric papillomavirus virus-like particles elicit antitumor immunity against the E7 oncoprotein in an HPV16 tumor model. Proc Natl Acad Sci USA 1998; 95: 1800-5.

Hagensee M, Galloway D. Growing human papillomaviruses and virus-like particles in the laboratory. Papillomavirus Report 1993; 4: 121-4.

Hagensee ME, Yaegashi N, Galloway DA. Self-assembly of human papillomavirus type 1 capsids by expression of the L1 protein alone or by coexpression of the L1 and L2 capsid proteins. J Virol 1993; 67: 315-22.

Harro CD, Pang YY, Roden RB, et al. Safety and immunogenicity trial in adult volunteers of a human papillomavirus 16 L1 virus-like particle vaccine. J Natl Cancer Inst 2001; 93: 284-92.

Hilleman MR. Overview of the pathogenesis, prophylaxis and therapeusis of viral hepatitis B, with focus on reduction to practical applications. Vaccine 2001; 19: 1837-48.

Ho GY, Bierman R, Beardsley L, et al. Natural history of cervicovaginal papillomavirus infection in young women. N Engl J Med 1998; 338: 423-8.

Hughes JP, Garnett GP, Koutsky L. The theoretical population-level impact of a prophylactic human papilloma virus vaccine. Epidemiology 2002; 13: 631-9.

Hunt S. Technology evaluation: HspE7, StressGen Biotechnologies Corp. Curr Opin Mol Ther 2001; 3: 413-7.

Kao JH, Chen DS. Global control of hepatitis B virus infection. Lancet Infec Dis 2002; 2: 395-403.

Kawana K, Kawana Y, Yoshikawa H, et al. Nasal immunization of mice with peptide having a cross-neutralization epitope on minor capsid protein L2 of human papillomavirus type 16 elicit systemic and mucosal antibodies. Vaccine 2001; 19: 1496-502.

Kawana K, Yoshikawa H, Taketani Y, et al. Common neutralization epitope in minor capsid protein L2 of human papillomavirus types 16 and 6. J Virol 1999; 73: 6188-90.

Kirnbauer R, Booy F, Cheng N, et al. Papillomavirus L1 major capsid protein self-assembles into virus-like particles that are highly immunogenic. Proc Natl Acad Sci USA 1992; 89: 12180-4.

Kirnbauer R, Chandrachud L, O'Neil B, et al. Virus-like particles of Bovine Papillomavirus type 4 in prophylactic and therapeutic immunization. Virology 1996; 219: 37-44.

Kirnbauer R, Taub J, Greenstone H, et al. Efficient self-assembly of human papillomavirus type 16 L1 and L1-L2 into virus-like particles. J Virol 1993; 67: 6929-36.

Kiviat N, Koutsky LA, Paavonen J. Cervical neoplasia and other STD-related genital tract neoplasias. In: Holmes KK, Sparling PF, Mardh P.-A, et al., eds. Sexually Transmitted Diseases. New York: McGraw-Hill, 1998, 811-31.

Kiviat NB, Koutsky LA. Do our current cervical cancer control strategies still make sense? J Natl Cancer Inst 1996; 88: 317-8.

Koutsky LA, Ault KA, Wheeler CM, et al. A controlled trial of a human papillomavirus type 16 vaccine. N Engl J Med 2002; 347: 1645-51.

Leder C, Kleinschmidt JA, Wiethe C, et al. Enhancement of capsid gene expression: preparing the human papillomavirus type 16 major structural gene L1 for DNA vaccination purposes. J Virol 2001; 75: 9201-9.

Liu WJ, Zhao KN, Gao FG, et al. Polynucleotide viral vaccines: codon optimisation and ubiquitin conjugation enhances prophylactic and therapeutic efficacy. Vaccine 2001; 20: 862-9.

Liu XS, Liu WJ, Zhao KN, et al. Route of administration of chimeric BPV1 VLP determines the character of the induced immune responses. Immunol Cell Biol 2002; 80: 21-9.

Lowe RS, Brown DR, Bryan JT, et al. Human papillomavirus type 11 (HPV11) neutralizing antibodies in the serum and genital mucosal secretions of African green monkeys immunized with HPV-11 virus-like particles expressed in yeast. J Infect Dis 1997; 176: 1141-5.

Lowy DR, Kirnbauer R, Schiller JT. Genital human papillomavirus infection. Proc Natl Acad Sci USA 1994; 91: 2436-40.

Mason HS, Warzecha H, Mor T, et al. Edible plant vaccines: applications for prophylactic and therapeutic molecular medicine. Trends Mol Med 2002; 8: 324-9.

Mays RM, Zimet GD, Winston Y, et al. Human papillomavirus, genital warts, Pap smears, and cervical cancer: knowledge and beliefs of adolescent and adult women. Health Care Women Int 2000; 21: 361-74.

Mestecky J, Russell MW. Induction of mucosal immune responses in the human genital tract. FEMS Imm. and Med. Micro. 2000; 27: 351-5

Muller M, Zhou J, Reed TD, et al. Chimeric papillomavirus-like particles. Virology 1997; 234: 93-111.

Nardelli-Haefliger D, Roden RBS, Benyacoub J, et al. Human papillomavirus type 16 virus-like particles expressed in attenuated Salmonella typhimurium elicit mucosal and systemic neutralizing antibodies in mice. Infect Immun 1997; 65: 3328-36.

Nardelli-Haefliger D, Wirthner D, Schiller JT, et al. Specific antibody levels at the cervix during the menstrual cycle of women vaccinated with human papillomavirus 16 virus-like particles. J Natl Cancer Inst 2003; 95:1128-37.

Nobbenhuis MA, Walboomers JM, Helmerhorst TJ, et al. Relation of human papillomavirus status to cervical lesions and consequences for cervical-cancer screening: a prospective study. Lancet 1999; 354: 20-5.

Parkin DM, Bray F, Ferlay J, et al. Estimating the world cancer burden: Globocan 2000. Int J Cancer 2001; 94: 153-6.

Pastrana DV, Vass WC, Lowy DR, et al. An HPV 16 VLP vaccine induces human antibodies that neutralize divergent variants of HPV16. Virology 2001; 279: 361-9.

Pilacinski WP, Glassman DL, Glassman KF, et al. Immunization against bovine papillomavirus infection. In Papillomaviruses: Ciba Foundation Symposium 120, pp. 136-156. Wiley, Chichester: Wiley, 1986.

Robbins JB, Schneerson R, Szu SC. Hypothesis: serum IgG antibody is sufficient to confer protection against infectious diseases by inactivating the inoculum. J Infect Dis 1995; 171: 1387-98.

Roden RB, Yutzy WI, Fallon R, et al. Minor capsid protein of human genital papilloma-viruses contains subdominant, cross-neutralizing epitopes. Virology 2000; 270: 254-7.

Roden RBS, Greenstone HL, Kirnbauer R, et al. In vitro generation and type-specific neutralization of a human papillomavirus type 16 virion pseudotype. J Virol 1996; 70: 5875-83.

Schiffman MH, Burk RD. Human Papillomaviruses. In: Evans AS, Kaslow R, eds. Viral infections in humans. New York: Plenum Medical Book Company, 1997, pp. 983-1023.

Schiller JT. Papillomavirus-like particle vaccines for cervical cancer. Mol Med Today 1999; 5: 209-215.

Shi W, Liu J, Huang Y, et al. Papillomavirus pseudovirus: a novel vaccine to induce mucosal and systemic cytotoxic T-lymphocyte responses. J Virol 2001; 75: 10139-48.

Stanberry LR, Spruance SL, Cunningham AL, et al. Glycoprotein-D-adjuvant vaccine to prevent genital herpes [comment]. New Engl J Med 2002; 347: 1652-61.

Stanley MA. Human papillomavirus vaccines. Curr Opin Mol Ther 2002; 4: 15-22.

Stoler MH, Schiffman M. Interobserver reproducibility of cervical cytologic and histologic interpretations: realistic estimates from the ASCUS-LSIL Triage Study. JAMA 2001; 285: 1500-5.

Stubenrauch F, Laimins LA. Human papillomavirus life cycle: active and latent phases. Semin Cancer Biol 1999; 9: 379-86.

Suzich JA, Ghim S, Palmer-Hill FJ, et al. Systemic immunization with papillomavirus L1 protein completely prevents the development of viral mucosal papillomas. Proc Natl Acad Sci USA 1995; 92: 11553-7.

Touze A, Coursaget P. In vitro gene transfer using human papillomavirus-like particles. Nucleic Acids Res 1998; 26: 1317-23.

Ulmer JB, Liu MA. Ethical issues for vaccines and immunization. Nat Reviews 2002;2:291-6.

Unckell F, Streeck RE, Sapp M. Generation and neutralization of pseudovirions of human papillomavirus type 33. J Virol 1997; 71: 2934-9.

Vandepapeliere P. Therapeutic vaccination against chronic viral infections. Lancet Infect Dis 2002; 2: 353-67.

White WI, Wilson SD, Bonnez W, et al. In vitro infection and type-restricted antibody-mediated neutralization of authentic human papillomavirus type 16. J Virol 1998; 72: 959-64.

Zhou J, Stenzel DJ, Sun XY, et al. Synthesis and assembly of infectious bovine papilloma-virus particles in vitro. J Gen Virol 1993; 74: 763-8.

Zimet GD, Mays RM, Winston Y, et al. Acceptability of human papillomavirus immunization. J Womens Health Gend Based Med 2000; 9: 47-50.

zur Hausen H. Immortalization of human cells and their malignant conversion by high risk human papillomavirus genotypes. Semin Cancer Biol 1999; 9: 405-11.

Chapter 13

Therapeutic Human Papillomavirus Vaccines

Morris Ling, B.A.[1] and T.-C. Wu, M.D., Ph.D.[1,2,3,4]
Departments of [1]Pathology, [2]Oncology, [3]Obstetrics and Gynecology, and [4]Molecular Microbiology and Immunology, The Johns Hopkins Medical Institutions

INTRODUCTION

Pre-existing HPV infection is a highly prevalent public health concern that is responsible for considerable morbidity and mortality. Evidence suggests that cellular immunity, particularly antigen-specific T cell-mediated immunity, is required for treatment of established HPV infection (Benton et al., 1992). It is therefore important to develop vaccines that induce cell-mediated immune responses specific for early viral proteins in order to effect regression of established HPV associated lesions and malignant tumors.

Most HPV therapeutic vaccines target carcinoma-associated HPV proteins, particularly E6 and E7, to generate antigen-specific cellular immunity. E6 and E7 are consistently expressed in most cervical cancers and their precursor lesions but are absent in normal tissue. While many tumor-specific antigens are derived from normal or mutated proteins, E6 and E7 are completely foreign viral proteins and may therefore harbor more antigenic peptides/epitopes than a mutant cellular protein. Furthermore, since E6 and E7 are required for the induction and maintenance of the malignant phenotype of cancer cells (Crook et al., 1989), cervical cancer cells are unlikely to evade an immune response through antigen loss. Finally, studies in animal models suggest that vaccination targeting papillomavirus early proteins such as E7 can generate therapeutic as well as protective effects (Campo et al., 1993). Thus, these viral oncoproteins represent potentially ideal targets for the development of antigen-specific vaccines to treat HPV associated cervical malignancies and their precursor lesions.

Various forms of HPV vaccines, such as peptide-based vaccines, protein-based vaccines, DNA-based vaccines, live vector-based vaccines, chimeric VLP-based vaccines, and cell-based vaccines have been described in experimental systems targeting HPV 16 E6 and/or E7 proteins (summarized in Table 1). Researchers typically focus on vaccines targeting E7 since it is more abundantly expressed and better characterized immunologically. Furthermore, its sequence is more conserved than that of the E6 gene (Zehbe et al., 1998). These experimental vaccines and their effects are illustrated in Figure 1, and will be discussed in the following sections.

1   LIVE VECTOR VACCINES

1.1   Viral vector vaccines

1.1.1   Vaccinia virus vaccines

Vaccinia viruses (vV) are members of the poxvirus family. Vaccinia vaccines offer several appealing features, including high efficiency of infection and high levels of recombinant gene expression (Moss, 1996). Infection with recombinant vV and expression of the desired gene product occurs quickly. Furthermore, the vaccinia genome can accommodate large recombinant gene insertions. The availability of replication-deficient recombinant poxvirus, such as canarypox virus, provides the opportunity to use this recombinant virus as a safe vector for gene transfer into host antigen-presenting cells (APCs). Productive viral replication is restricted to avian species and infection of mammalian cells fails to generate infectious viral particles (Sutter and Moss, 1992). Also, T cell responses against vaccinia antigens (present in most of the adult population immunized against smallpox) do not significantly cross-react with canarypox antigens (Plotkin et al., 1995), obviating the concern that pre-existing immunity would preclude immunization with canarypox virus. Finally, vaccinia is a lytic virus and thus the chance of integration of vaccinia genome into the host genome is extremely small.

Table 1. HPV Vaccine Strategies

LIVE VECTOR VACCINES

     Viral vector vaccines
          Vaccinia virus vaccines
          Adenovirus and adeno-associated virus vaccines
           Alphavirus vaccines
           HPV pesudovirion vaccines
     Bacterial vector vaccines
          Listeria vaccines
          Other bacterial vaccines (Salmonella, BCG)

PEPTIDE/PROTEIN VACCINES

     Peptide Vaccines
     Protein Vaccines

NUCLEIC ACID VACCINES

     DNA vaccines
          Intracellular targeting strategies
          Intercellular spreading strategies
          Prolonging DC survival
           Co-administration with cytokines or co-stimulatory molecules
          Enhancing protein degradation
     RNA vaccines

CELL-BASED VACCINES

     Dendritic cell-based vaccines
          DCs pulsed with peptides/proteins
          DCs transduced with genes
     Tumor cell-based vaccines

COMBINED APPROACHES

     Prime-boost vaccination strategies
     Co-administration with antiviral or anticancer drugs

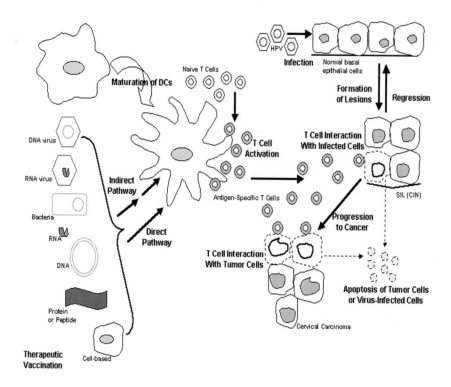

Figure 1. Immunologic effects of therapeutic vaccination. This diagram provides an overview of the immunologic effects of therapeutic vaccination with DNA virus vaccines (Vaccinia, Adenovirus), RNA virus vaccines (Alphavirus), bacterial vaccines (Listeria, Salmonella, BCG), RNA vaccines, DNA vaccines, protein or peptide vaccines, or cell-based vaccines (DC-based or tumor cell-based). DCs are the most potent professional APCs that prime helper and killer T cells *in vivo* (for review see (Cella et al., 1997; Liu, 2001; Steinman, 1991)). DCs also migrate to secondary lymphoid organs to select and stimulate antigen-specific T cells (Austyn, 1996). Thus, many therapeutic vaccine strategies have focused on targeting antigen to professional APCs, such as DCs, and enhancing antigen processing and presentation in DCs in order to augment T-cell mediated immune responses. Maturation of DCs can be induced by transduction/infection with antigen or uptake of antigen. Mature DCs are equipped to activate antigen-specific T cells, which may aid in lesion/tumor regression and induce apoptosis of tumor cells or virus-infected cells. Normal basal epithelial cells that are infected with HPV can lead to formation of squamous intraepithelial lesions (SIL; also referred to as cervical intraepithelial neoplasia, CIN), which can in turn progress to cervical cancer.

Several studies have shown that E6- and/or E7- specific immunotherapy using vaccinia vectors generates strong CTL activity (Boursnell et al., 1996; Gao et al., 1994) and antitumor responses in preclinical studies (Chen et al.,

2000b; Ji, et al., 1998; Lin, et al., 1996; Meneguzzi, et al., 1991). Results of phase I/II clinical trials using recombinant vV encoding HPV 16 and 18 E6/E7 (also called TA-HPV) indicated that some patients with advanced cervical cancer, CIN3, or early invasive cervical cancer developed T cell immune responses after vaccination (Borysiewicz et al., 1996; Adams et al., 2001). No significant complications or environmental spread of vV was noted in these trials.

vV has also been utilized to explore tumor vaccine strategies employing intracellular sorting signals. An increased understanding of intracellular pathways for antigen presentation has facilitated the design of novel strategies to enhance vaccine potency. For example, endosomal and lysosomal compartments are associated with MHC class II processing and presentation and characterized by the presence of a number of compartment-specific membrane proteins, including the lysosomal associated membrane protein (LAMP-1). A study by Wu et al. (1995) demonstrated that the linkage of the sorting signal of lysosome-associated membrane protein (LAMP-1) to the HPV 16 E7 antigen (creating recombinant Sig/E7/LAMP-1 vV) targets E7 to endosomal and lysosomal compartments and enhances MHC class II presentation to CD4+ T cells compared to vV expressing wild-type E7. Furthermore, the Sig/E7/LAMP-1 vV vaccine cures established E7-expressing tumors in mice while wild-type E7 vV shows no effect on established tumors (Lin, 1996). Another strategy for vaccinia vaccination against cervical cancer is the fusion of E7 to a nonhemolytic portion of listeriolysin O (LLO) (Lamikanra et al., 2001). Vaccination with LLO-E7 vaccinia induces a potent $CD8^+$ T cell-mediated immune response causing regression of established HPV 16 immortalized tumors in mice. This effect may be mediated by rapid proteolysis in the cytosol or enhanced trafficking to the proteasomes (Lamikanra, 2001). These studies suggest that strategies that reroute antigen or modify antigen processing may be able to improve the *in vivo* therapeutic potency of recombinant vaccinia vaccines against cervical cancer.

1.1.2   Adenovirus and adeno-associated virus vaccines

Recombinant adenoviruses (AdV) are widely employed vectors that have been used to treat a variety of illnesses, in particular cystic fibrosis (Wilson, 1995, Wilson, 1996). AdV vectors have a cloning capacity of approximately 8 kb, allowing for insertion of relatively large genes. They can be prepared easily in high titer and can efficiently transduce a wide range of cell types without integrating into the host genome. The major concern for immunization is the production of anti-AdV antibodies by the host, which may inhibit repeat vaccination and thereby compromise the therapeutic effect.

Recombinant AdV vectors encoding tumor-specific antigen such as P815A (Warnier et al., 1996), β-gal (Chen et al., 1996), or gp100 (Zhai et al., 1996) can induce an antigen-specific CTL response and antitumor effect. One study compared modified adenovirus (with Adv E1 oncogene deleted) and vaccinia virus expressing HPV 16 E6 or E7 and found that these vaccines enhanced antigen-specific $CD8^+$ and/or $CD4^+$ T cell immune responses and antitumor effects in a murine model (He et al., 2000). Another promising application of adenovirus is *ex vivo* preparation of dendritic cell (DC)-based vaccines. Adv vectors encoding E7 and targeted to CD40 by means of bispecific antibodies enhances E7 gene transfer to murine DCs (Tillman et al., 2000). Vaccination with Adv-modified E7-transduced DCs resulted in a CD8-dependent E7-specific therapeutic antitumor effect.

Adeno-associated virus (AAV) is a parvovirus that is non-pathogenic in humans. Replication-defective forms of AAV are useful as vectors for delivering therapeutic genes to a wide range of cell types (Flotte and Carter, 1995). One study found that vaccination of mice with AAV encoding HPV 16 E7 fused to heat shock protein 70 (HSP70) induced CD4- and CD8-dependent CTL activity and antitumor effects in vitro (Liu et al., 2000). HSPs are described in more detail in section 2.1. These studies indicate that Adv and AAV vectors may be safe and effective for the development of therapeutic HPV vaccines.

1.1.3   Alphavirus vaccines

Alphaviruses and their derivative vectors, i.e., Sindbis virus (Hariharan et al., 1998b; Xiong et al., 1989), Semliki Forest virus (Berglund et al., 1997; Ying et al., 1999) and Venezuelan equine encephalitis (VEE) virus (Pushko et al., 1997) are attractive candidates for vaccine development (naked alphavirus RNA replicon vaccines are discussed in section 3.2). Infectious alphavirus is highly efficient for introducing heterologous genes into target cells but has associated viral toxicity. Alphavirus replicon packaging cell lines can be used to produce replication-defective alphavirus replicon particles that are free of detectable replication-competent virus yet efficient at gene delivery (Polo et al., 1999; Velders et al., 2001a). The availability of these packaging cell lines allows for large-scale vector production of replication-defective virus that may be useful in vaccine applications. One study found that vaccination of mice with a replication-defective VEE virus replicon particle vector containing HPV 16 E7 RNA enhanced E7-specific $CD8^+$ T cell immune responses and eliminated established tumors (Velders, 2001a). Another study found that replication-defective Sindbis virus replicon particles encoding an unique intercellular spreading protein, herpes simplex virus type-1 (HSV 1) VP22 (described in section 3.1.3), linked to HPV 16 E7 generated improved E7-specific CD8$^+$ T cell immune responses and a potent antitumor effect in vaccinated mice (Cheng et al., 2002), and is more potent than HSV-1 VP22-containing vaccinia and DNA vaccines. The use of replication-defective alphavirus replicon particles thus holds promise for efficient delivery of antigen genes or immunogen/antigen fusion genes to target cells with low toxicity.

1.1.4   HPV pseudovirion vaccines

Naked DNA can be encapsulated in papillomavirus capsids using a variety of expression systems including recombinant vaccinia viruses (Zhao et al., 1998), Semliki Forest virus (Roden et al., 1996), and baculovirus (Touze and Coursaget, 1998) to form non-replicative pseudovirions. More recently, infectious virus particles containing a mammalian expressing DNA vector have been generated in *Saccharomyces cerevisiae* (Rossi et al., 2000). The target DNA plasmid can be packaged into HPV 16 VLPs expressed in yeast and transduced into different primary and established cells in culture and *in vivo* via receptor-mediated endocytosis, establishing a quantitative system to assess HPV 16 VLP infection. Non-replicative papillomavirus pseudovirions also allow for safe and improved delivery of therapeutic DNA to target cells. Touze and Coursaget have demonstrated higher frequency of gene transfer with HPV pseudovirions than with DNA alone or with liposome (Touze, 1998). Another study found that vaccination with papillomavirus-like particles containing mutated E7 DNA is able to induce mucosal and systemic E7-specific CTL responses (Shi et al., 2001). These studies demonstrate that it is possible to generate papillomavirus pseudovirions in an *in vitro* system and that such pseudovirions can deliver packaged DNA into different cell lines and induce antigen-specific CTL responses.

Several reasons may account for the ability of pseudovirions to enhance the delivery of DNA to professional APCs. The capsid can protect encapsulated DNA from nuclease activity and can also act as an adjuvant. In addition, $\alpha6$ integrin has been proposed as the cell surface receptor for HPV (McMillan et al., 1999) and is highly expressed by dendritic cells of the skin and lymph nodes (Price et al., 1997). Thus, pseudovirions may be useful for delivering therapeutic HPV DNA vaccines to DCs to prime HPV specific T cell immune responses.

1.2   Bacterial vector vaccines

1.2.1   Listeria vaccines

Listeria monocytogenes has emerged as a promising bacterial vector for use as a recombinant vaccine for human cancers. *L. monocytogenes* is a gram-positive intracellular bacterium that usually infects macrophages. When *L. monocytogenes* is phagocytosed by macrophages, it is taken up in a phagosome. However, unlike other intracellular bacteria, it escapes into the cytoplasm of the macrophage by secreting a listeriolysin O, a factor that disrupts the phagosomal membrane (Villanueva et al., 1995). Because of its presence in the endosomes and in the cytoplasm, *L. monocytogenes* can deliver its antigens or carry foreign antigens into both the MHC-I and MHC-II pathways, inducing strong cellular immune responses. A recent study found that vaccination with recombinant *L. moncytogenes* secreting HPV 16 E7 can lead to regression of pre-existing E7-expressing tumors using an E7-expressing murine tumor model, TC-1 (Gunn et al., 2001). Antigen-specific *L. monocytogenes* vaccines may also be administered orally in mice without losing efficacy (Pan et al., 1995).

1.2.2   Other bacterial vaccines

Mammalian expression vectors containing genes of interest can be transformed into attenuated bacteria, such as mutant strains of *Shigella, E. coli,* or *Salmonella,* which can serve as bacterial carriers to deliver plasmid encoding genes of interest to APCs. Among these mutant bacteria, *Salmonella* have already been used as live vaccines in humans. The advantage of using *Salmonella* as a carrier is its natural route of infection, which even allows oral vaccination (Darji et al., 1997). After leaving the intestinal lumen, *Salmonella* migrates into the lymph nodes and the spleen, where it encounters macrophages and DCs. The attenuated *Salmonella* then release multiple copies of antigen-coding plasmid inside phagocytes, which leads to expression of the antigen and elicits strong immune responses. Alternatively, genes of interest (i.e., antigen) can be cloned into a prokaryotic expression vector and transformed into *Salmonella* to induce expression of antigen in the bacteria. The bacteria can then be used as a carrier for the antigen in protein form as a vaccine. This approach has been used to deliver HPV 16 E7 (Krul et al., 1996) or E7 epitopes harbored in hepatitis B virus core antigen particles to generate E7-specific immune responses (Londono et al., 1996). Salmonella can also be engineered to express HPV 16 VLPs and used as a therapeutic vaccine against the development of HPV 16-expressing tumors in mice (Revaz et al., 2001). Another bacterial vaccine vector is Bacille Calmette-Guerin (BCG,

Mycobacterium bovis). BCG is safe as it is used for widespread vaccination against tuberculosis, and it may also induce prolonged immune responses. One study found that BCG encoding L1 and E7 induced E7-specific antibody and immune responses (Jabbar et al., 2000). Targeting to the right type of immune cells such as dendritic cells as well as the ability to enhance antigen presentation and prolong expression of antigen are the reasons to consider the use of bacterial carrier systems to deliver HPV vaccines.

2   Peptide/Protein Vaccines

2.1   Peptide vaccines

The identification and characterization of CTL epitopes for HPV has promoted the development of peptide vaccines against cervical cancer. For example, several HPV 16 E7-specific CTL epitopes have been characterized for the HLA-A.2 haplotype (Kast et al., 1993; Ressing et al., 1995). Immunization with a peptide derived from HPV 16 leads to protection of mice against a lethal dose of HPV 16 transformed tumor cells (Feltkamp et al., 1993). Peptide vaccines also have potential clinical applicability. At least three HLA-A2.1-restricted peptide CTL epitopes derived from HPV 16 E7, including aa 11-20 (YMLDLQPETT), aa 82-90 (LLMGTLGIV), aa 86-93 (TLGIVCPI), are able to induce CTL responses *in vivo* in HLA-A2.1 transgenic mice and lyse HPV 16 E7-containing HLA-A2.1 positive CaSki cells (Ressing, 1995). Peptides relevant to other HPV types (i.e., HPV 18) (Rudolf et al., 2001b) and other HLA backgrounds (i.e., HLA-B18) (Bourgault Villada et al., 2000), are also under investigation. In human studies, CTL responses were observed in some HPV associated cancer patients after vaccination with lipidated peptides derived from HPV 16 E7 (Steller et al., 1998). In one phase I/II study, no adverse side effects of peptide-based HPV vaccine were observed in patients (van Driel et al., 1999). In another study, HPV 16- and HLA-A.2-positive patients with high-grade cervical or vulvar intraepithelial neoplasia were vaccinated with epitopes aa 12-20 or aa 86-93; 10 of 16 patients exhibited measurable enhancement in cytokine release and cytolysis mediated by CTLs derived from PBMCs, and some patients had partial clearance of virus and regression of lesions (Muderspach et al., 2000). Studies have also identified human MHC class II-restricted T helper cell epitopes and T helper immune responses in response to peptide vaccination (Ressing et al., 2000; van der Burg et al., 2001b).

The potency of HPV 16 E7 peptide-based vaccines can be further enhanced by the use of adjuvants such as immune stimulatory complexes (ISCOMs) (Fernando et al., 1995) and immunostimulatory carriers (ISCAR)

(Tindle et al., 1995). Phase I clinical trials of HPV 16 peptide vaccines with adjuvant have been conducted using various adjuvants including incomplete Freund's adjuvant (Muderspach, 2000) and Montanide ISA 51 adjuvant (van Driel, 1999), leading to noticeable positive immunologic and pathologic effects. Cytokines such as IL-2 may boost the adjuvant effect in peptide-based vaccines according to a study using the gp100 melanoma-associated antigen (Rosenberg et al., 1998). Polycations, such as polylysine, can also act as adjuvants for peptide vaccines against cancer (Schmidt et al., 1997). Another adjuvant strategy involves the modification of CTL epitopes using lipid conjugation, tripalmitoyl-S-glycerylcysteinyl-seryl-serine (P3CSS) to form an immunogenic lipopeptide vaccine (Deres et al., 1989, Schild et al., 1991). Two similar strategies have been adapted for the treatment of HPV associated cancer including an E7 (aa 86-93) lipopeptide vaccine (Steller, 1998) and two dipalmitoyl-lysine-glycine-glycine (P2-KGG) lipid-tailed E6 and E7 peptide-based vaccines (Sarkar et al., 1995), both of which generated enhanced CTL responses.

Heat shock proteins are a family of chaperone proteins that facilitate delivery of noncovalently bound peptide to MHC class I molecules and induce peptide-specific CTL responses (Li, 1997; Srivastava, 1997; Suto and Srivastava, 1995). Immunization with HSP-peptide complexes isolated from tumor or virus-infected cells (Srivastava and Udono, 1994) or peptides fused with HSPs (Srivastava et al., 1998) can induce potent antitumor or antiviral immunity. HSPs thus serve as effective immunogens and have also been used in viral vaccines (see section 1.1), protein vaccines (see section 2.2), and DNA vaccines (see section 3.1.2). Another strategy to enhance the potency of peptide vaccines is to modify anchor residues in CTL epitope-bearing peptides. Anchor-modified peptide epitopes can efficiently induce CTL that are capable of recognizing wild-type epitope and can also protect against HPV 16 E7-expressing tumors (Vierboom et al., 1998). Modifications of epitopes may enhance the ability of peptide to be bound and transported by MHC class I and transporter associated with antigen (TAP).

Although vaccination with synthetic peptides containing CTL epitopes can induce protective CTL responses and effective antitumor immunity in several murine tumor model systems, this effect is not always seen. For example, vaccination with a CTL epitope derived from the human adenovirus type 5 E1A enhanced rather than inhibited the growth of Ad5E1A-expressing tumors (Toes et al., 1996a; Toes et al., 1996b). Interestingly, the same epitopes loaded onto DCs can generate protective immunity, indicating that it may not be the peptides *per se*, but rather the method of presenting the epitope to T cells that determines the outcome of immunization with peptide-based vaccines (Toes et al., 1998). It is therefore important to evaluate peptide-based vaccines using different adjuvants, routes of administration, and other conditions to determine their immunizing or tolerizing properties *in vivo* before clinical use.

2.2   Protein vaccines

The convenience of utilizing peptide-based vaccines is limited by MHC restriction and the necessity to define specific CTL epitopes. Most CTL epitopes of HPV 16 E6 and/or E7 in patients with HLA other than HLA-A.2 remain undefined, making it difficult to use peptide-based vaccines in such situations. In addition, the preparation of peptide-based vaccines for use on a large scale is inefficient and laborious. These limitations can potentially be overcome by using protein-based vaccines. Protein-based vaccines can present all possible epitopes of a protein to the immune system, thus bypassing the MHC restriction. In addition, protein vaccines offer certain safety advantages since insertional gene activation and transformation, a potential concern with certain recombinant virus vaccines and DNA vaccines, are not an issue.

A growing number of modified exogenous protein antigens, including HPV 16 E7, have been found to generate enhanced MHC-I restricted CTL responses. Association of E7 protein with adjuvants, such as PROVAX (Hariharan et al., 1998a), incomplete Freund's adjuvant (De Bruijn et al., 1998), saponin QS21, and monophosphoryl lipid A (MPL) (Gerard et al., 2001) is able to enhance E7-specific CTL activities. Studies have demonstrated that injection of heat-aggregated HPV 16 E7 antigen can prime CTLs (Schirmbeck et al., 1995). TA-GW fusion protein, which consists of HPV 6 L2 fused to E7 protein, has been tested for clinical treatment of genital warts (Lacey et al., 1999; Thompson et al., 1999) and TA-CIN fusion protein, which consists of HPV 16 L2/E6/E7 can induce E7-specific CD8$^+$ T cell immune responses and tumor protection (van der Burg et al., 2001a).

Various strategies have been developed to enhance the potency of protein-based vaccines or preparations, some of which have yet to be tested in the HPV context. The fusion of antigen with heat shock proteins (HSPs) is one such strategy for enhancing CTL priming (Suzue et al., 1997). This strategy has been tested using Mycobacterium bovis bacille Calmette-Guerin (BCG) HSP65 fused to HPV 16 E7, which led to CD8-dependent, CD4-independent regression of HPV 16 E7-expressing tumors in mice (Chu et al., 2000). Studies have demonstrated that GM-CSF linked to an antigen can target the antigen to dendritic cells and other GM-CSF-responsive cells after the chimeric molecule binds to the GM-CSF receptor, generating enhanced immune responses in these cells (Chen et al., 1994; Tao and Levy, 1993). Immunostimulatory CpG oligodeoxy-nucleotides (ODNs) that contain unmethylated CpG motifs are also able to enhance the potency of protein vaccines by inducing macrophages to secrete IL-12 and shifting cytokine profiles to Th1 type immunity (Chu et al., 1997; Roman et al., 1997). CpG ODNs are a promising alternative to complete Freund's adjuvant because they lack significant toxicity (Weiner et al., 1997), making them an attractive option for enhancing HPV protein-based vaccines.

Studies have elucidated potential mechanisms by which modified exogenous antigens are presented through the MHC class I pathway (Jondal et al., 1996; Rock, 1996). Exogenous antigens may be 1) taken up and transferred to the cytosol, allowing for processing via the MHC class I pathway (Kovacsovics-Bankowski and Rock, 1995); 2) taken up, digested, and secreted or "regurgitated" on the cell surface for binding to empty MHC class I molecules (Harding and Song, 1994); or 3) taken up in vesicular endosome/lysosome-like compartments, followed by transfer to MHC class I molecules (Gromme et al., 1999). It is likely that one or more of these mechanisms, and perhaps other as yet unrevealed processes, contribute to the processing and presentation of exogenous antigen via the MHC class I pathway.

Chimeric HPV virus-like particles (VLP) vaccines represent innovative protein-based HPV vaccines. Immunization with HPV VLPs induces high titer neutralizing antibodies in the serum and can protect animals from experimental papillomavirus infections. However, VLPs do not generate therapeutic effects for established or breakthrough HPV infections, which are prevalent in high-risk sexually active populations. Treatment of established infections requires the induction of T cell-mediated immune responses. This can be achieved using chimeric VLPs that carry E2 and/or E7 antigen (Greenstone et al., 1998; Jochmus et al., 1999; Peng et al., 1998; Schafer et al., 1999). E7 chimeric VLPs can also elicit high titers of neutralizing antibodies (Greenstone, 1998) and activate dendritic cells (Rudolf et al., 2001a). Currently, clinical grade HPV 16 L1/L2-E2-E7 chimeric VLPs, which contain four HPV-encoded proteins (L1, L2, E2 and E7) as target antigens, are being prepared for a future phase I clinical trial (J. Schiller, personal communication).

3   NUCLEIC ACID VACCINES

3.1   DNA vaccines

Naked DNA vaccines are useful because of their purity, simplicity of preparation, and stability. Preparation of DNA vaccines is also relatively inexpensive and can be carried out efficiently. DNA vaccines allow for sustained expression of antigen on MHC-peptide complexes compared to peptide or protein vaccines. Furthermore, the MHC restriction of peptide-based vaccines may be bypassed with approaches that directly transduce

DNA coding for antigen to APCs so that synthesized peptides can be presented by the patient's own HLA molecules. Since DNA vaccines targeting different HPV types can be administered together, DNA vaccines may be effective for treating a variety of HPV associated infections and tumors. These advantages have spurred interest in the development of DNA vaccines to treat cancers. DNA vaccines can be administered to the host by intramuscular injection, intradermal injection via hypodermic needle or gene gun (a ballistic device for delivering DNA-coated gold particles into the epidermis), intravenous injection, intranasal delivery or biojector delivery (for review, see Donnelly et al., 1997; Robinson and Torres, 1997b).

3.1.1   DNA vaccines and activation of T cells

Studies have investigated the mechanisms involved with intramuscular injection or gene gun delivery of DNA vaccines. Following intramuscular injection, myocytes can uptake DNA, allowing them to produce protein and transfer antigen to bone marrow-derived professional APCs (Corr et al., 1996). "Cross priming", the processing of exogenous antigen transferred from another cell (i.e., secreted from DCs or in apoptotic bodies) via the MHC class I pathway (Albert et al., 1998; Huang et al., 1994), provides an explanation for the transfer of antigen from cells initially transfected by intramuscular immunization (i.e., myocytes) to professional APCs.

After gene gun delivery, epidermal Langerhans cells uptake DNA and function as APCs. DCs in the skin carry antigen from the skin to the draining lymph nodes, where the antigen-loaded DCs activate naïve T cells (Condon et al., 1996). Intradermal vaccination with DNA facilitates direct priming, whereby antigen expressed in DCs is directly processed within the cell and presented on MHC class I molecules to CD8$^+$ T cells (Porgador et al., 1998). The method of DNA inoculation (gene gun versus intramuscular injection) and the form of the DNA-expressed antigen (cytoplasmic versus secreted) can also influence the type of T cell help (Th1 or Th2) (for review see Robinson, 1997a).

3.1.2   Intracellular targeting strategies to enhance MHC class I-restricted CD8$^+$ and MHC class II-restricted CD4$^+$ T cell responses

The delivery of DNA vaccines intradermally via gene gun allows for direct targeting of genes of interest into professional APCs *in vivo*. Gene gun immunization has been used to test several intracellular targeting strategies that enhance MHC class I and/or class II presentation of antigen. For example, MHC class I presentation of HPV 16 E7 can be significantly enhanced by linkage with *Mycobacterium tuberculosis* heat shock protein 70

(HSP70) (Chen et al., 2000a), calreticulin (Cheng et al., 2001b) or the translocation domain (domain II) of *Pseudomonas aeruginosa* exotoxin A (ETA(dII)) (Hung, et al., 2001b) in the context of a DNA vaccine. The linkage of these molecules to E7 results in augmentation of the E7-specific $CD8^+$ T cell immune response in vaccinated mice. (HSPs are described in more detail in section 2.1). Furthermore, the use of DNA encoding a signal sequence linked to E7 and the sorting signal of the lysosome associated membrane protein (LAMP-1) to create the Sig/E7/LAMP-1 chimera can enhance MHC class II antigen processing (Wu, 1995) (see section 1.1.1). Expression of this DNA vaccine *in vitro* and *in vivo* targets E7 to endosomal and lysosomal compartments and enhances MHC class II presentation to $CD4^+$ T cells compared to DNA encoding wild-type E7 (Ji et al., 1999). While chimeric E7/HSP70, ETA(dII)/E7 or CRT/E7 DNA generates potent $CD8^+$ T cell responses through enhanced MHC class I presentation, other constructs that target antigen to MHC class II presentation pathways may provide enhanced $CD4^+$ T cell responses. This realization raises the notion of co-administration of vaccines such as E7/HSP70 and Sig/E7/LAMP-1 in a synergistic fashion. Such an approach may directly enhance both MHC class I and class II presentation of E7 and lead to significantly enhanced E7-specific $CD4^+$ and $CD8^+$ T cell responses and potent antitumor effects.

Although DNA vaccines employing intracellular targeting strategies can significantly enhance MHC class I and class II presentation of antigen in transfected DCs, they may only generate a limited number of antigen-expressing DCs since naked DNA vaccines lack the intrinsic ability to amplify and spread *in vivo*. This significantly limits the potency of DNA vaccines. Therefore, a strategy that facilitates the spread of antigen to more DCs may significantly enhance the potency of naked DNA vaccines.

3.1.3 Intercellular spreading to enhance DNA vaccine potency

The potency of DNA vaccines may be enhanced through the use of herpes simplex virus (HSV 1) VP22, an HSV 1 tegument protein capable of intercellular transport and useful in spreading protein to surrounding cells (Elliott and O'Hare, 1997). HSV 1 VP22 (HVP22) is capable of enhancing intercellular spreading of the linked protein. Furthermore, mice vaccinated with HVP22/E7 DNA generate a significantly greater number of E7 specific $CD8^+$ T cell precursors (Hung et al., 2001a; Michel et al., 2002; Osen et al., 2001) and a stronger antitumor effect than wild-type E7 DNA (Hung, 2001a). The success of the chimeric HSV 1 VP22/E7 DNA vaccine warrants the consideration of other proteins with similar trafficking properties.

At least two other proteins with purported intercellular spreading properties have been reported, including bovine herpesvirus VP22 (BVP22) (Harms et al., 2000) and Marek's disease virus VP22 (MVP22)

(Koptidesova et al., 1995), both of which are VP22 homologues. Bovine herpesvirus VP22 shares about 22% amino acid identity to human herpesvirus VP22 (Harms, 2000). A previous study found that BVP22 trafficking may be more efficient than human VP22 trafficking after endogenous synthesis (Harms, 2000). Marek's disease virus VP22 (MVP22) shares about 17% amino acid identity to human herpesvirus VP22 and may be capable of intercellular transport after exogenous application (Dorange et al., 2000). MVP22/E7 DNA generates a significantly greater number of E7 specific $CD8^+$ T cell precursors and a stronger antitumor effect in vaccinated mice than wild-type E7 DNA (Hung et al., 2002).

3.1.4 Prolonging DC survival to enhance immune responses to DNA vaccines

Although E7-specific T cell-mediated immune responses and antitumor effects can be enhanced by the vaccine strategies mentioned in sections 3.1.2 and 3.1.3, vaccine efficiency may be limited since transduced dendritic cells may themselves become targets of effector cells through apoptosis via perforin/ granzyme B or death receptor pathways. One potential strategy to overcome this problem is to utilize DNA encoding inhibitors of apoptosis delivered to DCs in order to enhance the survival of DCs and prolong their ability to present the antigen of interest. Kim et al. have tested a variety of anti-apoptotic factors for their ability to enhance DC survival and E7-specific $CD8^+$ T cell immune responses including bclxL, bcl2, X-linked inhibitor of apoptosis protein (XIAP), and dominant negative (dn) caspase-9 and dn caspase-8. An examination of E7-specific immune responses, the antitumor effect, and the characteristics and kinetics of dendritic cell involvement, revealed that co-administration of E7-containing DNA with DNA encoding anti-apoptotic proteins enhanced DNA vaccine potency and efficacy (Kim et al., 2003).

3.1.5 Improving DNA vaccine potency with cytokines and costimulatory adjuvants

It is well known that costimulators are required to generate a CTL response. Methods that employ cytokines or costimulatory molecules may enhance the potency of DNA vaccines (Corr, et al., 1997; Irvine, et al., 1996; Tuting, 1999). Leachman et al. demonstrated that priming the E6 DNA vaccination site with a GM-CSF-expressing vector greatly enhances the effects of cottontail rabbit papillomavirus (CRPV) E6 vaccination, increasing tumor regression frequency and probability of rabbits remaining disease-free after CRPV challenge (Leachman et al., 2000). Tan et al. have shown that administration of IL-12 at the vaccination site of gene gun-administered plasmid DNA encoding E7 increased vaccine induced therapeutic efficacy (Tan et al., 1999). Thus, cytokines and costimulatory molecules may act as useful adjuvants for HPV DNA vaccines.

3.1.6   Enhancing protein degradation

The immune response elicited by DNA vaccines may be augmented by manipulating pathways for intercellular protein degradation. Ubiquitin, a small protein cofactor, targets conjugated protein for recognition and degradation within the proteasome. Velders et al. (2001b) have shown that a multi-epitope vaccine for HPV protected 100% of vaccinated mice against challenge with HPV 16, when ubiquitin and certain flanking sequences were included in the gene insert. Similarly, Liu et al. (2001) observed enhancement of E7-specific CTL activity and protection against E7-expressing tumors in mice given a DNA vaccine with a ubiquitinated L1-E7 gene insert. Although ubiquitin may be a useful molecule for expediting protein degradation and antigen processing, it is not the only means of enhancing intercellular protein degradation. Shi et al. (1999) engineered mutations into two zinc-binding motifs of an HPV 16 E7 DNA vaccine to generate a rapidly degraded E7 protein. This mutated E7 protein elicited a significantly enhanced E7-specific CTL response and better protection compared to a wild type E7 DNA vaccine. These studies suggest that the enhancement of intercellular degradation of the antigen of interest may increase the immunogenicity of DNA vaccines.

3.1.7   Safety of DNA vaccines

Although the efficacy of DNA vaccination is important, safety is also a critical issue. DNA present in the vaccine may integrate into the host genome, potentially inactivating tumor suppresser genes or activating oncogenes, thereby inducing malignant transformation of the host cell. Fortunately, it is estimated that the frequency of integration is much lower than that of spontaneous mutation and integration should not pose any real risk (Nichols et al., 1995). A second issue concerns potential risks associated with the presence of HPV 16 E7 protein in host cells. E7 is an oncoprotein that disrupts cell cycle regulation by binding to pRb, a tumor suppressor protein in nuclei (Lukas et al., 1994). The presence of E7 in the nuclei may lead to accumulation of genetic aberrations and eventual malignant transformation of the host cells. To avoid such problems, strategies such as the endosomal/lysosomal-targeting Sig/E7/LAMP-1 DNA vaccine may be employed to divert E7 away from the nucleus to regions such as the lysosomal and endosomal compartments to physically separate E7 from pRb. In addition, detailed mutational analysis of E7 has led to the identification of a number of mutations that abrogate the transformation activity of E7

(Edmonds and Vousden, 1989; Heck et al., 1992; Jewers et al., 1992; Phelps et al., 1992). One recent study demonstrated that a DNA vaccine encoding E7 with a mutation which inactivate Rb-binding site was able to enhance CTL activity and E7-specific antitumor effects compared to wild-type E7 (Shi, 1999). DNA vaccines using a shuffled E7 gene may also alleviate concerns of oncogenicity associated with E7 (Osen, 2001). Another strategy to avoid the problem of the oncogenicity of E7 is to use a DNA vaccine encoding a string of multiple epitopes surrounded by defined flanking sequences; this may be safe and promising for tumor protection and therapy, particularly if epitopes are targeted to the protein degradation pathway (Velders, 2001b). Ultimately, DNA vectors employed in human clinical trials may use a minimally mutated E7 gene or multiepitope gene approach in which critical epitopes are preserved while potential oncogenic activity is eliminated.

3.2 RNA replicon vaccines

Naked RNA is another strategy for cancer vaccine development, although RNA is typically less stable than DNA and often has lower transfection efficiency. To improve the immunogenicty of RNA vaccines, one can use self-replicating RNA replicon vectors. These non-infectious, self-replicating, and self-limiting RNA can be launched in RNA or DNA form, followed by transcription into RNA replicons in transfected cells or *in vivo* (Berglund et al., 1998). Self-replication allows for expression of the antigen of interest at high levels for an extended period of time, enhancing vaccine potency. Since RNA-launched or DNA-launched RNA replicons eventually cause lysis of transfected cells (Leitner et al., 2000; Ying, 1999), concerns about integration into the host genome associated with naked DNA vaccines are alleviated. This is particularly important for vaccine development targeting E6 and E7 since HPV 16 E6 and E7 are oncogenic proteins. The RNA replicon system has recently been applied to the development of HPV vaccines. Studies have demonstrated that the potency of HPV 16 E7-specific self-replicating RNA vaccines can be enhanced by applying the LAMP-1 targeting strategy (Cheng, et al., 2001d), the Mycobacterium tuberculosis HSP70 strategy (Cheng et al., 2001c), or the HSV 1 VP22 strategy (Cheng et al., 2001a) (see section 3.1.3). Self-replicating and self-limiting RNA replicon vaccines may be administered as DNA (Berglund, 1998). DNA-based RNA replicons, also known as 'suicidal' DNA, share the advantages of both RNA replicons and naked DNA vaccines without the disadvantages of either form of vaccine. Not only are they as stable and easily prepared as conventional naked DNA vaccines, they are also more potent than conventional naked DNA vaccines (Berglund, 1998). Since cells transfected with DNA-launched RNA replicons eventually undergo lysis (hence the term 'suicidal'), there is little concern for malignant transformation commonly associated with naked DNA vaccines. Hsu et al. recently employed DNA-launched RNA replicons for the development of HPV vaccines and have demonstrated significant E7-specific CTL activity and antitumor effects (Hsu et al., 2000). Thus, RNA- and DNA-launched RNA replicon vaccines are promising therapeutic options for the treatment of HPV associated cervical cancer.

4   CELL-BASED VACCINES

Cell-based vaccines for cancer immunotherapy can be conceptually divided into two broad categories: dendritic cell-based vaccines and cytokine-transduced tumor cell-based vaccines.

4.1   Dendritic cell-based vaccines

The generation of large numbers of DCs was previously hindered by a lack of information about DC maturation and the lineage-specific markers that define their cellular differentiation state. Recent advances have revealed the origin of DCs, their antigen uptake mechanisms, and the signals that stimulate their migration and maturation into immunostimulatory APCs (for review see Cella, 1997; Hart, 1997). Several strategies for the generation of large numbers of active DCs *ex vivo* focus on the use of cytokine factors to induce the differentiation of primitive hematopoietic precursors into DCs (Heufler et al., 1988; Inaba, et al., 1992; Witmer-Pack et al., 1987). DCs derived from cultured hematopoietic progenitors appear to have APC function similar to purified mature DCs. *Ex vivo* generation of DCs therefore provides a source of professional APCs for use in experimental immuno-therapy. There are several vaccine strategies using DCs prepared with HPV 16 E6/E7. Vaccine strategies using DCs generated *ex vivo* can be classified as follows: 1) DCs pulsed with peptides/proteins, and 2) DCs transduced with genes encoding HPV E6 and/or E7 through naked DNA or viral vectors.

4.1.1   Dendritic cells pulsed with peptides/proteins

Presentation of peptides derived from HPV E6 and/or E7 to the immune system by DCs is a promising method of circumventing tumor-mediated immunosuppression. Syngeneic spleen DCs pulsed with E7-specific T cell epitopes can generate protective E7-specific antitumor T cell mediated immunity (Ossevoort et al., 1995). Treatment of tumors with peptide-pulsed

DCs has resulted in sustained tumor regression in several different tumor models (for review, see Mayordomo et al., 1997). For example, Mayordomo et al. (1995) demonstrated in murine tumor models that bone marrow-derived DCs pulsed *ex vivo* with synthetic HPV 16 E7 peptide serve as an effective antitumor vaccine, protecting animals against an otherwise lethal tumor challenge. DCs pulsed with whole E7 protein can also generate an effective antitumor effect (De Bruijn, 1998). Another study demonstrated that DCs derived from patients can be pulsed with fusion proteins such as E6/E7 and used to generate E6/E7-specific CTLs *in vitro* (Murakami et al., 1999). DC-based vaccines are promising because they may be able to break peripheral tolerance; for example, DCs pulsed with E7 CTL epitope are able to overcome tolerance in the A2.1-K^b x K14 HPV 16 E7 transgenic mouse model (Doan et al., 2000).

4.1.2   Dendritic cells transduced with HPV E6 and/or E7 genes

Gene-transduced DC-based vaccines represent an attractive alternative to peptide-pulsed DC-based vaccines since MHC restriction may be bypassed by directly transducing genes coding for E6 and/or E7 inside DCs, allowing synthesized peptides to be presented by any given patient's HLA molecules. Gene transfer into DCs can be accomplished by a variety of methods involving either naked DNA or the use of viral vectors, such as adeno-associated virus (Chiriva-Internati et al., 2002, Liu et al., 2001). The major limitation to naked DNA transfer into DCs is poor transfection efficiency using various physical methods (Arthur et al., 1997). However, Tuting et al. (1997) have described the use of a gene gun for particle-mediated transfer of genes encoding HPV 16 E7 to generate DCs that express E7/MHC-I complexes. This vaccine not only generated an antigen-specific CTL response *in vivo*, it also promoted the rejection of an ordinarily lethal challenge with an HPV 16-transformed tumor cell line.

Route of administration may be important for the efficacy of DC-based vaccines. Wang et al. (2000) transduced HPV 16 E7 gene into a DC line by electroporation using an E7-expressing vector and demonstrated that intramuscular administration of DC-E7 generated the greatest anti-tumor immunity compared to subcutaneous and intravenous routes of administration. Furthermore, the study demonstrated that intramuscular administration of DC-E7 elicited the highest levels of E7-specific antibody and greatest numbers of E7-specific $CD4^+$ T helper and $CD8^+$ T cell precursors (Wang, et al., 2000). These findings indicate that the potency of DC-based vaccines may depend on the specific route of administration.

4.2   Tumor cell-based vaccines

The use of tumor cell-based vaccines may not be suitable for the treatment of early-stage, pre-cancerous HPV associated lesions because of the risks and controversy associated with administering modified tumor cells to these patients. Therefore, tumor cell-based vaccination is likely reserved for patients with advanced HPV associated cancer. Transduction of tumor cells with genes encoding co-stimulatory molecules or cytokines may enhance immunogenicity leading to T cell activation and antitumor effects after vaccination (for review, see Chen and Wu, 1998). Several HPV related tumor cell-based vaccines have been reported in preclinical model systems. For example, vaccines employing HPV transformed tumor cells transduced with cytokine genes such as IL-12 (Hallez et al., 1999) and IL-2 (Bubenik et al., 1999) have been demonstrated to generate strong antitumor effects in mice. Recently, it has been shown that an E7-expressing GM-CSF gene-transduced allogeneic tumor cell-based vaccine can generate E7-specific CTL activities and protective antitumor immunity in immunized mice (Chang et al., 2000). These preclinical data indicate that tumor cell-based vaccines may be useful for the control of minimal residual diseases in patients with advanced HPV associated cervical cancers.

5   COMBINED APPROACHES

Combining vaccine vehicles using a diverse prime-boost strategy has emerged as an attractive approach for cancer immunotherapy. The prime-boost regimen involves administering a primary vaccine to prime the immune system, followed by a second vaccine, the booster, to augment and maintain the immune response. A study conducted by Chen et al. (2000c) testing various combinations of viral vectors and nucleic acids in the prime-boost regimen, concluded that priming with a DNA vaccine followed by a recombinant vaccinia booster provided the most potent antitumor effects. Kowalczyk et al. (2001) found that priming with intramuscularly delivered L1-expressing DNA and boosting with adenoviral HPV 16 L1 induces antibodies in vaccinated mice, with Ig2a and Ig2b isotypes predominating in sera. Thus, prime-boost regimens may be a potent means of enhancing immune responses against HPV.

Another combinational approach involves the simultaneous administration of DNA vaccine and other antiviral or anticancerous agents. Combined administration of intralesional antiviral treatment and immune stimulation may be a feasible means of providing a long-lasting cure to persistent HPV infections (Christensen et al., 2001). Christensen et al. (2000) topically administered the antiviral agent cidofovir and intra-cutaneously administered via gene gun a DNA vaccine-encoding CRPV gene. Cures of large established CRPV-induced rabbit papillomas and reduced incidence of lesion recurrence were observed, suggesting that this combination may also be useful in treating persistent HPV infections.

CONCLUSION

In the past decade, significant progress has been made in the field of HPV vaccine development. The determination that HPV is the etiological agent for cervical cancer and its precursor lesions has paved the way for the development of preventive and therapeutic HPV vaccines that may lead to the control of HPV associated malignancies and their potentially lethal consequences. An understanding of the molecular progression of cervical cancer has led to the realization that HPV E6 and E7 are important targets for the development of HPV therapeutic vaccines for the control of established HPV infections and HPV associated lesions. Several experimental HPV vaccine strategies including vector-based vaccines, peptide-based vaccines, protein-based vaccines, nucleic acid-based vaccines, chimeric VLP-based vaccines, cell-based vaccines, pseudovirions, and RNA replicons have been shown to enhance HPV specific immune cell activity and antitumor responses in murine tumor systems. Several clinical trials are currently underway, based on encouraging preclinical results from these therapeutic HPV vaccines. A head-to-head comparison of these vaccines will help to identify the most potent therapeutic HPV vaccine with minimal negative side effects.

Clinical HPV vaccine trials provide a unique opportunity to identify the characteristics and mechanisms of immune response that best correlate with clinical vaccine potency. Such immunological parameters will help define protective immune mechanisms for controlling HPV infections and HPV related disease. Rational development of more effective vaccines for HPV infections would be greatly facilitated by comprehensive information on these protective immune mechanisms in humans. Therapeutic vaccines may be a practical option for patients with precancerous lesions or cervical cancer, with attention being paid to efficacy, safety, and cost. The higher prevalence of HPV associated cervical lesions and cancer in developing countries underlines the importance of developing safe and cost-effective vaccines and immunization regimens. With continued endeavors in HPV vaccine development, we may soon be able to implement a variety of safe and effective therapeutic vaccine strategies for the eventual control of HPV associated cervical cancer.

ACKNOWLEDGMENTS

This review is not intended to be an encyclopedic one and we apologize to the authors not cited. We would like to thank Drs. Keerti V. Shah, Michelle Moniz, Robert J. Kurman, Drew M. Pardoll, and Ken-Yu Lin for their helpful discussions. We also thank Drs. Richard Roden and Chien-Fu Hung for their critical review of the manuscript.

REFERENCES

Adams M, Borysiewicz L, Fiander A, et al. Clinical studies of human papilloma vaccines in pre-invasive and invasive cancer. Vaccine 2001;19:2549-56.

Albert ML, Sauter B, Bhardwaj N. Dendritic cells acquire antigen from apoptotic cells and induce class I- restricted CTLs. Nature 1998;392:86-9.

Arthur JF, Butterfield LH, Roth MD, et al. A comparison of gene transfer methods in human dendritic cells. Cancer Gene Ther 1997;4:17-25.

Austyn JM. New insights into the mobilization and phagocytic activity of dendritic cells. J Exp Med 1996;183:1287-92.

Benton C, Shahidullah H, Hunter JAA. Human papillomavirus in the immunosuppressed. In: Papillomavirus Report; 1992. p. 23-26.

Berglund P, Quesada-Rolander M, Putkonen P, et al. Outcome of immunization of cynomolgus monkeys with recombinant Semliki Forest virus encoding human immuno-deficiency virus type 1 envelope protein and challenge with a high dose of SHIV-4 virus. AIDS Res Hum Retroviruses 1997;13:1487-95.

Berglund P, Smerdou C, Fleeton MN, et al. Enhancing immune responses using suicidal DNA vaccines. Nat Biotechnol 1998;16:562-5.

Borysiewicz LK, Fiander A, Nimako M, et al. A recombinant vaccinia virus encoding human papillomavirus types 16 and 18, E6 and E7 proteins as immunotherapy for cervical cancer. Lancet 1996;347:1523-7.

Bourgault Villada I, Beneton N, Bony C, et al. Identification in humans of HPV-16 E6 and E7 protein epitopes recognized by cytolytic T lymphocytes in association with HLA-B18 and determination of the HLA-B18-specific binding motif. Eur J Immunol 2000;30:2281-9.

Boursnell ME, Rutherford E, Hickling JK, et al. Construction and characterisation of a recombinant vaccinia virus expressing human papillomavirus proteins for immunotherapy of cervical cancer. Vaccine 1996;14:1485-94.

Bubenik J, Simova J, Hajkova R, et al. Interleukin 2 gene therapy of residual disease in mice carrying tumours induced by HPV 16. Int J Oncol 1999;14:593-7.

Campo MS, Grindlay GJ, O'Neil BW, et al. Prophylactic and therapeutic vaccination against a mucosal papillomavirus. J Gen Virol 1993;74:945-53.

Cella M, Sallusto F, Lanzavecchia A. Origin, maturation and antigen presenting function of dendritic cells. Curr Opin Immunol 1997;9:10-6.

Chang EY, Chen CH, Ji H, et al. Antigen-specific cancer immunotherapy using an GM-CSF secreting allogeneic tumor cell-based vaccine. Int J Cancer 2000;86:725-30.

Chen C-H, Wang T-L, Hung C-F, et al. Enhancement of DNA vaccine potency by linkage of antigen gene to an HSP70 gene. Cancer Res 2000a;60:1035-42.

Chen CH, Suh KW, Ji H, et al. Antigen-specific immunotherapy for HPV-16 E7-expressing tumors grown in liver. J Hepatology 2000b;33:91-8.

Chen CH, Wang TL, Hung CF, et al. Boosting with recombinant vaccinia increases HPV-16 E7-specific T cell precursor frequencies of HPV-16 E7-expressing DNA vaccines. Vaccine 2000c;18:2015-22.

Chen CH, Wu TC. Experimental vaccine strategies for cancer immunotherapy. J Biomed Sci 1998;5:231-52.

Chen PW, Wang M, Bronte V, et al. Therapeutic antitumor response after immunization with a recombinant adenovirus encoding a model tumor-associated antigen. J Immunol 1996; 156:224-31.

Chen TT, Tao MH, Levy R. Idiotype-cytokine fusion proteins as cancer vaccines. Relative efficacy of IL-2, IL-4, and granulocyte-macrophage colony-stimulating factor. J Immunol 1994;153:4775-87.

Cheng WF, Hung CF, Chai CY, et al. Enhancement of sindbis virus self-replicating RNA vaccine potency by linkage of herpes simplex virus type 1 VP22 protein to antigen. J Virol 2001a;75:2368-76.

Cheng WF, Hung CF, Chai CY, et al. Tumor-specific immunity and antiangiogenesis generated by a DNA vaccine encoding calreticulin linked to a tumor antigen. J Clin Invest 2001b;108:669-78.

Cheng WF, Hung CF, Chai CY, et al. Enhancement of Sindbis virus self-replicating RNA vaccine potency by linkage of *Mycobacterium tuberculosis* heat shock protein 70 gene to an antigen gene. J Immunol 2001c;166:6218-26.

Cheng WF, Hung CF, Hsu KF, et al. Enhancement of sindbis virus self-replicating RNA vaccine potency by targeting antigen to endosomal/lysosomal compartments. Hum Gene Ther 2001d;12:235-52.

Cheng WF, Hung CF, Hsu KF, et al. Cancer immunotherapy using sindbis virus replicon particles encoding a VP22--antigen fusion. Hum Gene Ther 2002;13:553-68.

Chiriva-Internati M, Liu Y, Salati E, et al. Efficient generation of cytotoxic T lymphocytes against cervical cancer cells by adeno-associated virus/human papillomavirus type 16 E7 antigen gene transduction into dendritic cells. Eur J Immunol 2002;32:30-8.

Christensen ND, Han R, Cladel NM, et al. Combination treatment with intralesional cidofovir and viral-DNA vaccination cures large cottontail rabbit papillomavirus-induced papillomas and reduces recurrences. Antimicrob Agents Chemother 2001;45:1201-9.

Christensen ND, Pickel MD, Budgeon LR, et al. In vivo anti-papillomavirus activity of nucleoside analogues including cidofovir on CRPV-induced rabbit papillomas. Antiviral Res 2000; 48:131-42.

Chu NR, Wu HB, Wu T, et al. Immunotherapy of a human papillomavirus (HPV) type 16 E7-expressing tumour by administration of fusion protein comprising *Mycobacterium bovis* bacille Calmette-Guerin (BCG) hsp65 and HPV16 E7. Clin Exp Immunol 2000;121:216-25.

Chu RS, Targoni OS, Krieg AM, et al. CpG oligodeoxynucleotides act as adjuvants that switch on T helper 1 (Th1) immunity. J Exp Med 1997;186:1623-31.

Condon C, Watkins SC, Celluzzi CM, et al. DNA-based immunization by in vivo transfection of dendritic cells. Nat Med 1996;2:1122-8.

Corr M, Lee DJ, Carson DA, et al. Gene vaccination with naked plasmid DNA: mechanism of CTL priming. J Exp Med 1996;184:1555-60.

Corr M, Tighe H, Lee D, et al. Costimulation provided by DNA immunization enhances antitumor immunity. J Immunol 1997;159:4999-5004.

Crook T, Morgenstern JP, Crawford L, et al. Continued expression of HPV-16 E7 protein is required for maintenance of the transformed phenotype of cells co-transformed by HPV-16 plus EJ-ras. EMBO J 1989;8:513-9.

Darji A, Guzman CA, Gerstel B, et al. Oral somatic transgene vaccination using attenuated *S. typhimurium*. Cell 1997;91:765-75.

De Bruijn ML, Schuurhuis DH, Vierboom MP, et al. Immunization with human papillomavirus type 16 (HPV16) oncoprotein-loaded dendritic cells as well as protein in adjuvant induces MHC class I-restricted protection to HPV16-induced tumor cells. Cancer Res 1998;58:724-31.

Deres K, Schild H, Wiesmuller KH, et al. In vivo priming of virus-specific cytotoxic T lymphocytes with synthetic lipopeptide vaccine. Nature 1989;342:561-4.

Doan T, Herd KA, Lambert PF, et al. Peripheral tolerance to human papillomavirus E7 oncoprotein occurs by cross-tolerization, is largely Th-2-independent, and is broken by dendritic cell immunization. Cancer Res 2000;60:2810-5.

Donnelly JJ, Ulmer JB, Shiver JW, et al. DNA vaccines. Ann Rev Immunol 1997;15:617-48.

Dorange F, El Mehdaoui S, Pichon C, et al. Marek's disease virus (MDV) homologues of herpes simplex virus type 1 UL49 (VP22) and UL48 (VP16) genes: high-level expression and characterization of MDV-1 VP22 and VP16. J Gen Virol 2000;81:2219-30.

Edmonds C, Vousden KH. A point mutational analysis of human papillomavirus type 16 E7 protein. J Virol 1989;63:2650-6.

Elliott G, O'Hare P. Intercellular trafficking and protein delivery by a herpesvirus structural protein. Cell 1997;88:223-33.

Feltkamp MC, Smits HL, Vierboom MP, et al. Vaccination with cytotoxic T lymphocyte epitope-containing peptide protects against a tumor induced by human papillomavirus type 16-transformed cells. Eur J Immunol 1993;23:2242-9.

Fernando GJ, Stenzel DJ, Tindle RW, et al. Peptide polymerisation facilitates incorporation into ISCOMs and increases antigen-specific IgG2a production. Vaccine 1995;13:1460-7.

Flotte TR, Carter BJ. Adeno-associated virus vectors for gene therapy. Gene Ther 1995; 2: 357-62.

Gao L, Chain B, Sinclair C, et al. Immune response to human papillomavirus type 16 E6 gene in a live vaccinia vector. J Gen Virol 1994;75:157-64.

Gerard CM, Baudson N, Kraemer K, et al. Therapeutic potential of protein and adjuvant vaccinations on tumour growth. Vaccine 2001;19:2583-9.

Greenstone HL, Nieland JD, de Visser KE, et al. Chimeric papillomavirus virus-like particles elicit antitumor immunity against the E7 oncoprotein in an HPV16 tumor model. Proc Natl Acad Sci U S A 1998;95:1800-5.

Gromme M, Uytdehaag FG, Janssen H, et al. Recycling MHC class I molecules and endosomal peptide loading. Proc Natl Acad Sci U S A 1999;96:10326-31.

Gunn GR, Zubair A, Peters C, et al. Two *Listeria monocytogenes* vaccine vectors that express different molecular forms of human papilloma virus-16 (HPV-16) E7 induce qualitatively different T cell immunity that correlates with their ability to induce regression of established tumors immortalized by HPV-16. J Immunol 2001;167:6471-9.

Hallez S, Detremmerie O, Giannouli C, et al. Interleukin-12-secreting human papillomavirus type 16-transformed cells provide a potent cancer vaccine that generates E7-directed immunity. Int J Cancer 1999;81:428-37.

Harding CV, Song R. Phagocytic processing of exogenous particulate antigens by macrophages for presentation by class I MHC molecules. J Immunol 1994;153:4925-33.

Hariharan K, Braslawsky G, Barnett RS, et al. Tumor regression in mice following vaccination with human papillomavirus E7 recombinant protein in PROVAX. Int J Oncol 1998a; 12:1229-35.

Hariharan MJ, Driver DA, Townsend K, et al. DNA immunization against herpes simplex virus: enhanced efficacy using a Sindbis virus-based vector. J Virol 1998b;72:950-8.

Harms JS, Ren X, Oliveira SC, et al. Distinctions between bovine herpesvirus 1 and herpes simplex virus type 1 VP22 tegument protein subcellular associations. J Virol 2000; 74:3301-12.

Hart DN. Dendritic cells: unique leukocyte populations which control the primary immune response. Blood 1997;90:3245-87.

He Z, Wlazlo AP, Kowalczyk DW, et al. Viral recombinant vaccines to the E6 and E7 antigens of HPV-16. Virology 2000;270:146-61.

Heck DV, Yee CL, Howley PM, et al. Efficiency of binding the retinoblastoma protein correlates with the transforming capacity of the E7 oncoproteins of the human papillomaviruses. Proc Natl Acad Sci U S A 1992;89:4442-6.

Heufler C, Koch F, Schuler G. Granulocyte/macrophage colony-stimulating factor and interleukin 1 mediate the maturation of murine epidermal Langerhans cells into potent immunostimulatory dendritic cells. J Exp Med 1988;167:700-5.

Hsu KF, Hung KF, Cheng WF, et al. Enhancement of suicidal DNA vaccine potency by linking *Mycobacterium tuberculosis* heat shock protein 70 to an antigen. Gene Ther 2001; 8:376-83.

Huang AY, Golumbek P, Ahmadzadeh M, et al. Role of bone marrow-derived cells in presenting MHC class I-restricted tumor antigens. Science 1994;264:961-5.

Hung CF, Cheng WF, Chai CY, et al. Improving vaccine potency through intercellular spreading and enhanced MHC class I presentation of antigen. J Immunol 2001a;166:5733-40.

Hung CF, Cheng WF, Hsu KF, et al. Cancer immunotherapy using a DNA vaccine encoding the translocation domain of a bacterial toxin linked to a tumor antigen. Cancer Res 2001b; 61:3698-703.

Hung CF, He L, Juang J, et al. Improving DNA vaccine potency by linking Marek's disease virus type 1 VP22 to an antigen. J Virol 2002;76:2676-82.

Inaba K, Inaba M, Romani N, et al. Generation of large numbers of dendritic cells from mouse bone marrow cultures supplemented with granulocyte/macrophage colony-stimulating factor. J Exp Med 1992;176:1693-702.

Irvine KR, Rao JB, Rosenberg SA, et al. Cytokine enhancement of DNA immunization leads to effective treatment of established pulmonary metastases. J Immunol 1996;156:238-45.

Jabbar IA, Fernando GJ, Saunders N, et al. Immune responses induced by BCG recombinant for human papillomavirus L1 and E7 proteins. Vaccine 2000;18:2444-53.

Jewers RJ, Hildebrandt P, Ludlow JW, et al. Regions of human papillomavirus type 16 E7 oncoprotein required for immortalization of human keratinocytes. J Virol 1992;66:1329-35.

Ji H, Chang EY, Lin KY, et al. Antigen-specific immunotherapy for murine lung metastatic tumors expressing human papillomavirus type 16 E7 oncoprotein. Int J Cancer 1998;78:41-5.

Ji H, Wang T-L, Chen C-H, et al. Targeting HPV-16 E7 to the endosomal/lysosomal compartment enhances the antitumor immunity of DNA vaccines against murine HPV-16 E7-expressing tumors. Human Gene Therapy 1999;10:2727-2740.

Jochmus I, Schafer K, Faath S, et al. Chimeric virus-like particles of the human papillomavirus type 16 (HPV 16) as a prophylactic and therapeutic vaccine. Arch Med Res 1999; 30:269-74.

Jondal M, Schirmbeck R, Reimann J. MHC class I-restricted CTL responses to exogenous antigens. Immunity 1996;5:295-302.

Kast WM, Brandt RM, Drijfhout JW, et al. Human leukocyte antigen-A2.1 restricted candidate cytotoxic T lymphocyte epitopes of human papillomavirus type 16 E6 and E7 proteins identified by using the processing-defective human cell line T2. J Immunother 1993;14:115-20.

Kim TW, Hung CF, Ling M, et al. Enhancing DNA vaccine potency by coadministration of DNA encoding antiapoptotic proteins. J Clin Invest 2003;112:109-17.

Koptidesova D, Kopacek J, Zelnik V, et al. Identification and characterization of a cDNA clone derived from the Marek's disease tumour cell line RPL1 encoding a homologue of alpha- transinducing factor (VP16) of HSV-1. Arch Virol 1995;140:355-62.

Kovacsovics-Bankowski M, Rock KL. A phagosome-to-cytosol pathway for exogenous antigens presented on MHC class I molecules. Science 1995;267:243-6.

Kowalczyk DW, Wlazlo AP, Shane S, et al. Vaccine regimen for prevention of sexually transmitted infections with human papillomavirus type 16. Vaccine 2001;19:3583-90.

Krul MR, Tijhaar EJ, Kleijne JA, et al. Induction of an antibody response in mice against human papillomavirus (HPV) type 16 after immunization with HPV recombinant Salmonella strains. Cancer Immunol Immunother 1996;43:44-8.

Lacey CJ, Thompson HS, Monteiro EF, et al. Phase IIa safety and immunogenicity of a therapeutic vaccine, TA-GW, in persons with genital warts. J Infect Dis 1999;179:612-8.

Lamikanra A, Pan ZK, Isaacs SN, et al. Regression of established human papillomavirus type 16 (HPV-16) immortalized tumors in vivo by vaccinia viruses expressing different forms of HPV-16 E7 correlates with enhanced CD8(+) T-cell responses that home to the tumor site. J Virol 2001;75:9654-64.

Leachman SA, Tigelaar RE, Shlyankevich M, et al. Granulocyte-macrophage colony-stimulating factor priming plus papillomavirus E6 DNA vaccination: effects on papilloma formation and regression in the cottontail rabbit papillomavirus--rabbit model. J Virol 2000;74:8700-8.

Leitner WW, Ying H, Driver DA, et al. Enhancement of tumor-specific immune response with plasmid DNA replicon vectors. Cancer Res 2000;60:51-5.

Li Z. Priming of T cells by heat shock protein-peptide complexes as the basis of tumor vaccines. Semin Immunol 1997;9:315-22.

Lin K-Y, Guarnieri FG, Staveley-O'Carroll KF, et al. Treatment of established tumors with a novel vaccine that enhances major histocompatibility class II presentation of tumor antigen. Cancer Research 1996;56:21-26.

Liu DW, Tsao YP, Kung JT, et al. Recombinant adeno-associated virus expressing human papillomavirus type 16 E7 peptide DNA fused with heat shock protein DNA as a potential vaccine for cervical cancer. J Virol 2000;74:2888-94.

Liu WJ, Zhao KN, Gao FG, et al. Polynucleotide viral vaccines: codon optimisation and ubiquitin conjugation enhances prophylactic and therapeutic efficacy. Vaccine 2001; 20: 862-9.

Liu Y, Chiriva-Internati M, Grizzi F, et al. Rapid induction of cytotoxic T-cell response against cervical cancer cells by human papillomavirus type 16 E6 antigen gene delivery into human dendritic cells by an adeno-associated virus vector. Cancer Gene Ther 2001;8:948-57.

Liu YJ. Dendritic cell subsets and lineages, and their functions in innate and adaptive immunity. Cell 2001;106:259-62.

Londono LP, Chatfield S, Tindle RW, et al. Immunisation of mice using Salmonella typhimurium expressing human papillomavirus type 16 E7 epitopes inserted into hepatitis B virus core antigen. Vaccine 1996;14:545-52.

Lukas J, Muller H, Bartkova J, et al. DNA tumor virus oncoproteins and retinoblastoma gene mutations share the ability to relieve the cell's requirement for cyclin D1 function in G1. J Cell Biol 1994;125:625-38.

Mayordomo JI, Zorina T, Storkus WJ, et al. Bone marrow-derived dendritic cells pulsed with synthetic tumour peptides elicit protective and therapeutic antitumour immunity. Nat Med 1995;1:1297-302.

Mayordomo JI, Zorina T, Storkus WJ, et al. Bone marrow-derived dendritic cells serve as potent adjuvants for peptide-based antitumor vaccines. Stem Cells 1997;15:94-103.

McMillan NA, Payne E, Frazer IH, et al. Expression of the alpha6 integrin confers papillomavirus binding upon receptor-negative B-cells. Virology 1999;261:271-9.

Meneguzzi G, Cerni C, Kieny MP, et al. Immunization against human papillomavirus type 16 tumor cells with recombinant vaccinia viruses expressing E6 and E7. Virology 1991;181:62-9.

Michel N, Osen W, Gissmann L, et al. Enhanced immunogenicity of HPV 16 E7 fusion proteins in DNA vaccination. Virology 2002;294:47-59.

Moss B. Genetically engineered poxviruses for recombinant gene expression, vaccination, and safety. Proc Natl Acad Sci U S A 1996;93:11341-8.

Muderspach L, Wilczynski S, Roman L, et al. A phase I trial of a human papillomavirus (HPV) peptide vaccine for women with high-grade cervical and vulvar intraepithelial neoplasia who are HPV 16 positive. Clin Cancer Res 2000;6:3406-16.

Murakami M, Gurski KJ, Marincola FM, et al. Induction of specific CD8+ T-lymphocyte responses using a human papillomavirus-16 E6/E7 fusion protein and autologous dendritic cells. Cancer Res 1999;59:1184-7.

Nichols WW, Ledwith BJ, Manam SV, et al. Potential DNA vaccine integration into host cell genome. Ann N Y Acad Sci 1995;772:30-39.

Osen W, Peiler T, Ohlschlager P, et al. A DNA vaccine based on a shuffled E7 oncogene of the human papillomavirus type 16 (HPV 16) induces E7-specific cytotoxic T cells but lacks transforming activity. Vaccine 2001;19:4276-86.

Ossevoort MA, Feltkamp MC, van Veen KJ, et al. Dendritic cells as carriers for a cytotoxic T-lymphocyte epitope-based peptide vaccine in protection against a human papillomavirus type 16-induced tumor. J Immunother Emphasis Tumor Immunol 1995;18:86-94.

Pan ZK, Ikonomidis G, Pardoll D, et al. Regression of established tumors in mice mediated by the oral administration of a recombinant *Listeria monocytogenes* vaccine. Cancer Res 1995; 55:4776-9.

Peng S, Frazer IH, Fernando GJ, et al. Papillomavirus virus-like particles can deliver defined CTL epitopes to the MHC class I pathway. Virology 1998;240:147-57.

Phelps WC, Munger K, Yee CL, et al. Structure-function analysis of the human papillomavirus type 16 E7 oncoprotein. J Virol 1992;66:2418-27.

Plotkin SA, Cadoz M, Meignier B, et al. The safety and use of canarypox vectored vaccines. Dev Biol Stand 1995;84:165-70.

Polo JM, Belli BA, Driver DA, et al. Stable alphavirus packaging cell lines for Sindbis virus and Semliki Forest virus-derived vectors. Proc Natl Acad Sci U S A 1999;96:4598-603.

Porgador A, Irvine KR, Iwasaki A, et al. Predominant role for directly transfected dendritic cells in antigen presentation to CD8+ T cells after gene gun immunization. J Exp Med 1998; 188:1075-82.

Price AA, Cumberbatch M, Kimber I, et al. Alpha 6 integrins are required for Langerhans cell migration from the epidermis. J Exp Med 1997;186:1725-35.

Pushko P, Parker M, Ludwig GV, et al. Replicon-helper systems from attenuated Venezuelan equine encephalitis virus: expression of heterologous genes in vitro and immunization against heterologous pathogens in vivo. Virology 1997;239:389-401.

Ressing ME, Sette A, Brandt RM, et al. Human CTL epitopes encoded by human papillomavirus type 16 E6 and E7 identified through in vivo and in vitro immunogenicity studies of HLA-A*0201-binding peptides. J Immunol 1995;154:5934-43.

Ressing ME, van Driel WJ, Brandt RM, et al. Detection of T helper responses, but not of human papillomavirus-specific cytotoxic T lymphocyte responses, after peptide vaccination of patients with cervical carcinoma. J Immunother 2000;23:255-66.

Revaz V, Benyacoub J, Kast WM, et al. Mucosal vaccination with a recombinant Salmonella typhimurium expressing human papillomavirus type 16 (HPV16) L1 virus-like particles (VLPs) or HPV16 VLPs purified from insect cells inhibits the growth of HPV16-expressing tumor cells in mice. Virology 2001;279:354-60.

Robinson HL. Nucleic acid vaccines: an overview. Vaccine 1997a;15:785-7.

Robinson HL, Torres CA. DNA vaccines. Semin Immunol 1997b;9:271-283.

Rock KL. A new foreign policy: MHC class I molecules monitor the outside world. Immunol Today 1996;17:131-7.

Roden RB, Hubbert NL, Kirnbauer R, et al. Assessment of the serological relatedness of genital human papillomaviruses by hemagglutination inhibition. J Virol 1996;70:3298-301.

Roman M, Martin-Orozco E, Goodman JS, et al. Immunostimulatory DNA sequences function as T helper-1-promoting adjuvants. Nat Med 1997;3:849-54.

Rosenberg SA, Yang JC, Schwartzentruber DJ, et al. Immunologic and therapeutic evaluation of a synthetic peptide vaccine for the treatment of patients with metastatic melanoma. Nat Med 1998;4:321-7.

Rossi JL, Gissman L, Jansen K, et al. Assembly of infectious human papillomavirus type 16 virus-like particle in Saccharomyces cerevisae. Hum Gene Ther 2000;11:1165-76.

Rudolf MP, Fausch SC, Da Silva DM, et al. Human dendritic cells are activated by chimeric human papillomavirus type-16 virus-like particles and induce epitope-specific human T cell responses in vitro. J Immunol 2001a;166:5917-24.

Rudolf MP, Man S, Melief CJ, et al. Human T-cell responses to HLA-A-restricted high binding affinity peptides of human papillomavirus type 18 proteins E6 and E7. Clin Cancer Res 2001b;7:788s-795s.

Sarkar AK, Tortolero-Luna G, Nehete PN, et al. Studies on in vivo induction of cytotoxic T lymphocyte responses by synthetic peptides from E6 and E7 oncoproteins of human papillomavirus type 16. Viral Immunol 1995;8:165-74.

Schafer K, Muller M, Faath S, et al. Immune response to human papillomavirus 16 L1E7 chimeric virus-like particles: induction of cytotoxic T cells and specific tumor protection. Int J Cancer 1999;81:881-8.

Schild H, Deres K, Wiesmuller KH, et al. Efficiency of peptides and lipopeptides for in vivo priming of virus- specific cytotoxic T cells. Eur J Immunol 1991;21:2649-54.

Schirmbeck R, Bohm W, Melber K, et al. Processing of exogenous heat-aggregated (denatured) and particulate (native) hepatitis B surface antigen for class I-restricted epitope presentation. J Immunol 1995;155:4676-84.

Schmidt W, Buschle M, Zauner W, et al. Cell-free tumor antigen peptide-based cancer vaccines. Proc Natl Acad Sci U S A 1997;94:3262-7.

Shi W, Bu P, Liu J, et al. Human papillomavirus type 16 E7 DNA vaccine: mutation in the open reading frame of E7 enhances specific cytotoxic T-lymphocyte induction and antitumor activity. J Virol 1999;73:7877-81.

Shi W, Liu J, Huang Y, et al. Papillomavirus pseudovirus: a novel vaccine to induce mucosal and systemic cytotoxic T-lymphocyte responses. J Virol 2001;75:10139-48.

Srivastava PK. Purification of heat shock protein-peptide complexes for use in vaccination against cancers and intracellular pathogens. Methods 1997;12:165-71.

Srivastava PK, Menoret A, Basu S, et al. Heat shock proteins come of age: primitive functions acquire new roles in an adaptive world. Immunity 1998;8:657-65.

Srivastava PK, Udono H. Heat shock protein-peptide complexes in cancer immunotherapy. Curr Opin Immunol 1994;6:728-32.

Steinman RM. The dendritic cell system and its role in immunogenicity. Ann Rev Immunol 1991;9:271-96.

Steller MA, Gurski KJ, Murakami M, et al. Cell-mediated immunological responses in cervical and vaginal cancer patients immunized with a lipidated epitope of human papillomavirus type 16 E7. Clin Cancer Res 1998;4:2103-9.

Suto R, Srivastava PK. A mechanism for the specific immunogenicity of heat shock protein-chaperoned peptides. Science 1995;269:1585-8.

Sutter G, Moss B. Nonreplicating vaccinia vector efficiently expresses recombinant genes. Proc Natl Acad Sci U S A 1992;89:10847-51.

Suzue K, Zhou X, Eisen HN, et al. Heat shock fusion proteins as vehicles for antigen delivery into the major histocompatibility complex class I presentation pathway. Proc Natl Acad Sci USA 1997;94:13146-51.

Tan J, Yang NS, Turner JG, et al. Interleukin-12 cDNA skin transfection potentiates human papillomavirus E6 DNA vaccine-induced antitumor immune response. Cancer Gene Ther 1999; 6:331-9.

Tao MH, Levy R. Idiotype/granulocyte-macrophage colony-stimulating factor fusion protein as a vaccine for B-cell lymphoma. Nature 1993;362:755-8.

Thompson HS, Davies ML, Holding FP, et al. Phase I safety and antigenicity of TA-GW: a recombinant HPV6 L2E7 vaccine for the treatment of genital warts. Vaccine 1999;17:40-9.

Tillman BW, Hayes TL, DeGruijl TD, et al. Adenoviral vectors targeted to CD40 enhance the efficacy of dendritic cell-based vaccination against human papillomavirus 16-induced tumor cells in a murine model. Cancer Res 2000;60:5456-63.

Tindle RW, Croft S, Herd K, et al. A vaccine conjugate of 'ISCAR' immunocarrier and peptide epitopes of the E7 cervical cancer-associated protein of human papillomavirus type 16 elicits specific Th1- and Th2-type responses in immunized mice in the absence of oil-based adjuvants. Clin Exp Immunol 1995;101:265-71.

Toes RE, Blom RJ, Offringa R, et al. Enhanced tumor outgrowth after peptide vaccination. Functional deletion of tumor-specific CTL induced by peptide vaccination can lead to the inability to reject tumors. J Immunol 1996a;156:3911-8.

Toes RE, Offringa R, Blom RJ, et al. Peptide vaccination can lead to enhanced tumor growth through specific T-cell tolerance induction. Proc Natl Acad Sci U S A 1996b;93:7855-60.

Toes RE, van der Voort EI, Schoenberger SP, et al. Enhancement of tumor outgrowth through CTL tolerization after peptide vaccination is avoided by peptide presentation on dendritic cells. J Immunol 1998;160:4449-56.

Touze A, Coursaget P. In vitro gene transfer using human papillomavirus-like particles. Nucleic Acids Res 1998;26:1317-23.

Tuting T. The immunology of cutaneous DNA immunization. Curr Opin Mol Ther 1999;1:216-25.

Tuting T, DeLeo AB, Lotze MT, et al. Genetically modified bone marrow-derived dendritic cells expressing tumor-associated viral or "self" antigens induce antitumor immunity in vivo. Eur J Immunol 1997;27:2702-7.

van der Burg SH, Kwappenberg KM, O'Neill T, et al. Pre-clinical safety and efficacy of TA-CIN, a recombinant HPV16 L2E6E7 fusion protein vaccine, in homologous and heterologous prime-boost regimens. Vaccine 2001a;19:3652-60.

van der Burg SH, Ressing ME, Kwappenberg KM, et al. Natural T-helper immunity against human papillomavirus type 16 (HPV16) E7-derived peptide epitopes in patients with HPV16-positive cervical lesions: identification of 3 human leukocyte antigen class II-restricted epitopes. Int J Cancer 2001b;91:612-8.

van Driel WJ, Ressing ME, Kenter GG, et al. Vaccination with HPV16 peptides of patients with advanced cervical carcinoma: clinical evaluation of a phase I-II trial. Eur J Cancer 1999;35:946-52.

Velders MP, McElhiney S, Cassetti MC, et al. Eradication of established tumors by vaccination with Venezuelan equine encephalitis virus replicon particles delivering human papillomavirus 16 E7 RNA. Cancer Res 2001a;61:7861-7.

Velders MP, Weijzen S, Eiben GL, et al. Defined flanking spacers and enhanced proteolysis is essential for eradication of established tumors by an epitope string DNA vaccine. J Immunol 2001b;166:5366-73.

Vierboom MP, Feltkamp MC, Neisig A, et al. Peptide vaccination with an anchor-replaced CTL epitope protects against human papillomavirus type 16-induced tumors expressing the wild-type epitope. J Immunother 1998;21:399-408.

Villanueva MS, Sijts AJ, Pamer EG. Listeriolysin is processed efficiently into an MHC class I-associated epitope in Listeria monocytogenes-infected cells. J Immunol 1995;155:5227-33.

Wang T-L, Ling M, Shih I-M, et al. Intramuscular administration of E7-transfected dendritic cells generates the most potent E7-specific anti-tumor immunity. Gene Ther 2000;7:726-33.

Warnier G, Duffour MT, Uyttenhove C, et al. Induction of a cytolytic T-cell response in mice with a recombinant adenovirus coding for tumor antigen P815A. Int J Cancer 1996;67:303-10.

Weiner GJ, Liu HM, Wooldridge JE, et al. Immunostimulatory oligodeoxynucleotides containing the CpG motif are effective as immune adjuvants in tumor antigen immunization. Proc Natl Acad Sci USA 1997;94:10833-7.

Wilson JM. Gene therapy for cystic fibrosis: challenges and future directions. J Clin Invest 1995;96:2547-54.

Wilson JM. Adenoviruses as gene-delivery vehicles. N Engl J Med 1996;334:1185-7.

Witmer-Pack MD, Olivier W, Valinsky J, et al. Granulocyte/macrophage colony-stimulating factor is essential for the viability and function of cultured murine epidermal Langerhans cells. J Exp Med 1987;166:1484-98.

Wu T-C, Guarnieri FG, Staveley-O'Carroll KF, et al. Engineering an intracellular pathway for MHC class II presentation of HPV-16 E7. Proc Natl Acad Sci 1995;92:11671-5.

Xiong C, Levis R, Shen P, et al. Sindbis virus: an efficient, broad host range vector for gene expression in animal cells. Science 1989;243:1188-91.

Ying H, Zaks TZ, Wang RF, et al. Cancer therapy using a self-replicating RNA vaccine. Nat Med 1999;5:823-7.

Yoon H, Chung MK, Min SS, et al. Synthetic peptides of human papillomavirus type 18 E6 harboring HLA-A2.1 motif can induce peptide-specific cytotoxic T-cells from peripheral blood mononuclear cells of healthy donors. Virus Res 1998;54:23-9.

Zehbe I, Wilander E, Delius H, et al. Human papillomavirus 16 E6 variants are more prevalent in invasive cervical carcinoma than the prototype. Cancer Res 1998;58:829-33.

Zhai Y, Yang JC, Kawakami Y, et al. Antigen-specific tumor vaccines. Development and characterization of recombinant adenoviruses encoding MART1 or gp100 for cancer therapy. J Immunol 1996;156:700-10.

Zhao KN, Sun XY, Frazer IH, et al. DNA packaging by L1 and L2 capsid proteins of bovine papillomavirus type 1. Virology 1998;243:482-91.

Chapter 14

Policies for Implementing Cervical Cancer Preventive and Control Strategies

Robert A. Hiatt, M.D., Ph.D. and Jon F. Kerner, Ph.D.
Division of Cancer Control and Population Sciences, National Cancer Institute

INTRODUCTION

Research on cervical cancer is rapidly generating fundamental knowledge that is increasing our understanding of this disease. Effective control of cervical cancer requires that this new knowledge be translated into interventions that reach all populations at risk for developing and dying of this disease. However, the application of effective interventions in diverse medical and public health settings usually requires policy decisions by responsible authorities. By 'policy', we refer to the various courses of action that can be taken by governments, organized medical systems (e.g. health plans), and professional entities that have the power to influence decision-making with regard to health and cancer-related programs. For example, policies may be made by governments to cover payment for the early detection of cervical neoplasia, by professional societies in generating guidelines for care, or by organized health care systems that adopt evidence-based protocols for behavioral interventions. This chapter will examine cervical cancer control policies that are already in place as well as opportunities for new policies anticipated in the near future.

Cervical cancer can claim to be the first neoplasm for which a cancer control policy was ever established. Gynecologic surgeons, motivated by a deep concern over the often fatal outcomes for women with invasive cervical cancer and the dismal treatment options available, formed the American Society for the Control of Cancer (later the American Cancer Society) in New York City in 1913. Their first actions as a society were to make recommendations for cancer case registration, the analysis of vital statistics and the study of the geographic distribution of the disease, as well as for educational programs about the 'accepted cancer facts' (Hoffman, 1913 quoted by Hiatt and Rimer, 1999).

The 'policy' of regular Pap smear screening recommended by all screening guidelines and almost universally accepted as part of good preventive medicine in developed countries, is a prime example of the translation of fundamental knowledge into an effective intervention. Adoption of routine Pap smear screening in the U.S. has been associated with a stunning 70% decrease in cervical cancer mortality following its introduction in the 1930s (Papanicolaou, 1941) and a 53% decrease from 1973 through 1999 (Ries et al., 2002). However, despite this success, the task of eliminating avoidable cervical cancer morbidity and mortality remains incomplete. In order to reach the goal of making cervical cancer an increasingly uncommon and easily treatable disease, new modes of prevention, early detection and treatment are needed. New policies will be required to ensure their effective application.

To explain how policy decisions influence cancer control, we draw on a framework (Figure 1) that has been adopted by the U.S. National Cancer Institute (NCI) (Hiatt and Rimer, 1999) from earlier work by the Advisory Committee on Cancer Control, National Cancer Institute of Canada (Adv Comm, 1994). This framework has been highly effective in setting the national agenda in cancer control research in both countries since the mid 1990s (Best et al., 2003). The framework delineates the inter-relationships between basic or fundamental research, which answers 'what do we know', intervention research, which tells us 'what works', and surveillance research, which answers the question 'where are we?'. After a process of knowledge synthesis and decision-making that tells us 'where we need to go next', effective intervention approaches can be disseminated through new or available channels to the service delivery entities that will make use of them. It is at this point in the process, in the application and delivery of evidence-based interventions, that policy setting becomes critical. All these processes draw on the principles of accountability, empowerment, ethics, and efficiency with regard to the communities served.

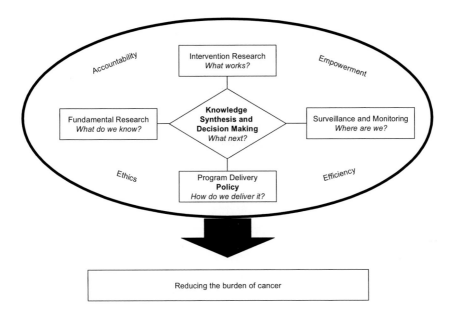

Figure 1: Cancer Control Research Framework. Adapted from the 1994 Advisory Committee on Cancer Control, National Cancer Institute of Canada. Policy is critical in the delivery of synthesized knowledge from cancer control research.

Taking a broader international perspective in policy making, one must be mindful of the stark contrast between the cervical cancer burden in developed countries, like the U.S., and that of many developing countries. Whereas in the U.S cervical cancer is the 10th most common cause of new cases of cancer and the 14th most common cause of death from cancer (estimated at 13,000 new cases and 4,100 deaths in 2002) (Reis et al., 2002), among women worldwide it is second for new cases and fifth for deaths, with an estimated 471,000 new cases and 233,000 deaths annually (Parkin et al., 2001). Maps of cervical cancer mortality internationally (Figure 2) illustrate a marked geographic variation in rates (Ferlay et al., 2001). As can be seen, there is, on average, more than a two-fold excess burden of the disease in the less developed world compared to that in the developed world and as much as an 8-fold contrast between specific regions such as Western Europe and East Africa or Southeast Asia.

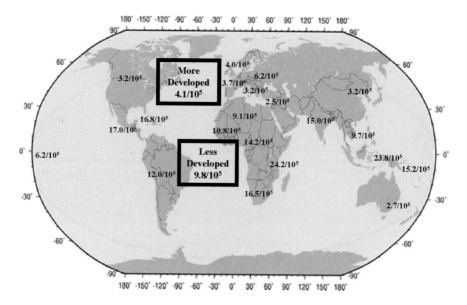

Figure 2: International Cervical Cancer Mortality Variation.   Adapted from data in GLOBOCAN 2000, Ferlay et al., 2001.

While it would be ideal if a single intervention could be effective everywhere, clearly this is not the case and policies need to be adjusted to take into consideration both the prevalence of disease and the available resources in any specific country or region. Furthermore, even within some countries, a uniform approach to the control of cervical cancer could be misguided because it would not take into account what we know about variation in the geographic and social class distributions of incidence, mortality and health care resources. It is quite apparent that a lack of resources for early detection and treatment has a major impact on the health burden associated with cervical cancer. In many developing countries it is prohibitively expensive to conduct Pap smears, or follow-up on abnormal findings (Goldie et al., 2001; Goldie, 2002).

For the U.S. (Figure 3), mortality maps reflect considerable geographic disparities. For whites, the high mortality counties extend from rural Maine down through Appalachia to the Texas/Mexico border, while for African Americans (not shown), the high mortality counties are concentrated in the southeastern and mid-Atlantic states. The majority of these counties are rural or suburban, and have high proportions of low income and low education populations. It should also be noted that approximately 95% of the white population in the counties along the Texas/Mexico border are of Latin American origin (Devesa et al., 1999).

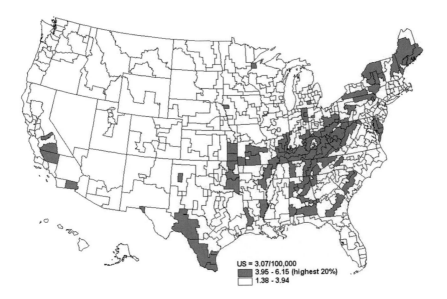

Figure 3. Cancer Mortality Rates by State Economic Area*, Cervix Uteri: White Females, 1970-98. Shaded area indicates the SEAs with the highest 20% of mortality rates. The map was constructed utilizing 1970-98 mortality data from the National Center for Health Statistics and population estimates from the US Census Bureau. Rates per 100,000 person-years were directly standardized using the 1970 U.S. population.

Surveys often reveal additional variation within geographic areas that prove useful in setting intervention policies. Research in the San Francisco Bay Area that has simultaneously evaluated race, ethnicity and socio-economic variables, has shown that race and ethnicity tend not be as strong a predictor of screening behavior as socio-economic factors. Whether an individual is insured, has regular medical care, or is a recent immigrant were the more powerful predictors of screening (Hiatt et al., 2001). In Appalachia, historically a medically underserved area of the U.S., women with the lowest education and income report substantially lower Pap smear rates in the previous 3 years (67.4 and 71.2%, respectively) compared to women overall (82.4% in 1996-98) (Hall et al., 2002). These observations suggest policy approaches that would redirect services to very high-risk groups within the larger population of women at risk.

Given these introductory considerations on the variability of cervical cancer mortality in relation to geographic area, race or ethnicity, and

---

* A State Economic Area (SEA) is an individual county or group of counties that are relatively homogeneous with respect to various demographic, economic, and cultural factors. The 508 SEAs do not cross state lines.

socioeconomic status, we now review policies specific to both those diagnosed with and those at risk of cervical cancer. As an organizing principle we will discuss policies along what has been called the 'cancer control continuum' (NCI, DCCPS, 2003), which goes from the pre-clinical state through diagnosis and treatment, to the end-of-life. Different interventions and policy decisions are needed for each phase of this continuum from prevention, to early detection, to treatment and long-term care, examples of which we illustrate in Figure 4.

THE CERVICAL CANCER CONTROL CONTINUUM

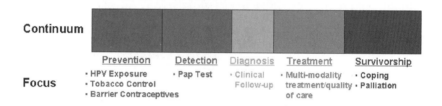

Figure 4. The Cervical Cancer Control Continuum

1   POLICIES FOR PRIMARY PREVENTION

The first phase of the cancer control continuum is that of primary prevention. While it is clear that certain social factors such as sexual practices, low income, and tobacco use play a significant role as determinants of cervical cancer, there is little literature on the impact of interventions that focus on these factors specifically in regard to cervical cancer (see Chapter 9), and therefore policies with respect to these factors, will not be discussed here.

1.1   Barrier contraceptives

The sexually transmissible oncogenic human papillomavirus (HPV) is now considered a necessary cause of cervical cancer (Munoz et al., 1992; Walboomers et al., 1999; Chapter 7) and this central etiologic role of HPV has been found to be true throughout the world (Bosch et al., 1995). However, unlike most other sexually transmitted diseases, mechanical or barrier methods are not reliable methods for the prevention of anogenital

HPV infections, because the virus in commonly present at external genital sites not covered by the barrier (zur Hausen, 2002). A policy that encourages barrier contraceptives may be justified for its value in preventing other sexually transmissible diseases, but their use in cervical cancer control requires further study. There is some indication that proper hygiene in routine gynecologic examinations can minimize inoculation of the cervix with HPV, and the establishment of higher standards of hygienic practice among gynecologists and obstetricians may be beneficial (zur Hausen, 2002).

1.2 Preventive vaccines

Recent research on HPV vaccines looks very promising and vaccines for both preventive and therapeutic uses may be available within the next 10 years (Harro et al., 2001; Chapters 12 and 13). A recent controlled trial demonstrated that a monovalent HPV-16 vaccine was highly efficacious against new, persistent infections in 16 to 23 year old women (Koutsky et al., 2002). If future studies confirm and expand this result and if the impact is anything close to that of vaccines against hepatitis B infection in Taiwan (Huang et al., 2000), the impact of HPV preventive vaccines could be substantial in the near future. Such vaccines could be expected to substantially decrease the frequency of abnormal Pap smears soon after their introduction, and could substantially reduce the health care burden on both women and their physicians. An innovative change of this magnitude and significance will require new policy decisions. A determination will have to be made regarding the age at which such a vaccine should be administered, and to whom. At least 20 different genital types of HPV are associated with cervical cancer worldwide (Bosch et al., 1995). Decisions regarding which of these are significant enough to merit inclusion in preventive vaccines must be made, but multivalent vaccines that include at least types 16, 18, 31, 33, and 45 will undoubtedly be developed and tested for their public health effectiveness. The costs of HPV vaccines are likely to be high initially, and perhaps prohibitive in developing countries (Goldie, 2002), and this will undoubtedly generate policy debate. Recommendations regarding how frequently screening should occur will have to change when the incidence of new HPV infections and abnormal screening tests is markedly lower. Finally, the availability of vaccines for a sexually transmitted disease is likely to provoke some psychosocial resistance to their full and appropriate use in certain political and cultural circles. Like oral contraceptives before them, they may be seen as implying permissiveness with regard to sexual activity. While research in this area has not yet begun, there is a window of opportunity during the vaccine development and testing phase, to explore some of the possible sociocultural and psychological barriers to adoption of an HPV vaccine. Preventive HPV vaccines have not yet led to policy decisions, but it seems inevitable that they will.

2   EARLY DETECTION POLICIES

The second place along the cancer control continuum where policy has a great impact is in the early detection of cervical cancer and its precursors. Since traditional screening, using the Pap smear, detects pre-malignant as well as invasive lesions, it has been credited with markedly reducing the incidence of, and morbidity and mortality from cervical cancer since its introduction in the 1930s (Papanicoloau et al., 1941).

U.S. surveillance data clearly show that the use of Pap smears has continued to increase in a steady trend over time (Figure 5). The most recent estimate from the National Health Interview Survey (NHIS) in 2000 indicates that overall 82.4% of women over 25 years of age have had a Pap smear within the last three years (Swan et al., 2003). However, there are certain subgroups within the U.S. population that continue to have substantially lower rates of screening. Lack of access to screening services is one factor, but the group with the lowest reported rate (58.3%) are those with no health care coverage (Swan et al., 2003). A comparison of white and African American women shows that there is very little difference between them in adherence to screening guidelines and, that in fact, African American women report slightly higher rates (Swan et al., 2003).

The NHIS data are the most reliable information available nationally on cervical cancer screening rates. However, policy makers, who base decisions on self-reported data, must be aware of an overestimation bias in the absolute values of screening in even well conducted surveys. Validation studies have repeatedly shown that self-reported data on Pap smears overestimate the true value based on rates documented in medical records for the same individuals (Hiatt et al., 1995; McPhee et al., 2002). Therefore, screening prevalence rates may need to adjusted downward by as much as one third for low-income, ethnic women (McPhee et al., 2002).

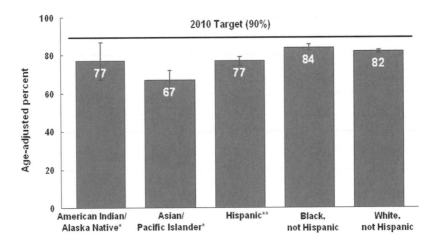

| 95% confidence interval.
* Includes persons of Hispanic and non-Hispanic origin.
** Persons of Hispanic origin may be of any race.
Note: Data are age adjusted to the 2000 standard population.
Source: National Health Interview Survey (NHIS), CDC, NCHS.

Figure 5. Pap tests received within past 3 years: Females 18 and over, by race/ethnicity, 2000

2.1   Current practices and policy issues

2.1.1   Access to early detection services

Access to screening services is a key issue in determining overall Pap smear screening rates. Factors determining access vary widely by country depending on whether there is universal access from national health systems, piecemeal access dependent on insurance coverage, or little access because of a lack of resources. Policies that provide coverage for Pap smears have been established in the U.S. by the Centers for Medicare and Medicaid (CMS). Medicaid, the state-based program that covers persons below a set level of income, offers coverage of Pap smear screening either routinely or upon a physician's recommendation. Medicare, which provides services for persons over age 65 years of age and certain special groups below that age, covers Pap smears every three years routinely or every year, if a woman has had an abnormal Pap smear in the preceding three years.

Data from the National Survey of America's Families shows that for low-income women, having some sort of insurance is strongly associated with receiving a recent Pap smear (Almeida et al., 2001). It did not matter if that insurance coverage was from Medicaid, since both privately insured and

Medicaid insured women reported a test in the last year more frequently than uninsured women (56.5% and 64.5%, respectively compared to 42.5% for uninsured women) (Almeida et al., 2001). Similar findings were documented among 55,278 women enrolled in the Women's Health Initiative's Observational Study (Hsia et al., 2000).

The main governmental policy program in the U.S. designed to rectify the lack of access and coverage beyond that provided by Medicaid and Medicare and to provide cervical cancer screening is the Center for Disease Control and Prevention's (CDC) National Breast and Cervical Cancer Early Detection Program (NBCCEDP) (Henson et al., 1996; Lawson et al.,1998). Established in 1991 by the passage of the Breast and Cervical Cancer Prevention Act, the NBCCEDP operates in all 50 states, the District of Columbia, six U.S. territories and 14 tribal organizations. By 2000 the NBCCEDP had screened over 1.5 million women, provided 3.5 million screening exams, and diagnosed more than 48,000 pre-cancerous cervical lesions and over 800 invasive cervical cancers (Lawson et al., 2000).

In recent years, the NBCCEDP has been working with state and local programs to focus more effort and resources on screening women who have never been screened, or who had not screened in the past 5 years. A policy that resulted from this new focus was the CDC requirement that women with three or more consecutive negative annual Pap smears be moved to a triennial screening schedule. This policy met with resistance because many programs originally built their recruitment around annual visits, both because it is an easy schedule to promote and monitor, and because it made it possible to coordinate mammogram and Pap smear screening schedules. However, the NBCCEDP has only received enough funds in its annual Congressional appropriation to screen approximately 15% of the uninsured or underinsured women who are eligible. Therefore, it makes better use of these limited resources to focus efforts on reaching more women at less frequent intervals and on those who have never or only rarely been screened, rather than on annual Pap screens for all women. A broader policy approach is reflected in the integration of Pap smear screening into programs that expand access to preventive services in primary care settings. Thus, the recent expansion of the Health Resources and Services Administration (HRSA) Community Health Center Program in the U.S. provides new opportunities for unscreened and under-screened women to gain access to testing. A critical issue to the success of this program as it expands is the need to develop the means to insure that those screened are also provided with clinical follow-up and access to care.

Within health care systems where access to screening is a covered benefit, variation may still remain in the use of screening. For example, diagnosis of late stage cervical cancer is less common among enrollees of organized health care systems such as health maintenance organizations (HMOs) than it is among persons who receive health care on a fee-for-service basis (Riley et al., 1994). However, within HMOs invasive cervical cancer continues to be diagnosed even in the most comprehensive systems. In such settings the majority of cases of invasive disease have been documented among women who, for whatever reason, were not screened in the previous three years despite continuous membership, even when they had been seen for other medical conditions (Sung et al., 2000). Obviously, strategies to improve the use of screening by following recommended guidelines remain a challenge even where access is not an issue.

2.1.2   Guideline policies

Recommendations regarding screening are generated both by professional medical organizations and governmental agencies. Key issues are those regarding the age at which a woman should start being screened, how to determine what the screening interval should be, and the age at which screening should stop. In the U.S. there are currently several different guidelines for cervical cancer screening which, although close to each other in what they recommend, are not in complete harmony. Those currently in circulation in the U.S. have been summarized in a number of publications (Rimer et al., 2000). The most recent guideline recommendations were released by the American Cancer Society (ACS) in late 2002 (Saslow et al., 2002) and by the U.S. Preventive Services Task Force in early 2003 (USPSTF, 2003).

The question of what age a woman should be when she begins screening is difficult because it is related to human behavior and the acquisition of HPV infections. Women quickly acquire HPV infections when they begin to be sexually active. However, most infections clear within 24 months (Sawaya et al., 2001a) and aggressive diagnostic evaluations and treatment of the cytologic abnormalities that can result from HPV infection may lead to physical harm, emotional distress and increased costs. The use of cone biopsy is associated with undesirable outcomes related to future pregnancy, although the precise level of risk conferred by cryotherapy and the loop electrosurgical excision procedure requires further study. In light of this, policy makers in the U.S. have generally recommended that screening begin either at the age of 18, or with the onset of sexual activity and at least by age 21 (Saslow et al., 2002; USPSTF, 2003). However, in European countries, such as the U.K. and Finland screening is not initiated until 21 and 30 years of age, respectively, without consideration of the onset of sexual activity (Sawaya et al., 2001a). There has also been a long-standing debate about the appropriate interval for Pap smear screening (Saslow et al., 2002; Sawaya et al., 2001). This is particularly significant in light of the cost of Pap smear tests and follow-up care, which is now part of routine care for women in industrialized countries. Savings that might be realized through less frequent screening and its attendant reduction in further medical visits and procedures make this of pressing interest to health care systems and government payers. A recent large study that used a retrospective case-control study design in a stable health plan population, has provided the most accurate data thus far on this topic. It demonstrated that two and three year intervals between Pap smears as compared to annual screening increased the odds of invasive cervical cancer to 1.7 and 2.1, respectively (Miller et al., 2002). The difference between one and either two or three year intervals was statistically significant, but still rather small in absolute terms. Thus, decisions regarding the recommended interval between Pap tests must weigh the increased costs of more frequent screening against the marginal increased benefit of preventing invasive cervical cancer, and the even smaller benefit of reduced mortality. Most guidelines now recommend screening every three years if there is evidence of three or more previous consecutive normal tests (Saslow et al., 2002; USPSTF, 2003).

Another critical issue has been the question of the age at which Pap smear screening can be safely stopped, if ever. In developed countries mortality from cervical cancer continues to rise with age. Even though there has been a dramatic reduction in mortality overall and for each age group, in the U.S. mortality remains the highest for women over 65 years of age (Figure 6). In the U.S., 38% of all women who die from cervical cancer are over 65 years of age even though they account for only 21% of the new cases (Reis et al., 2002).

Although HPV infection is usually acquired early in a woman's reproductive life, the manifestations of repeated and persistent exposure over time are seen most starkly in the older age group. While Pap smear screening has become an accepted part of a woman's regular gynecologic and obstetrical care during the reproductive years, the number of tests declines after the menopause (Sawaya et al., 2001b). To some extent this is because post-menopausal women visit obstetricians and gynecologists less often as part of routine healthcare.

Despite the fact that mortality is highest in older women, policies directed toward keeping older women on a regular screening schedule may be misguided. While older women have the highest mortality and lowest screening rates, they are also at the lowest risk of new HPV infections. Thus, the policy that makes the most sense for this population group is to recommend screening both for those who have not had Pap smears recently and those with a previous abnormal result, and less frequent or no screening over age 65 years, if consecutive previous Pap smears have been normal (Sawaya et al., 2001b; Colgan et al., 2002; Saslow et al., 2002; USPSTF, 2003).

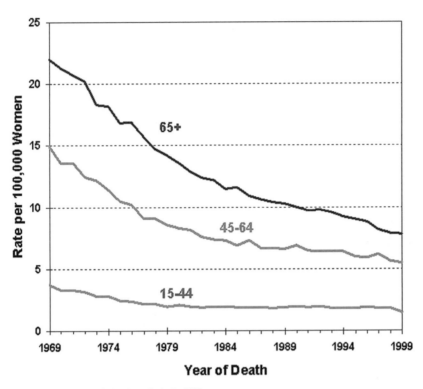

Source: NCHS Mortality Data. Age-adjusted to 2000.

Figure 6. U.S. time trends in cervical cancer mortality by age, 1969-99

2.1.3   Behavioral interventions

Effective behavioral interventions to improve adherence to recommended screening practices may be the basis of policy decisions by health care systems. Such interventions are most often directed at those who have never had a Pap smear, and to encourage regular or maintenance screening among those who have begun the practice.

Follow-back studies of women with invasive cervical cancer have shown that the largest subgroup among such women are those women who have never been screened or have not been screened within the past five years despite access and opportunities for screening (Janerich et al., 1995; Sung et al., 2000). Many of those who have never been screened in the U.S. are minority and new immigrant populations (Hiatt et al., 2001).

A Cochrane Library systematic review has been conducted of effective interventions in improving cervical cancer screening. Reviewers looked for good quality, randomized controlled trial evidence of invitations to screening, reminders, educational programs, message framing, counseling, risk factor assessment, facilitation of the procedure and the removal of economic barriers (Forbes et al., 2000). They concluded that only invitation letters, and possibly the benefits from educational interventions, were efficacious. A more recent review has found additional evidence of efficacy from targeted interventions, like telephone reminders, sociocultural and organizational health systems interventions (Yabroff et al., 2003). Individual studies of interventions have been successful in a number of settings and with a variety of audiences. For example, the use of patient and provider reminders has been successful (Somkin et al., 1997), although they are generally only incorporated into medical practices with the aid of computer systems, and, therefore, more often found in the context of well-established medical care systems. Challenges of a different nature are faced by providers and patients in opportunistic situations where women come in contact with medical care in emergency rooms or urgent care settings. Studies have documented that in situations where women require pelvic examinations for sexually transmitted diseases, and who are given Pap testing, rather high rates of pre-invasive and invasive cervical cancer are detected (Engelstad et al., 2001). Whether certain settings, like inner-city county hospitals should rely on performing opportunistic preventive care in emergency rooms as a matter of policy, however, is an open question. Efforts to improve adherence to screening recommendations through the use of lay health workers in community public health settings have also been studied. Lay health workers are non-professional persons, frequently from the communities they serve, who are trained to promote health care and preventive practices and to facilitate access to services. Although such interventions can be successful (Bird et al., 1998), the establishment of policies to provide this service await data on costs and cost-effectiveness, which have not been well studied.

Modern behavioral science intervention approaches have begun to make use of 'tailored' messages with the help of information technology (Rimer et al., 1999). These interventions make use of known factors such as age, race and ethnicity, past screening history, and a person's readiness to change to frame messages in such a way so as to make them more effective. The efficacy of this approach has been documented for both breast and cervical cancer (Rimer et al., 1999) and offers new options for screening programs for organized systems of care in settings such as health plans and government supported clinics. Unfortunately, the cost burden of obtaining the kind of demographic and individual data needed in order to tailor messages of this kind may limit the adoption of this very promising innovation in health behavior change because those settings that would benefit the most are frequently resource poor.

A recent systematic review of the evidence for effective behavioral interventions at the community level was conducted under the auspices of the U.S. Centers for Disease Control and Prevention to be published in the Guide to Community Preventive Services (Briss et al., 2000). This review will update the general understanding of the evidence currently available and, in addition, point out the need to consider issues of informed decision making (Austoker, 1999) and cost-effectiveness ratios as part of the development of policies that advance cervical cancer screening in public health settings. Thus, the evidence on the effectiveness of various behavioral interventions has been well evaluated and this evidence is sound enough to support policy decisions on strategies to improve screening adherence.

2.1.4   Follow-up of abnormal Pap tests

For a screening test to be effective, an abnormal result must be followed up promptly and appropriately and, if necessary, treatment must be administered. However, there is substantial evidence that women do not always follow-up after abnormal Pap smears. One review of studies found that 10 to 40% of women were not adherent to recommended procedures, although the definition of non-adherence was not standard across studies (Khanna and Phillips, 2001). Common barriers to follow-up included lack of understanding of the purpose of colposcopy, fear of cancer, forgetting appointments, and lack of time, money, or childcare (Khanna and Phillips, 2001). Policies to minimize the problem of incomplete or inadequate follow-up may take the form of practice guidelines for providers that suggest steps to take when a patient receives an abnormal result, or how to improve access and coverage for the kind of care needed by women in such situations. Among the strategies that have proven successful is telephone counseling prior to an appointment for repeat testing or diagnostic follow-up (Lerman et al., 1992; Miller et al., 1997). Case-management interventions have been found successful in emergency rooms as well as in urban hospital urgent care settings that serve women at high-risk of cervical cancer (Engelstad et al., 2001). There have also been pilot tests of programs that use same day screening and follow-up (Holschneider et al., 1999; Prislin et al., 1997), and patient navigator systems (Freeman et al., 1995), but these have not been systematically evaluated. In a review, personalized reminders to women from their physicians, and case management were found to be the most effective methods of improving adherence (Khanna and Phillips, 2001; Engelstad et al., 2001). While interventions to improve the likelihood that women with abnormal cervical cytology will get to colposcopy appear to have the potential to be extremely effective, more systematic research is needed to elucidate the most cost-effective approaches to clinical follow-up in diverse health care settings

As screening rates continue to rise, the emphasis in health policies may need to be shifted from persuading women to be screened in the first place, to interventions that assure follow-up. More health services and health policy research will be needed to determine how to ensure that the promise of early detection is realized through timely clinical follow-up of abnormal findings, and access to appropriate care when needed.

2.2   New technologies and revised terminology

Liquid based cytologic screening and HPV DNA testing are two new technologies with the potential to substantially improve the effectiveness of cervical cancer screening. In 2002, the ACS guidelines recommend that liquid-based cytology may be performed every two years (Saslow et al., 2002), but the impact of this policy on rates of detection is not yet known. The superiority of liquid cytology over the traditional Pap smear is still being debated (Hartmann et al., 2001; Moseley and Paget, 2002) and the current policy of the federal government in the CDC's BCCEDP is to reimburse providers no more than the cost of a Pap smear, even if more expensive liquid cytologic methods are used.

HPV DNA testing, frequently used in conjunction with liquid cytology, also holds much promise as an efficient triage strategy for some low-grade Pap smears. In the recently completed ASCUS/Low-grade Squamous Intra-epitheal Lesion (LSIL) Triage Study (ALTS) of women whose Pap smear showed atypical squamous cells of unknown significance (ASCUS), three alternative strategies were evaluated, but results have not been published (Solomon et al., 2001). The 2002 ACS guideline makes a 'preliminary recommendation' for HPV DNA testing for primary cervical cancer screening in conjunction with cytology, after pointing out that the U.S. Food and Drug Administration has not yet approved it. The ACS recommended that HPV DNA testing could be considered in combination with conventional cytology as an alternative to conventional cytologic screening alone for women over age 30 years, but not more frequently than every 3 years (Saslow et al., 2002). The U.S. Preventive Services Task Force, on the other hand, concluded that evidence was insufficient to recommend for or against either new technologies, such as liquid-based cytology, or routine HPV testing (USPSTF, 2003). Appropriate and optimal strategies for monitoring women with positive HPV tests and normal cytologic tests have not been devised.

Policy makers will have to consider cost effectiveness and system capacity as changes in current recommendations are considered as a result of these new technologies. In 2001, the American Society for Colposcopy and Cervical Pathology sponsored an international conference in Bethesda to reach consensus on the management of cervical cytological abnormalities using these new technologies (Wright et al., 2002). For the critical group of women with ASCUS, the consensus was that management could either be a program of two repeat cytology tests, immediate colposcopy, or DNA testing for high-risk HPV types. Testing for HPV DNA was the preferred strategy when liquid-based cytology was used (Wright et al., 2002), and reflex HPV DNA testing provided the best ratio of cost to years of life saved. Liquid-based cytology with HPV DNA testing that used samples collected at the same time as conventional cytology and done every three years, had a cost of $59,000 per year of life saved (compared to $20,300 per year of life saved for every 5 years) (Kim et al., 2002). The authors concluded that adoption of such a strategy could save over $15 billion for a cohort of U.S. women aged 18 to 24 years (Goldie 2002). These conclusions from the Bethesda conference await the publication of results from the ALTS trial, and policies based on them would be premature as of this writing.

The evolution of scientific knowledge and these newer technologies has also stimulated a need to update and revise the terminology for reporting the results of cervical cytology (Solomon et al., 2002). A 2001 Bethesda Workshop was convened to establish recommendations on terminology that would be accepted and utilized by all those involved in cervical cytology. The policy on terminology, reached on the basis of an evaluation of the scientific literature, expert opinion, and the use by participants of an internet bulletin board was intended to promote effective communication of cytologic results from the laboratory to clinicians (Solomon et al., 2002).

2.3 Policies in low-resource settings

For many developing countries, cervical cancer is more common than in industrialized countries, and may even be one of the greatest causes of cancer mortality (Figure 3). Unfortunately, in many such countries the resources and personnel necessary to conduct traditional cytologic screening are often not available and low technology approaches may be the wisest strategies. Current methods include aided visualization, cervicography, computer-assisted screening devices, optical probe devices, self-collected vaginal samples for HPV DNA testing, and spectroscopy/electronic detection devices. If conventional cytology is considered, the relative benefits of testing no more than a few times, or even just once during a lifetime, need to be considered (Goldie et al., 2002).

An analysis of one example of an alternative strategy in a low-resource country used a mathematical model and data from South Africa, where cervical cancer mortality is approximately 5-fold that in the U.S. (Ferlay et al., 2001; Goldie et al., 2001). A comparison of the cost per year of life saved when screening was conducted once or twice in a lifetime, compared to annual or even every three-year testing in the U.S. is striking. This analysis showed that once in a lifetime screening could reduce the incidence of invasive cervical cancer 20-30% for a cost of less than $50 per year of life saved. This was in contrast to a 90% reduction for every three-year Pap test screening with reflex HPV DNA testing, at a cost $60,000 per year of life saved. Stated in another way, these data demonstrated that for every $50,000 invested in the U.S., there would be an overall 15-week average life expectancy gain, whereas in South Africa, a comparable investment would produce a life expectancy gain of 1000 years (Goldie, 2002).

Investigators also considered direct visual inspection (DVI) of the cervix, conventional cytologic screening, and DNA testing for high-risk types of HPV (Goldie et al., 2001; Mandelblatt et al., 2002). For a hypothetical cohort of 30-year old black South African women, HPV testing followed by treatment of screen-positive women at a second visit cost only $39 per year of life saved and resulted in a reduction of 27% in cancer incidence. However, almost as effective was DVI with a reduction in incidence of 26% and this approach was actually more cost effective. The conclusion from this study was that strategies that incorporate either DVI or HPV DNA testing and eliminate colposcopy were superior to conventional cytology in low-resource settings (Goldie et al., 2001).

In another analysis using a population-based simulation model and data from Thailand, visual inspection after the application of acetic acid performed every five years in women aged 35-55 years with immediate treatment of abnormalities was the least expensive ($517 per year of life saved) and saved the most lives of seven low technology screening approaches evaluated (Mandelblatt et al., 2002). In the same evaluation, a combination of Pap smear and HPV testing at 5-year intervals for women aged 20-70 achieved more than a 90% reduction in mortality for $1,683 per year of life saved (Mandelblatt et al., 2002).

These examples are based on data from developing countries, but as was pointed out at the beginning of this chapter, there are also marked differences in the burden of cervical cancer even within developed countries like the U.S. (Figure 3). Exploring more cost-effective approaches to cervical cancer control within the underserved populations of developed countries like the U.S. might produce intervention approaches and policies with more relevance to the developing world. Working against such an approach, however, may be the inequity suggested by promoting low-tech solutions for the poor while providing high-tech ones for the wealthy.

3   TREATMENT

3.1   Access to treatment

The discussion about the control of cervical cancer has revolved primarily around questions of improved screening. However, it is clear that screening alone is not effective unless women with abnormal results have access to appropriate treatment. 'Treatment' must include both procedures to ablate preinvasive lesions, which are the key to successful sceening programs, and those appropriate for invasive neoplasia. Unfortunately, access even to follow-up testing and initial therapy seems to be limited in both industrialized and developing countries (Khanna and Phillips, 2001). Furthermore, treatment options for invasive cervical cancer may not be applied uniformly among populations in the U.S. Evidence from 62 randomly selected institutions documented less aggressive radiotherapy treatment among minority women from low-income neighborhoods who received care in large institutions that primarily serve those populations compared to a randomly chosen national sample (Katz et al., 2000). Recent advances in the multi-modality therapy for regional and metastatic disease have been dramatic and the results are highly encouraging for those women who have access to it, but a lack of resources to support such a multi-modality approach on a wider scale makes access a real issue. There have been efforts in the U.S. to establish policies that would centralize the purchase and provision of expensive medical technology, but these have not been highly successful in the past due to the desire of many medical facilities to have their own equipment. Policies related to access and quality of care for cervical cancer with currently available treatment are badly needed for both preinvasive and invasive disease.

As other new forms of treatment appear, they will also need to be taken into consideration when decisions are made regarding how to allocate scarce resources for testing and treatment of an increasingly uncommon disease. Preventive vaccines have begun to show promise (Koutsky et al., 2002; Chapter 12), however, therapeutic vaccines that can reverse established HPV infection are still in early development (Crum, 2002; Chapter 13).

3.2   Measures of quality of care and monitoring systems

The fundamental question, 'What is good quality of care for cervical cancer?', is central to all policy decisions that must be made in order to achieve high standards in treatment, as well as in the prevention, screening and long-term care of women with this disease.

The National Cancer Policy Board (NCPB) of the Institute of Medicine (IOM) in the U.S. has released a series of reports and recommendations related to this question for cancer in general. The first of these was entitled Ensuring Quality of Cancer Care (Hewitt and Simone, 1999) and the second, Enhancing Data Systems to Improve the Quality of Cancer Care (Hewitt and Simone 2000). These reports call for efforts to achieve consensus on the identification of measures of quality care, the development of data systems to monitor these measures, and specific recommendations for how improvement in the quality of care might be achieved. The National Cancer Institute, its partners in cancer research and practice, as well as payers and consumers have engaged in a project with the National Quality Forum (NQF, 2003) to develop a consensus on a core set of measurements of quality of care that includes quality of life among cancer survivors, communications between patients and their providers, and screening. The results of this project are expected to be available in late 2004, and are intended to improve the assessment of quality for cervical cancer, as well as for cancer in general.

Quality measures for cervical cancer care have been introduced only for screening by the National Committee for Quality Assurance (NCQA). This was done through the Health Plan Employer Data and Information Set (HEDIS), a standardized method of assessing health plan performance that is issued to consumers and purchasers of health care (NCQA, 2003). NCQA is interested in developing additional measures of quality related to treatment. Other organizations such as the Joint Commission on Accreditation of Healthcare Organizations (JCAHO), and the Foundation for Accountability (FACCT), have also developed performance measurement systems to evaluate quality of care in population-based studies. Other approaches that use a case-based measurement system are also being developed (Malin et al., 2000). The limitation of these measure sets is that they are directed at a particular audience (e.g., HEDIS to health plans only) and a broader consensus on core measures of quality of care is needed.

4   ADDITIONAL POLICY IMPLICATIONS

Currently, no one organization or sector of society is responsible for establishing policies related to cervical cancer control. A more coordinated effort that brings together a large number of interested parties is called for. In the U.S. these include the NCI, CDC, HRSA, CMS, state health departments, providers and health plans. Recent efforts to bridge the gap that exists between research discovery and program delivery have led to new collaborative efforts that may be effective in speeding up the process by which policy is made and interventions put into place. Some examples of these federal collaborations include: 1) NCI, CDC, and HRSA are developing cancer screening service protocols within the HRSA-funded community health centers; 2) CDC, NCI, and the U.S. Department of Agriculture (USDA) are developing a collaborative training program for CDC NBCCEDP outreach staff, USDA cooperative extension agents, NCI Cancer Information Service outreach and partnership staff, and ACS regional cancer control staff. The intent is to adopt evidence-based approaches to promoting Pap smear screening to women who have never been screened and who live in high mortality counties; and 3) a new web-portal being developed by NCI, CDC, ACS and SAMSHA (the Cancer Control PLANET (Plan, Link, Act, Network with Evidence-based Tools)), which is intended to facilitate access to web-based comprehensive cancer control planning and program tools for cancer control service providers.

These and other similar collaborations, especially in less developed countries, will be needed to further insure that effective interventions are translated into policies that will make cervical cancer an increasingly uncommon and easily treatable disease worldwide.

CONCLUSION

We have placed policies for implementing cervical cancer prevention and control strategies into a conceptual framework that illustrates how they relate to other elements of cancer control. In addition, we have described policies, both existing and anticipated, along the cancer continuum from prevention, through early detection, to treatment and follow-up. Policies can and have to be implemented at multiple levels, including the national, state and local government levels, as well as by health plans and individual providers of care. Existing policies are primarily focused on early detection, but a new understanding of the role of the human papillomavirus in cervical cancer will result in new policies for primary prevention as well. Additionally, policies that define the quality of cervical cancer care are in development, and consensus is being sought on recommendations for coverage, reimbursement, guideline development, and further research. Strategies at any point along the cancer continuum should be based on evidence that relates not just to the biology of the disease and co-morbid conditions, but to the realities of the health care system (e.g., insurance coverage, lack of follow-up) and epidemiologic factors, such as age, race/ethnicity, and social class. Thus, strategies for implementing cervical cancer prevention and control must take into account the capacity of low-resource settings. Likewise, where resources are more abundant, coordination between the multiple entities involved in the care of women at risk of or diagnosed with cervical cancer is needed to more effectively reduce the burden of this disease.

RECOMMENDATIONS

To take advantage of the many new discoveries in the biology of cervical cancer, policies should take into account the epidemiology of cervical cancer and consider available resources in the geographic area where strategies are to be introduced. The adoption of newer technologies (e.g., HPV DNA testing and HPV vaccination) will require thoughtful consideration of costs and benefits to assure optimum implementation. Behavioral aspects of prevention and screening interventions must be considered to ensure that they are widely disseminated and adopted, and measures of the quality of care of cervical cancer patients should be developed relevant to the setting in which the care is delivered. The monitoring of these measures should become a part of national cancer data systems. Finally, to the extent possible, all women should be assured access to cervical cancer care, including screening, follow-up, and treatment, independent of their ability to pay.

ACKNOWLEDGEMENTS

We appreciate the critical reviews kindly provided by George Sawaya and Robin Yabroff, the timely editing assistance of June Hiatt, and the expert support with graphics and manuscript formatting from Dan Grauman.

REFERENCES

Advisory Committee on Cancer Control. Bridging research to action: a framework and decision-making process for cancer control. Advisory Committee on Cancer Control, National Cancer Institute of Canada. Can Med Assoc J 1994;151:1141-6.

Almeida RA, Dubay LC, Ko G. Access to care and use of health services by low-income women. Health Care Financing Review 2001;22: 27-47.

Austoker J. Editorial. Gaining informed consent for screening. Brit Med J 1999;319:722-3.

Best A, Hiatt RA, Cameron R, et al. The evolution of cancer control research: an international perspective from Canada and the United States. Cancer Epidemiol Biomarkers Prev 2003; 12:705-12.

Bird JA, McPhee SJ, Ha NT, et al. Opening pathways to cancer screening for Vietnamese-American women: lay health workers hold a key. Prev Med 1998;27:821-9.

Bosch FX, Manos M, Munoz N, et al. Prevalence of human papillomavirus in cervical cancer: a worldwide perspective. International biological study on cervical cancer (IBSCC) Study Group. J Natl Cancer Inst 1995;87:796-802.

Briss PA, Zaza S, Pappaioanou M, et al. Developing an evidence-based guide to community preventive services--methods. The Task Force on Community Preventive Services. Am J Prev Med 2000;18(1 Suppl):35-43.

Colgan TJ, Clarke A, Hakh N, Seidenfeld A. Screening for cervical disease in mature women. Strategies for improvement. Cancer (Cervical Cytopathol) 2002;96:195-203.

Crum CP. The beginning of the end for cervical cancer? (Editorial) N Engl J Med 2002; 347:1703-5.

Devesa SS, Grauman DJ, Blot WJ, et al. Atlas of cancer mortality in the United States. 1950-94. National Institutes of Health, National Cancer Institute. NIH Publication No. 99-4564, September, 1999.

Engelstad LP, Stewart SL, Nguyen BH, et al. Abnormal Pap smear follow-up in a high-risk population. Cancer Epidemiol Biomarkers Prev 2001;10:1015-20.

Ferlay J, Bray F, Pisani P, Parkin DM. GLOBOCAN 2000: Cancer incidence, mortality and prevalance worldwide, Version 1.0.IARC CancerBase No. 5. Lyon, IARC Press, 2001.

Forbes C, Jepson R, Martin-Hirsch P. Interventions targeted at women to encourage the uptake of cervical screening. Cochrane Library. http://www.cochranelibrary.com. Accessed 12/30/02.

Freeman HP, Muth BJ, Kerner JF. Expanding access to cancer screening and clinical follow-up among the medically underserved. Cancer Pract 1995; 3:19-30.

Goldie SJ, Kuhn L, Denny L, et al. Policy analysis of cervical cancer screening strategies in low-resource settings: clinical benefits and cost-effectiveness. JAMA 2001;285:3107-15.

Goldie SJ. Health economics and cervical cancer prevention: a global perspective. Virus Res 2002; 89:301-9.

Hall HI, Uhler RJ, Coughlin SS, Miller D. Breast and cervical screening among Applalachian women. Cancer Epidemiol Biomarkers Prev 2002;11:137-42.

Harro CD, Pang Y-YS, Roden RB, et al. Safety and immunogenicity trial in adult volunteers of a human papillomavirus 16 L1 virus-like partical vaccine. J Natl Cancer Inst 2001;93:284-92.

Hartmann KE, Nanda K, Hall S, Myers E. Technologic advances for evaluation of cervical cytology: Is newer better? Obstet Gynecol Survey 2001;56:765-74.

Henson RM, Wyatt SW, Lee NC. The National Breast and Cervical Cancer Early Detection Program: a comprehensive public health response to two major health issues for women. J Public Health Manag Pract 1996;2:36-47.

Hewitt M, Simone JV. Eds. Ensuring Quality Cancer Care. National Cancer Policy Board, Institute of Medicine and National Research Council. 1999. Washington, DC: National Academy Press.

Hewitt M, Simone JV. Eds. Enhancing Data Systems to Improve the Quality of Cancer Care. National Cancer Policy Board, Institute of Medicine and National Research Council. 2000. Washington, DC: National Academy Press.

Hiatt RA, Perez-Stable EJ, Quesenberry D Jr, et al. Agreement between self-reported early cancer detection practices and medical audits among Hispanic and non-Hispanic white health plan members in Northern California. Prev Med 1995;24:278-85.

Hiatt RA, Pasick RJ, Stewart S, et al. Community-based cancer screening for underserved women: design and baseline findings from the Breast and Cervical Cancer Intervention Study. Prev Med 2001;33:190-203.

Hiatt RA, Rimer BK. A new strategy for cancer control research. Cancer Epidemiol Biomarkers Prev 1999;8:957-64.

Hoffman FL. The menace of cancer. In: Transactions of the American Gynecologic Society. Vol 38. pp 397-452. Philadelphia: William J. Dornan Publishing, 1913.

Holschneider CH, Ghosh K, Montz FJ. See-and-treat in the management of high-grade squamous intraepithelial lesions of the cervix: A resource utilization analysis. Obstet Gynecol 1999; 94:377-85.

Hsia J, Kemper E, Kiefe C, et al. The importance of health insurance as a determinant of cancer screening: evidence from the Woman's Health Initiative. Prev Med 2000;31:261-70.

Huang K, Lin S. Nationwide vaccination: a success story in Taiwan. Vaccine 2000; 18 (Suppl 1):S35-S38.

Janerich DT, Hadjimichael O, Schwartz PE, et al. The screening histories of women with invasive cervical cancer, Connecticut. Am J Pub Health 1995;85:791-4.

Katz A, Eifel PJ, Moughan J, Owen JB, Mahon I, Hanks GE. Socioeconomic characteristics of patients with squamous cell carcinoma of the uterine cervix treated with radiotherapy in the 1992 to 1994 patterns of care study. Int J Radiation Oncology Biol Phys 2000;47:443-50.

Khanna N, Phillips M. Adherence to care plan in women with abnormal Papanicolaou smears: A review of barriers and interventions. J Am Board Fam Pract 2001;14:123-30.

Kim JJ, Wright TC, Goldie SJ. Cost-effectiveness of alternative triage strategies for atypical squamous cells of undetermined significance. JAMA 2002;287:2428-9.

Koutsky LA, Ault KA, Wheeler CM, et al., for the Proof of Principle Study Investigators. A controlled trial of human papillomavirus type 16 vaccine. N Engl J Med 2002;347:1645-51.

Lawson HW, Lee NC, Thames SF, et al. Cervical care screening among low-income women: results of a national screening program, 1991-1995. Obstet Gynecol 1998;92:745-52.

Lawson HW, Henson R, Bobo JK, Kaeser MK. Implementing recommendations for the early detection of breast and cervical cancer among low-income women. Oncology 2000; 14:1528-30.

Lerman C, Hanjani P, Caputo C, et al. Telephone counseling improves adherence to colposcopy among lower-income minority women. J Clin Oncol 1992;10:330-3.

Malin JL, Asch SM, Kerr EA, McGlynn EA. Evaluating the quality of cancer care: development of cancer quality indicators for a global quality assessment tool. Cancer 2000; 88:701-7.

Mandelblatt JS, Lawrence WF, Gaffikin L, et al. Costs and benefits of different strategies to screen for cervical cancer in less-developed countries. J Natl Cancer Inst 2002;94:1469-83.

McPhee SJ, Nguyen TT, Shema SJ, et al. Validation of recall of breast and cervical cancer screening by women in an ethically diverse population. Prev Med 2002;35:463-73.

Miller M, Sung H-Y, Sawaya GS, et al. Screening interval and risk of invasive squamous-cell cervical cancer: a case-control study among long-term members of a large prepaid health plan. Obstet Gynecol 2003;101:29-37.

Miller SM, Siejak KK, Schroeder CM, et al. Enhancing adherence following abnormal Pap smears among low-income minority women: a preventive telephone counseling strategy. J Natl Cancer Inst 1997;89:703-8.

Moseley RP, Paget S. Liquid-based cytology: is this the way forward for cervical screening? Cytopath 2002;13:71-82.

Munoz N, Bosch FX, de Sanjose S, et al. The causal link between human papillomavirus and invasive cervical cancer: a population-based case-control study in Columbia and Spain. Int J Cancer 1992;52:743-9.

National Cancer Institute. Division of Cancer Control and Population Sciences. Cancer Control Continuum. National Cancer Institute

Website. http://dccps.nci.nih.gov/od/ continuum.html.

National Committee for Quality Assurance (NCQA)

Website. http://www.ncqa.org/Programs/HEDIS/ Accessed January 12, 2003.

National Quality Forum. 'Cancer Quality Measures Project'. Website http://www.qualityforum.org/txNQFprojectsummarycancer_SteerComm6-12-02.pdf. Accessed January 12, 2003.

Papanicolaou GN, Traut HF. The diagnostic value of the vaginal smears in carcinoma of the uterus. Am J Obstet Gynecol 1941;42:193-206.

Parkin DM, Bray FI, Devesa SS. Cancer burden in the year 2000: The global picture. Eur J Cancer 2001;37: Suppl 8:S4-S66.

Prislin MD, Dinh T, Giglio M. On-site colposcopy services in a family practice residency clinic: Impact on physician test-ordering behavior, patient compliance, and practice revenue generation. J Am Board Fam Pract 1997; 10:259-64.

Ries LAG, Eisner MP, Kosary CL, et al (eds). SEER Cancer Statistics Review, 1973-1999, National Cancer Institute. Bethesda, MD, http://seer.cancer.gov/csr/1973_1999/, 2002.

Riley GF, Potosky AL, Lubitz JD, Brown M. Stage of cancer at diagnosis for Medicare HMO and fee-for-service enrollees. Am J Pub Health1994;84:1598-604.

Rimer BK, Schildkraut J, Hiatt RA. Cancer Screening, Chapter 25. In: Cancer: Principles and Practice in Oncology. 6th Ed. Devita VT Jr, Hellman S, Rosenberg SA. Eds. 2000.

Rimer BK, Conaway M, Lyna P, et al. The impact of tailored interventions on a community health center population. Patient Education Counseling 1999;37:125-40.

Saslow D, Runowixcz CD, Solomon D, et al. American Cancer Society guideline for the early detection of cervical neoplasia and cancer. CA Cancer J Clin 2002;52:342-62.

Sawaya GF, Brown AD, Washington AE, Garber AM. Current approaches to cervical-cancer screening. N Engl J Med 2001a;344:1603-7.

Sawaya GF, Sung HY, Kearney KA, et al. Advancing age and cervical cancer screening and prognosis. J Am Geriatr Soc 2001b;49:1499-504.

Schneider DL, Burke L, Wright TC, et al. Can cervicography be improved? An evaluation with arbitrated cervicography interpretations. Am J Obstet Gynecol 2002:187:15-23.

Sedlacek TV. Cost effectiveness in new technology in cervix cancer screening. Epidemiology 2002; 13:26-9.

Solomon D, Schiffman M, Tarone R; ALTS Study Group. Comparison of three management strategies for patients with atypical squamous cells of undetermined significance: baseline results from a randomized trial. J Natl Cancer Inst 2001;93:293-9.

Solomon D, Davey D, Kurman R, et al: The Forum Group Members; The Bethesda 2001 Workshop. The 2001 Bethesda System: terminology for reporting results of cervical cytology. JAMA 2002;287:2140-1.

Somkin CP, Hiatt RA, Hurley LB, et al. The effect of patient and provider reminders on mammography and Papanicolaou smear screening in a large health maintenance organization. Arch Int Med 1997;157:1658-64.

Sung HY, Kearney KA, Miller M, et al. Papanicolaou smear history and diagnosis of invasive cervical carcinoma among members of a large prepaid health plan. Cancer 2000; 88:2283-9.

Swan J, Breen N, Coates RJ, et al. Progress in cancer screening practices in the United States: results from the 2000 National Health Interview Survey. Cancer 2003; 97:1528-40.

U.S. Preventive Services Task Force. Screening for Cervical Cancer. January 2003. Agency for Healthcare Research and Quality, Rockville, MD. http://www.ahrq.gov/clinic/3rduspstf/cervicalcan/cervcanrr.htm. Accessed January 22, 2003.

Walboomers JM, Jacobs MV, Manos MM, et al. Human papillomavirus is a necessary cause of invasive cervical cancer worldwide. J Pathol 1999;189:12-9.

Wright TC Jr, Cox JT, Massad LS, et al. 2001 Consensus guidelines for the management of women with cervical cytological abnormalities. ASCCP-sponsored consensus conference. JAMA 2002;287:2120-9.

Yabroff KR, Mangan P, Mandelblatt JS. Effectiveness of interventions to increase Pap smear use. J Am Board Fam Pract 2003;16:188-203.

zur Hausen H. Papillomaviruses and cancer: from basic studies to clinical application. Nature Reviews 2002;2:342-50.